EXPLORING THE DANGEROUS TRADES

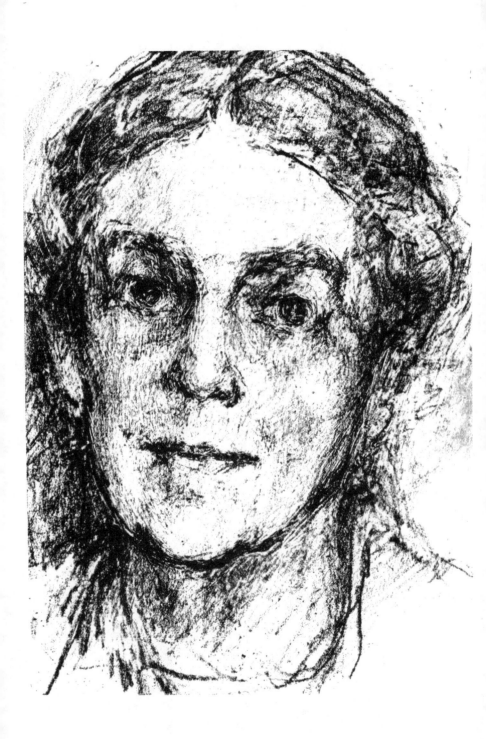

EXPLORING THE DANGEROUS TRADES

The Autobiography

of

ALICE HAMILTON, M.D.

With a Foreword by
Jean Spencer Felton, MD

With Illustrations by Norah Hamilton

OEM PRESS
Beverly, Massachusetts

The author is indebted to the *Atlantic, Harper's,* the *American Mercury,* and *Survey Graphic* for permission to use certain material which appeared originally in the pages of those magazines.

OEM Press Edition 1995

ISBN 1-883595-04-5

Printed in the United States of America

To My Three Sisters
And My Brother

Contents

Contents

$\mathcal{I}llustrations$

Foreword

GREAT WOMEN in history have appeared in each millennium, but until the end of the nineteenth century they were best known in the arts, in the houses of royalty, and as amorous companions of world leaders. With the century's turn, though, new distaff voices began to be heard in intelligent, keenly sensitive protest. From these emerging leaders came the creative growth of strong social reforms. Public health nursing, social casework, settlement house groupwork, women's suffrage, women's trade unions, and the protective philosophy culminating in the formation of the Women's and Children's Bureaus are all traceable to the molding of the public conscience by spirited women who demanded to be heard.

Concomitant with these early changes in many lifestyles was greater participation in the sciences by capably trained women. Medicine, chemistry, physics, and biology began to attract young graduates who were later to make illustrious contributions in research and practice. With considerable hardship, some of these perceptive, socially aware, fearless practitioners ventured into areas previously occupied only by men.

Such a person was Alice Hamilton, MD, whose career began in research and academic medicine. Through her medical activity she soon saw social inequities, the social pathology, and the industrially-caused morbidity and mortality that were products of early twentieth century commercial and manufacturing expansion. With vocational capability in laboratory research together with avocational skills in reaching the hearts of oppressed peoples, Dr. Hamilton joined these two operational areas to give shape to the future specialty of occupational medicine as it is known today.

Not only did this physician assume a giant's place in medicine; she entered industry, first on behalf of the Illinois Commission on Occupational Diseases in 1910, and later for the US Department of Labor, to conduct surveys of the poisonous trades. Hardened managers and foremen found this "little lady" informed in the area of occupationally incurred illnesses and also fully capable of defending her viewpoint verbally and in writing of considerable strength.

Her contributive sharing in the protest movement was not limited to spotlighting dangerous and dusty workplaces, for Dr. Hamilton rose to be counted while some of the country's most heated issues were being argued at the highest levels. As her writings well testify, she fought for peace, for strikers when they were justified in their demands, for women's participation in the labor movement, for fairness in the judging of Sacco and Vanzetti, and against poverty, hunger, child labor, and ill health in both friendly and enemy countries abroad. Hers was a vigorous voice in the United States at a time when dissent was unpopular and unwelcome.

Dr. Hamilton's prime identification is with occupationally-caused diseases, although the beginnings of her lengthy career were in pathology and infectious diseases. It was in this new field in the United States that she began her "exploring," for apart from a sparse article or two in the American literature, the bulk of information was to be found in European writings. While her autobiography covers most of the educational and professional aspects of Dr. Hamilton's life from birth in 1869 to 1942, the most fascinating trail to be followed is that of the recognition, both immediate and long-continuing, of the worth of her studies. Her initial publication on lead poisoning appeared in 1910 and was cited in the first comprehensive text on occupational diseases, prepared by W. Gilman Thompson, MD [1].

Writings on lead toxicity continued, with a presentation given in Washington, DC, at the Fifteenth International Congress on Hygiene and Demography. At that time, in 1912, Alice Hamilton had been living some 15 years at Chicago's Hull House, headed by Jane Addams, and had had contact with immigrants from all over Europe. It was these associations that further aroused her interest in the use of the burgeoning labor force. It was only with great difficulty that she could identify affected workers, for records were almost nonexistent and there was no mandating legislation pertinent to the lead trades. Tracing afflicted workers proved baffling at times because of inconsistencies in the use and spelling of foreign surnames. That Hamilton's reputation had begun to have meaning is seen in the simultaneous appearance at the 1912 conference in Washington of the newcomer, Dr. Hamilton, and the senior Sir Thomas Oliver of Great Britain, author of the text *Dangerous Trades* [2], which she had used to learn about occupational diseases. Nearly every significant monograph that followed in the century's early years either cited Hamilton's writings or quoted directly from them.

In those beginning decades, many reports were produced for the Bureau of Labor, and in their preparation Dr. Hamilton was left to her own resources in locating manufacturing plants and arranging for the method of investigation. Her reports covered investigations into lead manufacturing, commercial painting, the rubber industry, the printing trades, and the explosives, dyes, and viscose rayon industries.

Her work for the US Department of Labor was not merely to determine the extent of a particular substance's toxicity as it related to its handlers, for Dr. Hamilton always carried on additional correspondence to guide managerial personnel toward the introduction of various modes of illness prevention.

Alice Hamilton's writings were numerous, so that between 1911 and 1945 some 55 articles were published in a variety of journals, many in the *Journal of the American Medical Association* as well as in the *Journal of Industrial Hygiene*, established in 1919. Through the 1970s her work continued to be cited in publications related either directly to occupational diseases or to the general field of occupational health. In more recent monographs, in the 1980s, her activities were discussed from a sociological point of view.

With the passage of the mid-twentieth century years, Dr. Hamilton became part of the history of occupational medicine, credit being given for her early study, on-site, of a variety of industries. Her role has been described in a number of writings, several carrying a photograph of Dr. Hamilton taken at the peak of her career.

While originators of new thought in the United States do not always meet with acceptance in Western Europe, Dr. Hamilton had been an exception. In a 1923 British text her work was recognized by Dr. Donald Hunter, the dean of occupational medicine in Great Britain, who included her photograph and quoted extensively from *Exploring the Dangerous Trades;* that material was carried through from the first edition of *The Diseases of Occupations* in 1955 [3] to the eponymous 1987 printing.

Richard Schilling, also a "great" in England, cites the early work of Dr. Hamilton, recalling: "She had to face opposition from both employers and members of her own profession, one of whom described her report on lead poisoning as false, malicious, and slandering" [4].

That the eminence of Alice Hamilton remains is evident in two current publications. In what has become a "standard" — Zenz's *Occupational Medicine* (1994) — two of the contributors, writing on occupational vibration, quote from her 1918 report on stone cutters, observing: "To this day, Hamilton's description of the signs and symptoms of HAVS [Hand-arm vibration syndrome] have not been surpassed in the literature" [5].

In a recent textbook, in oversized format, descriptive of occupational health in the US Army, over three pages are devoted to Dr. Hamilton's work, one full page containing a photograph with a lengthy legend offering a brief biography [6].

In 1929 she produced her first book, *Industrial Poisons in the United States*, a text of nearly 600 pages [7]. Current writers in occupational medicine continue to emphasize the need of a complete occupational history when one sees a patient presenting with a possible occupational illness. Among Dr. Hamilton's prefatory remarks in her initial monograph is her chiding of healthcare personnel who neglect this aspect of the patient's past: "If the recording intern would only treat the poison from which the man is suffering with as much interest as he gives to the coffee the patient has drunk and the tobacco he has smoked, if he would ask as carefully about the length of time he was exposed to the poison as about the age at which he had measles, the task of the searcher for the truth about industrial poisons would be made so very much easier." [8] This reproof, penned 70 years ago, still holds.

In her first hardback publication, Dr. Hamilton ended her Preface with the statement, "The literature up to January 1, 1924, has been included." It must be remembered that most of the early literature stemmed from Europe, so that translation into English was needed. All the Hamiltons, parents and siblings, knew Greek and Latin as well as French and German, and Dr. Hamilton taught herself Italian, so that the literature unquestionably could be covered.

A second monograph appeared in 1934, "a short review of modern industrial toxicology rather than a logically planned textbook" [9]. This work was smaller and part of a series the publisher was directing toward "the general practitioner." But the principle of thorough search persisted, for in the Preface to this work Dr. Hamilton concluded: "The literature up to January, 1933, has been covered." One can be certain that *all* writings were pursued, for some 655 references were cited, published originally in seven different languages.

While there were occasional light episodes in Dr. Hamilton's long life, there were also sad elements, as Barbara Sicherman, the eminent historian, has indicated, in that *Exploring the Dangerous Trades* is the quietly understated work of a woman who refused to see either her life or herself as unusual; thus, the autobiography was short of truly personal reminiscences. As Sicherman put it, Dr. Hamilton's books lacked intimacy although they nevertheless were deeply personal [10].

There is a great feeling of self-deprecation throughout her letters to family members and friends. The present writer had occasion to send Dr. Hamilton a copy of *Man, Medicine, and Work — Historic Events in Occupational Medicine*, published in 1964 [11]. While commenting favorably about the book, Dr. Hamilton continued in her letter of response, "I recognized, of course, Hippocrates, Pliny and Paracelsus and Ramazzini, but nobody else. But why put me in? It's like a sparrow in a flock of eagles." [12] The following November she wrote to Dr. Clara Haas, a Rhode Island psychiatrist, "The 'Historic Events in Occupational Medicine' lies on my desk . . . I enjoyed it, especially the illustrations, but was disgusted to find myself coupled with Hippocrates and Ramazzini" [13].

The sense of self-deprecation appears frequently, as Sicherman points out through several instances. In her early sixties, Dr. Hamilton called a laudatory article "a beautiful fiction which overwhelms me with shame. I feel myself a bluffer of the worst kind," and, again, "I simply cannot believe that I am a person of more than ordinary ability, though I know that chance has given me a more than ordinarily interesting life" [14].

In parallel with these self-views is the memory of a visit made by the present writer to Dr. Hamilton in Hadlyme in 1962. After a pleasant lunch, she was asked as to the whereabouts of the many awards she had received. She indicated they were in the attic, and in order to get there, one had to climb a vertical ladder attached to a wall. In the attic, the plaques were all there, but scattered about the floor as though a giant hand had flipped them randomly about the room.

Dr. Hamilton's awards and honors were many, most being given in the years following publication of *Exploring the Dangerous Trades*. All were received with the humility that characterized her professional life. When named the recipient of the Knudsen Award, occupational medicine's highest honor from the then Industrial Medical Association (now the American College of Occupational and Environmental Medicine), she responded in part:

> It is indeed an honor and a deep pleasure to be offered the Knudsen Award. Of course I wish to express my gratitude to the old friends who have chosen me to receive it. Now that I am an old woman, living in retirement in a tiny country village, it is especially gratifying to know that my

former comrades still remember me. I still . . . look back with nostalgia to the days when I too was in active work. [15].

Noteworthy writings continued in the 1940s. With Dr. Rutherford T. Johnstone of Los Angeles, she wrote a section on industrial toxicology for *The Oxford Medicine*, published later as a separate volume in 1945 [16]. Her earlier work *Industrial Toxicology* was enlarged, with Dr. Harriet L. Hardy as co-author, in 1949. Its third edition appeared in 1974, four years after Dr. Hamilton's death, but the designation of the original authors remained, showing Hamilton as "Late Assistant Professor Emerita of Industrial Medicine, Harvard School of Public Health, Boston, Massachusetts."

In 1967 Dr. Madeleine P. Grant's book *Alice Hamilton — Pioneer Doctor in Industrial Medicine* was published, aimed at a younger readership [17].

The name of this eminent lady has been memorialized in the Alice Hamilton Laboratory in Cincinnati, a dormitory at Connecticut College named for Alice and her sister Edith, and the creation of the Alice Hamilton Fund for Occupational Medicine at the Harvard School of Public Health. On the occasion of her one-hundredth birthday, President Richard Nixon wrote to Dr. Hamilton, in part:

> [Your achievements] speak better than any words of your brave, dynamic leadership in this vital area of human endeavor. I know of no one who can look with greater satisfaction on as many decades of selfless, ungrudging service to humanity. [18].

Many of the thoughts expressed in *Exploring the Dangerous Trades* forecast the future. Dr. Hamilton was "strong for the English worship of tea" and believed that if American workers in offices and factories "took five minutes off morning and afternoon . . . it would make work easier and less tiring, [and] more efficient." [19] In this country, the coffee break at the workplace has since become standard. She wrote of miners who not only became "poisoned themselves, but carried home so much quicksilver in their overalls that their wives contracted poisoning through washing the clothes" [20]. This transfer of a toxic material was to be recalled in the 1970s with the attention paid to asbestos workers.

In looking ahead, Dr. Hamilton observed that even if the point were reached when all harmful work substances were to be brought under control, one would "still have to deal with that much more baffling and widespread industrial evil, fatigue of 'mind, body and soul.'" [21] The term "burnout" was not to be used in this sense until the early 1970s. Her prognostication concerning the future, as expressed midway through World War II, read "The medical profession will never again neglect industrial diseases, the employer will never again refuse to assume responsibility toward them. Our progress in this field has been great and it will keep on." [22] In part, this change has been seen.

That Dr. Hamilton's recorded life should be shared with a newer generation was seen in the reprinting of *Exploring the Dangerous Trades* in 1985 [23]. In the Foreword, Barbara Sicherman wrote:

> She lived on for nearly three decades after completing her autobiography, continuing to express herself on the issues of her times with singular grace and integrity. In old-old age, the issues that concerned her had changed somewhat, but the passionate intensity of her beliefs had not. The need to make her life count remained undimmed. [23]

And now, 10 years later, Alice Hamilton's first 73 years' experiences are being made available once again. With the beginning of the Occupational Safety and Health Act coinciding with the end of this pioneer's life, and with the gains made in occupational health over the past 25 years, we are, indeed, still gathering the rewards accruing from the work of this early explorer of the dangerous trades.

Jean Spencer Felton, MD
Mendocino, California

REFERENCES

1. Thompson WS. *The Occupational Diseases: Their Causation, Symptoms, Treatment and Prevention.* New York, NY, D. Appleton, 1914, pp. 65–6, 204–5.
2. Oliver T. *Dangerous Trades: The Historical, Social, and Legal Aspects of Industrial Occupations as Affecting Health, by a Number of Experts.* London, John Murray, 1902.
3. Hunter D. *The Diseases of Occupations.* Boston, MA. Little, Brown, 1955.
4. Schilling RSF, ed. *Occupational Health Practice.* London, Butterworth, 1973, pp. 16–7.
5. Taylor WA, Wasserman DE. Occupational Vibration. In Zenz C, Dickerson OB, Horwath EP Jr., eds. *Occupational Medicine*, 3rd ed. St. Louis, Mosby, 1994, p. 299.
6. Gaydos JC. Occupational Health in the U.S. Army, 1775–1990, in Deeter DP, Gaydos JC. *Occupational Health — The Soldier and the Industrial Base.* Washington, DC, Office of the Surgeon General, US Department of the Army, Borden Institute, Walter Reed Army Medical Center, 1993, pp. 3–6.
7. Hamilton A. *Industrial Poisons in the United States.* New York, NY, Macmillan, 1925. (Reprinted in 1929.)
8. Ibid., p. v.
9. Hamilton A. *Industrial Toxicology.* New York, NY, Harper & Brothers, 1934, p. vii.
10. Sicherman B. *Alice Hamilton: A Life in Letters.* Cambridge, MA, Harvard University Press, 1984, p. 373.
11. Felton JS, Newman JP, Read DL. *Man, Medicine, and Work - Historic Events in Occupational Medicine.* Washington, DC, US Department of Health Education, and Welfare, Public Health Service, Division of Occupational Health, 1964.
12. Alice Hamilton to J. S. Felton, March 26, 1964.
13. Sicherman B, p. 413.
14 Sicherman B, p. 9.
15. Alice Hamilton to H. A. Vonachen, January 29, 1953.
16. Sicherman B, p. 377.
17. Grant MP. *Alice Hamilton — Pioneer in Industrial Medicine.* New York, NY, Abelard-Schuman, 1967, dust-jacket legend.
18. Richard Nixon to A. Hamilton, February 27, 1969.

19 Hamilton A. *Exploring the Dangerous Trades.* Boston, MA, Little Brown, 1943, pp. 238–9 [EDT].
20. Hamilton A. *EDT,* p. 280.
21. Hamilton A. *EDT,* pp. 417–8.
22. Hamilton, A. *EDT,* p. 419.
23. Hamilton A. *Exploring the Dangerous Trades.* Boston, MA, Northeastern University Press, 1985.
24. Sicherman B, in Foreword, *ibid,* pp. xix–xx.

EXPLORING THE DANGEROUS TRADES

I

Introduction

THIRTY–TWO years ago, in 1910, I went as a pioneer into a new, unexplored field of American medicine, the field of industrial disease. This book is a record of what I found there thirty-two years ago, of the changes that have taken place in that region through the years that have followed, and of what still remains to be done before we can say that the wilderness has been conquered and the country completely civilized.

It was while I was living in Hull-House and working in bacteriological research that the opportunity came to me to investigate the dangerous trades of Illinois [1] — not those where violent accidents occurred, but those with the less spectacular hazard of sickness from some industrial poison. It was a voyage of exploration that we undertook, our little group of physicians and student assistants, for nobody in Illinois knew even where we should make our investigations, beyond a few notorious lead trades. American medical authorities had never taken industrial diseases seriously, the American Medical Associations had never held a meeting on the subject, and while European journals were full of articles on industrial poisoning, the number published in American medical journals up to 1910 could be counted on one's fingers.

For a surgeon or physician to accept a position with a manu-

[1] A State Commission was appointed by Governor Deneen in 1910 to report on "occupational diseases in Illinois."

facturing company was to earn the contempt of his colleagues as a "contract doctor"; as for factory inspection and control, we never discovered a trace of it.

This ignorance and indifference was not confined to the medical profession — employers and workers both shared it. The employers could, if they wished, shut their eyes to the dangers their workmen faced, for nobody held them responsible, while the workers accepted the risks with fatalistic submissiveness as part of the price one must pay for being poor.

As I look back, some striking pictures come to me of that anarchic period. One is the picture of the works manager of a big white-lead plant, a gentleman of breeding and something of a philanthropist. He is looking at me indignantly and exclaiming, "Why, that sounds as if you think that when a man gets lead poisoning in my plant I ought to be held responsible!" Another is that of a Hungarian woman at Hull-House, telling me of a terrible accident in a steel mill on the South Shore in which her husband had been injured. He and the other victims were being held incommunicado in the company hospital. No one was allowed to see them, she knew nothing except that her husband was not dead. It took a formal protest from the Austro-Hungarian Consul to the State Department to change that system.

It was not that employers were brutal. They really did not know what was happening in their plants, for there was no system of workmen's compensation to open their eyes to the hazards and to force safety measures. The workman might sue for damages, and that fact led to the sort of secrecy the steel industry and other big concerns practised. But even if he was seriously injured, it was hard for him to get past the strong defenses erected by law for the employer: the "assumption of risk," which meant that he had deliberately chosen to run the risk inherent in the job; or the "negligence of a fellow workman," which meant that he, not the employer, was responsible for the carelessness of the other employees. When we wonder why the workers did not rebel, we must remember that big industry employed almost exclusively immigrant labor at that time. In the heavy industries especially, the rule was to work the men as hard as possible — the seven-day week and twelve-hour day continued in steel until 1922 — pay them as low wages as possible, and then, when American ideas began to penetrate and revolt to raise its head, to put it down with force, discharge and blacklist the trouble-makers, and start afresh with a new lot of immigrants. In this, it must be added, the heavy industries were greatly helped by the courts of law and by the state constabulary forces.

Many times in those early days I met men who employed foreign-born labor because it was cheap and submissive, and then washed their hands of all responsibility for accidents and sickness in the plant, because, as they would say: "What can you do with a lot of ignorant Dagoes, Wops, Hunkies, Greasers? You couldn't make them wash if you took a shotgun to them." They deliberately chose such men because it meant no protest against low wages and wretched housing and dangerous work, no trouble with union agents; but rather a surplus of eager, undemanding labor. They wanted to have men whom they could deal with as if they were children, but in that case they should have treated them with the protective care and patient guidance that children are entitled to. They had all the advantages of the system; they took, for the most part, none of the responsibilities that it entailed.

Another defense used by the employer was alcoholism. The men were sick because they drank, and the employer did not need to prove it. He never went through the list of employees and showed that the ones who suffered from lead poisoning were the alcoholics. He just asserted it and it quieted his conscience. There is no form of industrial poisoning, from lead to dinitrobenzol, from mercury to carbon tetrachloride and nitric acid, which I have not heard some man attribute to whiskey. Yet a hundred years ago, Tanquerel des Planches, the great French authority on plumbism, declared that the men who succumbed to lead poisoning were not by any means only the drunkards; some of his severest cases were men who led sober and frugal lives. I used to suggest gently to my medical colleagues that it would be useful to have actual figures showing how alcoholism favored plumbism, but none of them seemed to be interested in collecting such proof, although they held to the theory firmly.

Through these thirty-odd years I have seen great changes in the attitude of labor, very deep changes, because the influence of American ideas has had time to work on the generation of men and women who now make up the labor force. But back in those early years I used to despair of relief for the overworked, underpaid immigrant laborers, who took with hopeless submission whatever was given them, who rarely ever dreamed of protesting, much less rebelling. It was they who did the heavy, hot, dirty, and dangerous work of the country. In return for it they met little but contempt from more fortunate Americans. The men killed in the mines or in construction work or in the steel mills would almost all be foreigners. Immigration was pushed with great diligence after the Civil War, and the labor supply was so abundant that the Chicago stockyards boasted that their gates were besieged each morning by a crowd of five or six hundred men, clamoring for the few available jobs. The Carnegie Company's principle of a high tariff to shut out cheap foreign-made goods, and a wide-open door to let in cheap foreign labor, resulted in the building up of great fortunes; but measured in terms of human welfare it was cruel and ruthless.

Yet in spite of the neglect of the doctors and the medieval backwardness of the lawmakers, the picture of that period is not all black, it is lightened by some remarkable instances of wise and humane employers, who were far in advance of their times, as I discovered when I first went into this field.

Our procedure in the Illinois survey and in the work that I carried on later for the Federal government was completely informal. We had no authority to enter any plant, we had no instructions as to which we should visit, we simply explored the state. When we found a place which seemed to belong in our field, we asked permission to enter it. Never were we refused, never did I, at least, meet with anything but courtesy in those very early days. Sometimes it was because the manager was proud of his plant and eager to show it (even when it was outrageously bad); sometimes it was because he had a strong suspicion that all was not well with his men and he really wanted more light. As to the way we should deal with the conditions we found, that was a question for each of us to settle. The Illinois Commission expected me to report back to it and in such a way that no factory described in the report could be identified. That I did, of course, but I could not feel that my whole responsibility was thereby discharged. I was the only one who had seen the men working on the Scotch hearths in the smelters, emptying the baghouse and flues, sandpapering the lead-painted ceilings of Pullman cars, shoveling the white lead from the drying pans. How could I hope that a cold, printed report which would satisfy the Commission would serve to do away with these pressing dangers?

There was no use in going to the factory inspectors: they were ignorant and powerless.

So, from the first, I made it a rule to try to bring before the responsible man at the top the dangers I had discovered in his plant and to persuade him to take the simple steps which even I, with no engineering knowledge, could see were needed. As I look back on it now from this changed world of "safety first," expert factory inspection, the National Safety Council, industrial insurance companies, strict compensation laws, it astonishes and amuses me to see how very well this primitive method often worked. I must recite a few instances, for they redound so much to the credit of the American manufacturer. Was it not Santayana who said that "it is by his kindness that one recognizes an American"? I cannot go so far as that; I have some bitter memories and they involve not the small and struggling manufacturer, but so-called captains of industry. Still, I insist they are few compared to my pleasant memories, for the arrogant and cold-blooded employer has, in my experience, made up a very small minority.

First to mind comes my experience with a beautiful new white-lead works which had been carefully planned to provide as much protection for the men as possible. But when I visited it I found that it was already, after a few months of operation, in a wretched way. This was, as is so often the case, simply a matter of bad housekeeping — heaps of dry white lead lying where they had no business to be, and other lots trucked about and dumped with no care at all. The manager was deeply vexed and hurt by my criticism; I could do nothing with him. The head of the company lived in an Eastern city; I might write to him, but he was old and no longer in active charge. Then I remembered that his daughter was a friend of one of my Farmington schoolmates, and I wrote to her, telling her frankly of my dilemma and asking her if I should appeal to her father or, if not, to whom. Only a short time later I received a formal letter saying that a representative of the firm would call on me. And that settled it; the plant was put in shape and I was asked to check up on it from time to time.

Across the river from St. Louis, in East St. Louis, I had a pleasant experience. I met a man who — even in 1910 — was genuinely concerned about the evil of lead poisoning in that industry, and had a feeling of personal responsibility toward it. This was Frank Hammar, of Hammar Brothers' White Lead. He was struggling with the problem, assisted not very helpfully by a doctor who advised him to make the men wear rubber gloves. We kept in touch with each other for many years after that visit. It was Mr. Hammar who, when I was at Harvard, induced the Lead Institute to endow a three-year research on the action of lead in the animal body, and entrusted the Harvard Medical School with the task. This endowment made possible the studies of Joseph C. Aub and his colleagues — studies which are still our best source of knowledge of how lead operates and how lead poisoning can be prevented.

Even more important reforms followed my contact with the National Lead Company which had several white-lead and lead-oxide works in and near Chicago. I visited them and found much dangerous work going on in all of them. One of the vice-presidents, Edward Cornish, later president, came to Chicago and I went to see him in the Sangamon Street works. He was both indignant and incredulous when I told him I was sure men were being poisoned in those plants. He had never heard of such a thing; it could not be true; they were model plants. He went to the door and shouted to a pass-

ing workman to come in. "Did the lead ever make you sick?"
he demanded. The man, a badly scared Slav, stammered, "No,
no, never sick." "Any other men sick?" demanded Mr. Cornish.
"No, no, all good," and the poor man escaped quickly. "There,"
said Mr. Cornish, "you see!" "But I do not see," I answered.
"Your men are breathing white-lead dust and red lead and
litharge and the fumes from the oxide furnaces. They are no
different from other men; a poison is a poison to them as it
is to any man." He thought a moment and then he said, "Now,
see here. I don't believe you are right, but I can see you do.
Very well then, it is up to you to convince me. Come back
here with proof that my men are being leaded and I give you
my word I will follow all your directions, even to employing
plant doctors."

It was not an easy task I faced, tracking down actual, proved
cases of lead poisoning among men who came from the
Serbian, Bulgarian, and Polish sections of West and Northwest Chicago, and were known to the employing office only
as Joe, Jim, or Charlie, with no record of their street and
number! It meant digging up hospital records, for I had to
be sure of the diagnosis, then a search for the home, and finally an interview with the wife to discover where the man
had been working, for of course no hospital interne ever noted
where the victim of plumbism had acquired the lead. Hospital
history sheets noted carefully all the facts about tobacco, alcohol, and even coffee consumed by the leaded man, though
obviously he was not suffering from those poisons; but curiosity as to how he became poisoned with lead was not in the
interne's mental make-up.

In the end I was able to present Mr. Cornish with authentic
records of twenty-two cases of plumbism severe enough to
require hospital care. He was better than his word. Begin-

ning with the Sangamon Street works, he went on to reform
all the plants in the Chicago region, and this meant dust and
fume prevention, often by methods which had never before
been worked out. There were no models to follow; the engineers faced new problems. As each was solved, Mr. Cornish
sent the blueprints to the plants in other states and later on,
when I visited these, invariably I found the same changes being introduced. I had told Mr. Cornish he could never fully
protect his men unless he employed doctors to keep strict
watch over their condition, to make at least a brief inspection
of each lead worker once a week. He accepted this recom-
mendation without protest and before our report was published there was a medical department in each plant of the
National Lead Company in Illinois. I have met many admirable men in industry throughout these thirty-two years,
but my warmest gratitude and admiration goes to Edward
Cornish.

In 1911, one year after the publication of the *Survey of
Occupational Diseases*, Illinois passed a law providing compensation for industrial diseases caused by poisonous fumes, gases,
or dusts (a good law till the lawyers got at it and messed it up
so that a new one had to be framed in 1938). The reforms
that followed the passage of this law were swift and drastic.
Employers found they must insure against possible claims
and the insurance companies saw to it that the causes for
such claims were removed. One by one, but slowly, other
states passed similar laws, until by 1937 almost all the important industrial states and a few of the nonindustrial ones had
passed legislation providing compensation for industrial diseases. Invariably reforms in the dangerous trades followed.

Two great industrial states held out for years: Michigan
waited till 1937, Pennsylvania till 1938. Pennsylvania's law

is still a meager concession to the pressure of modern progress. No compensation is to be paid to the widow and orphans of a workman killed in industry if they live in a foreign country. Moreover, the compensation provided is pretty niggardly. I have before me a letter about an award recently granted by a court of appeal in that state to a widow for whose husband's death carbon disulphide[2] was claimed to be responsible. The award is for only $1.50 a week. Yet a great Pennsylvania company has fought the claim for three years, refusing to admit that carbon disulphide is an industrial poison.

It is a pity that I cannot recall any instance of help from the organized industrialists to obtain for American workmen the sort of protection provided years ago in European industrial countries. But the truth is that the National Association of Manufacturers has fought the passage of occupational-disease compensation as it has fought laws against child labor, laws establishing a minimum wage for women and a maximum working day.[3] Yet members of the N.A.M. are many of them humane and benevolent employers. But as an organization they have shown themselves to be as devoid of a sense of responsibility to the public as the most self-seeking of the trade-unions. I have gone before legislative committees in

[2] See Chapter XXI.

[3] This does not apply to compensation for accidental injury or to accident prevention by means of safety devices. Organized industrialists have been very active in this field and have often favored protective legislation. Enlightened self-interest alone would have dictated such action, but besides that, accidents in industry are striking, dramatic, and the cause is clear, while occupational disease comes on slowly and insidiously, and the responsibility is more easily evaded. The attitude of industrialists toward accidents has been excellent; toward the other less dramatic evils, sickness, child labor, long hours, low wages, it has been quite different.

Illinois, New York, and Massachusetts and I have invariably found the salaried representative of the manufacturers there in opposition.

Perhaps it is our instinctive American lawlessness that prompts us to oppose all legal control, even when we are willing to do of our own accord what the law requires. But I believe it is more the survival in American industry of the feudalistic spirit, for democracy has never yet really penetrated into many of our greatest industries. England affords a striking contrast. When I was there in 1928 the Home Office was making a new set of rules for the control of lead poisoning in storage-battery plants. Representatives of the manufacturers and of the trade-union sat in with the factory inspection experts and had equal voting power. In our country I had just been through the painful experience of seeing the best-managed storage-battery plant in the United States pass under the control of a company with which I had struggled for fourteen years in a vain effort to get decent protection for its employees against lead poisoning. I thought how impossible it would be to copy that English procedure. We had no trade-union, no organization of employers which could speak for the industry, and, in the particular state I have in mind, no factory inspectors expert and courageous enough to deal with the situation.

Yet great changes have come in these thirty-two years, great reforms in industrial hygiene have been brought about by the joint effort of physicians and legislators. Far from being ignored, industrial medicine is now one of the most important medical branches, and hundreds of doctors choose it as their specialty. The Public Health Service has a large division devoted to industrial medicine; the Department of

Labor has its Division of Labor Standards, which acts as a guide to state factory inspection services. There are even a few state Labor Departments that are free from political interference and do a good job.

Labor too has changed. It is no longer willing to submit to preventable ills. Workmen now are graduates of our public schools, where they have been taught that all men are created equal, that any boy has a chance to be President, that America is the land of opportunity, and all the rest. Naturally such a lad faces his employer with a different spirit from that of his peasant father from the Old World. He steps from a world of democratic ideals in school to a feudalistic industrial world, and he takes the adjustment with difficulty. I think we are now just at the dividing line: feudalism still holds sway in much of the industrial world while all the rest of our American world proclaims democracy. No wonder there is unrest — more unrest even than there was under the old, bad system, for the submissive spirit is gone. And though the conspicuous evils in industrial work have been removed to a great extent, there are still evils against which the modern American rebels.

Even under short hours and fair wages there is unrest. But we must not forget that modern work is different from what our race has been used to for aeons. We cannot adjust ourselves to it all of a sudden. Compare the sort of work a man on a punch press does with the work his ancestors did for centuries. Work used to be heavy and hard, but there was enough sameness in it to provide for a growing skill and enough variety to keep a man interested. You cannot fell two trees in exactly the same way, nor dig two ditches exactly alike. Then, too, a man could set his own pace, speed up for a bit, then slow down. Now a great deal of work requires no skill, and the machine sets the pace and makes the man feel he is its slave, not its master. He loses pride in his work and he loses his sense of individual importance.

The studies of the Fatigue Laboratory of Harvard and the investigation made at the Western Electric Company in Chicago of what makes men and women work well [4] have given a scientific foundation to the truth some of us discovered years ago: that factors more important than wages or conditions of work influence the temper of the worker. In Chicago, I once talked to a group of girls who looked as if they were all suffering from hay fever of a severe form because they had been working in a room where the air was full of strongly alkaline soap powder. I asked them why they stood it. "Well," one of them said, "we're always saying we'll quit, but then Tom comes along. He's the foreman and he's a swell guy and he jollies us along and we stay." Out in the Arizona copper country I found that one of the very worst mines, with its dust and poor lighting and lack of safety devices, was the one that stood highest in the estimation of the miners because the manager was "white, square." You could talk to him. Soon after I had returned East I found myself sitting next to Sam Lewisohn at a dinner. I told him of my visit to his admirably run mine, the Inspiration in Miami, and of my astonishment to find it was rated lower by the men than one that was vastly inferior. We discussed the labor troubles out there and he told me how they had distressed him and his brother. "But what can one do?" he asked. "One hires men to get out copper, and finds that they are experts in that job but idiots when it comes to handling men. Yet one can't oust them and put in experts in human relations

[4] See *Fatigue of Workers. Its Relation to Industrial Production*, by The Committee on Work in Industry of the National Research Council, Summarized by George Homans. Reinhold Publishing Corporation, 1941.

because they know nothing about copper. The institutes of technology simply must face this fact and begin to teach engineers psychology." That is now a commonplace, but Sam Lewisohn may have started the movement to introduce this new subject into the curricula of schools of engineering.

The Harvard investigators have no doubt at all that the economic motive is not the strongest one governing industrial workers. They say that it is entirely possible for an industrial company to give good wages and to provide in every way for the welfare of the men and yet have strikes — because the men in charge fail to understand the psychology of their employees: they believe that wages and hours are all-important; they ignore men's tendency to form social groups with codes and loyalties for mutual defense, all of which help to make a man feel he is a personality, that he has some control. Let him be tied to a machine which sets his pace and determines every action, and you produce in him an "experience of personal futility," of "heavy preoccupation, pessimistic revery." To join with his fellows in an organization is the only escape from this humiliating position — and that organization may be quite informal, but effective. This point should be illuminating to the large section of the public that has no patience with strikes carried on "only" for the right to organize.

Protection of workers in the dangerous trades is the chief but not the only subject of this book. Other things have played a great part in my life. I should never have taken up the cause of the working class had I not lived at Hull-House and learned much from Jane Addams, Florence Kelley, Julia Lathrop, and others. Hull-House is not an episode of the past; its influence still lives, and it deserves a tribute from one of its devoutest followers. The years from 1914 to 1942 have been full of issues more tremendous than the struggle of labor for its rights and, living as I did with Jane Addams, I could not escape being drawn into the peace movement and the efforts to reconstruct Europe after the Armistice. So that too enters into the picture. And childhood and student life, the men I worked under in school and laboratory, the background of Fort Wayne, Mackinac, Chicago, later on of Boston and Hadlyme — these are all significant parts of the picture I have tried to paint: a picture of life as I have seen it under the period of passionate and hopeful idealism in the nineties; of slowly increasing disillusion culminating in the shock of war in 1914; of the war years with their intolerance and bitterness and wave of reaction; of the "giddy twenties" when, underneath the surface froth, I saw unemployment and exploitation; the soberer thirties with the increasing movement toward social justice. Russia, the League of Nations, the Sacco-Vanzetti case, the starvation blockade in Germany and Austria, Hitler's Germany, France and Germany during the "Munich betrayal" — all these go to make up the record of my life.

II

The Old House

M Y CHILDHOOD home was Fort Wayne, Indiana, where my father's father had come as a young man from the North of Ireland and his father had joined him later, so that my generation was the fourth to live in what we called the Old House. I should have been born there as my two younger sisters were, but my mother went home to her mother in New York to have her second baby. I always have to give New York City as my birthplace, most inappropriately, for I left it at the age of six weeks and I really belong to Indiana.

We were four sisters born within six years' time, which was hard on our mother but made for close intimacy from our earliest childhood. Years later, when I was just seventeen, there was an aftermath in the shape of the first boy, my brother Arthur, who is always known as Quint because we dubbed him that when an old German gentleman said to my father, "You should call your son Primus, Mr. Hamilton." "Indeed no," we said, "he is only Quintus" — and Quintus he has been ever since. Edith, the first-born, though only eighteen months older than I, seemed much more mature, partly because she was a passionate reader while I was a reluctant one, partly because she went with the older cousins and I joined the younger group. Edith read everything she could lay her hands on, except the few forbidden books in my father's library: the *Decameron* of Boccaccio, the *Heptameron* of Marguerite of Navarre, Eugène Sue's *Wandering Jew*, and a few others I have forgotten. She was a natural storyteller, and on the long walks my mother insisted on our taking every day, Edith would give us résumés of Scott and Bulwer-Lytton and De Quincey. She could not understand my childish tastes in books and she would stop at an exciting spot, such as Amy Robsart's death in *Kenilworth*, and say, "Now you've got to finish it yourself." Sometimes I did, but sometimes I slipped back to the "Katy" books, to her infinite disgust. She also loved to learn poetry by heart, and as we walked to and from our daily music lesson, she would recite to me Macaulay's *Lays of Ancient Rome*, "Naseby," and "Ivry" till I knew them by heart. Then came Shelley, Keats, and Byron. I am sure I learned "The Eve of St. Agnes" just by listening to her recite it.

Edith and Margaret were born readers. Norah and I were not, but family pressure made us too into bookworms finally; and since we saw so little of any children outside our own family, the people we met in books became real to us. First they were the children in the "Franconia" books of Jacob Abbott and in Sophie May's "Susy and Prudy" books; then Susan Coolidge's "Katy" books, which we liked much better than Louisa Alcott's; then the Schönberg-Cotta books, and Charlotte Yonge's May and Underwood families, who still are more vivid to me than any real people I met in those years.

Margaret is two and a half years younger than I, but because she was the only one of us who had ill health as a child, she did not seem really younger. Today, her sore throat and rheumatic pains and listlessness would be traced to infected tonsils, the source would be removed, and she would emerge from chronic ill health; but in those days the old family doctor had no remedy except quinine, and all my mother could offer was sea-salt baths and long hours on the sofa. This meant reading and thinking for Margaret, while the rest of us were playing football and climbing trees, and it made her the quiet, stable, thoughtful one among us. I cannot remember fits of temper or deliberate teasing and tormenting on Margaret's part, such as the rest of us were sometimes guilty of.

Norah, the youngest, was my father's special pet and pride. When she early showed her talent for drawing, he used to call her his genius. We never felt jealous because we were not geniuses; indeed the relations between us four were so intimate and understanding that when one of us would be singled out for admiration by a not too discerning parent, it would only amuse both the praised and the unpraised. Norah was as vivid and intense as Margaret was steady — with her it was rapture or tragedy, and so of course she was terribly vulnerable to the sort of teasing and baiting that children love to inflict when they find an easy victim.

Fort Wayne was an attractive little city in those days. The streets were shaded by elms and maples; the sidewalks were of mellowed red brick, for asphalt had not yet spread its ugly way across our cities. The shops were too quiet and uniform to be really ugly, the show windows did not attempt any original stunts, and I remember as the most exciting thing on Calhoun Street a drugstore which displayed in the window two tall graceful flasks filled with colored water, each of them flanked by a pair of smaller flasks, also brightly colored. Edith and I would race for this store, and the one who reached the window first might "choose" the combination she liked best; then it belonged to her. I suppose the swiftly moving automobile has made merchants think they must scream aloud their wares with violent red and green paint and crowded show windows or nobody will notice them. But when everybody screams at once, there are only confusion and ugliness. There were a number of fine old houses dating back before the Civil War, some of them showing the Southern tradition which was strong in Fort Wayne's early days. Our most important street was Calhoun Street, and we had others named for Clay, Douglas, Breckinridge, but none for Lincoln. The Civil War split the Presbyterian Church in two and must have caused deep division between citizens.

My Hamilton grandfather's house, which we called the Old House, was large and substantial. It was of brick and had been built in 1840 with three stories and a two-storied ell and a basement kitchen. Like most houses of a hundred years ago, it was built for beauty, space, dignity, not for comfort and convenience. The ceilings were fourteen feet high, the rooms were spacious, and a wood-burning furnace made little impression on the cold of our Indiana winter. There were open fires in every room. Nobody thought of the endless carrying of wood, coal, ashes, up and down the long stairways, for there was always a "hired man," who had little else to do in winter. There were also plenty of housemaids to carry clean water upstairs and dirty water downstairs in those pre-plumbing days. On top of the house was what we called the "cupalo," a square little room, big enough for a crowd of us and never disturbed by the grownups. To reach it we passed a forbidden door which led into a room we were told had no floor. It was a horrible thought, that bottomless pit of darkness, and we never ventured to turn the handle.

Our frame house was the White House, my uncle's in the same grounds was the Red House, and of brick. Neither was so big as the Old House, and the ceilings were somewhat lower; the furnaces burned coal and there were running water and a bathroom, so much had comfort progressed between 1840 and 1873. But space and dignity were still the first desiderata. Our hall was vast, and the rooms — library, parlor, dining room — opened into it by triple doors of black walnut, but as it could never be heated in winter, those doors had to be kept shut. The wide stairs were also black walnut. Of a winter's night, when the house was very still, a ghost might start at the attic door and come creaking down the two flights to the hall. This happened one evening when I was quite alone in the library, reading the fearsome tale of black magic in *The Lay of the Last Minstrel*.

There was one great advantage in our big house — one that more than made up for the inadequate furnace — and that was the opportunity for escape, for solitude. One could curl up in the big armchair in the library or hide in the parlor — or, if the others were persistent, there was a refuge at the top of the attic stairs and, in warm weather, out on a bit of flat roof which could be reached from the billiard-room window. In spring and fall there were endless hiding places in lilac hedges or up in the thick leaves of an apple tree.

Allen Hamilton, my grandfather, the pioneer ancestor, came to Fort Wayne when it was still very primitive, an outpost in a land of Indians. His career was typical of America in those days. He dealt with Indians at first, and the tales that have come down to us show that his fairness won their confidence and respect. He played a large part in the development of the city and was one of a small group of men who put through the Pittsburgh, Fort Wayne, and Chicago railroad. He was ambitious for his family, sending his sons not only to college but to Göttingen and Jena Universities, his daughters to Miss Porter's School in Farmington, Connecticut. He was Scotch-Irish and my father always stressed the first word,

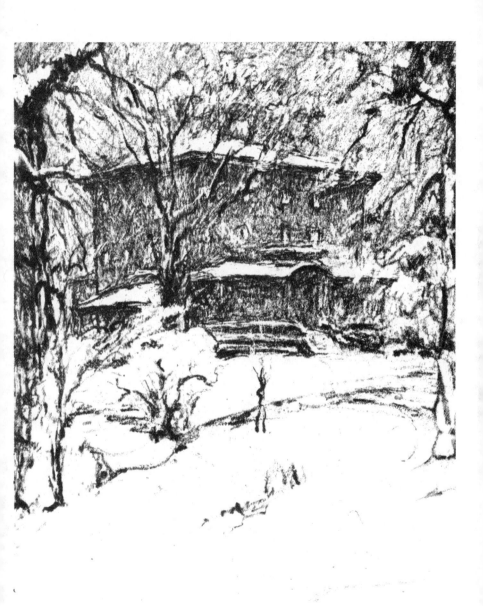

but we children were fascinated by the Irish part and loved to hear tales of an old Irish Katy who came over with the family and who saw fairies and heard the banshee wail when our grandfather died.

He found his bride in Aurora, an older, more settled community on the Ohio River, not far from Cincinnati. My grandmother always spoke of "going in" when she went home and "going out" when she returned to what in her youth had been the frontier. She was only seventeen when she went with her young husband to that distant spot where somehow she learned to preside over a large household and where she bore eleven children. The first four years of my life were spent in that house; and although after that we lived in a house of our own, it was on the same big place and the Old House with its orchard and cow pasture and extensive "yard" (nobody had "grounds" in those days) was as important a background for my life as our own place. My grandfather died before any of the younger generation were born, but my grandmother lived on till we older ones were in our teens. She was descended from English emigrants who settled first in Virginia, then moved on to Kentucky and to Southern Indiana.

My grandmother was a fascinating person to all of us, but we never knew her intimately; there was something elusive about her; and her affection, which embraced all seventeen of us cousins, was quite impersonal. I always felt I was "Montgomery's second daughter" to her. She was a tiny person, quick and wiry, and her mind was as quick as her body. She loved reading passionately. I can remember often seeing her in the library of the Old House, crouched over the fireplace where the soft-coal fire had gone out without her knowing it, so deep had she been in her book. Once she was perched on the top of a ladder, level with the last shelf of the bookcase. She had meant to dust the books but had come upon one so fascinating that she lost herself in it and forgot where she was. She could enthrall us children with Scott's poems, telling us the story in prose and suddenly dropping into long passages of the poetry, as, for instance, the trial and walling up of Constance de Beverley in the monastery of Lindisfarne from *Marmion*. She was an ardent advocate of the temperance movement and, chiefly through it, of woman's suffrage. Those two valiant crusaders, Frances Willard and Susan B. Anthony, were her personal friends and used to stay at the Old House when they came to Fort Wayne. It took a good deal of courage in those days to come out for such causes, especially for woman's suffrage.

My mother's father, Loyal Sylvester Pond, came from Vermont to New York and was a sugar importer dealing with Cuba chiefly. He died when I was still a child and I only remember him as white-haired, with very bright blue eyes and something about him which did not encourage real intimacy. My grandmother lived to a great age and played a large part in our lives. She was of Dutch descent, with English and Irish admixture, but to us, steeped as we were in Motley's *Dutch Republic*, the Dutch part of our ancestry was much the most interesting. Her education was typical of mid-Victorianism and so was her outlook on life. She had gone to Miss Lucy Green's School in New York, where she had learned the most correct morals and manners, where she had come to adore Byron but had promised Miss Lucy never to read *Don Juan*, where her belief in the literal inspiration of the Bible and the complete iniquity of the Roman Catholic Church had been strengthened so that she never lost it, and her attitude toward social questions might be summed up by two state-

ments I remember her making in later years. One was on
the question of Negro slavery. "Doubtless it was hard on the
slaves, but we had to have cotton." Another was on Lincoln. "My dear, what was the name of our President during
the war, a most uncouth person I always heard, though well-
meaning in his way?" While I was at Hull-House she used
to send me garments for poor children which she herself made,
but the stuff she bought was always gray or brown or dark
blue, for she felt that bright colors were not fitting for the
poor. Yet she was the sweetest, gentlest soul; I never remember her impatient or censorious, but always serene and kindly.

She had been in Europe with her children throughout the
Civil War and her husband was a Southern sympathizer who
wrote her that "that damned rail splitter" had actually been
nominated for the Presidency. The result of all this was that
the Civil War was never very real to my mother; and though
my father ran away from Princeton to enlist at the age of nineteen and served till he was invalided home, he never idealized
it — in fact, he hardly ever spoke of it except to excoriate the
profiteers who had sold paper boots and rotten food to the
Army. He believed that the South had a right to secede and
he never claimed that anything but boyish love of adventure
had carried him into the war. So we children knew little
of the enthusiasm for that conflict that New England children had, which I think was something of a loss.

There were eleven cousins living in the same big place. We
needed no "outsiders," having our own games, our own traditions and rules of conduct. Eight of us played together, being
near enough of an age. In those days children invented their
own games, grownups looked after health, studies, manners and
morals, but amusement was not their responsibility. We played
long-continued games, Robin Hood and his band, the Knights

of the Round Table, the siege of Troy, with the carriage
house as Troy and our woodhouse the Greek camp.

Once we were out of doors we were free, except for a few
prohibitions which we always observed, for we were obedient.
We were also truthful; that is, we told nothing but the truth.
We did not always tell the whole truth, for we argued that
the less the impulsive and incalculable grownups knew, the
better for them and us. Thus, when Allen's wooden sword
cut my forehead I ran to the pump and struck the place
against the iron handle so that I could truthfully say that
the handle had hit me, and not risk the chance of having
tournaments forbidden. We lived in our own world, a child's
world which we left only briefly to enter the far less real one
of the grownups. Three of us were very close in age, born
within five months — Agnes Hamilton, Allen Hamilton Williams, and I, who were known in the family circle as the three
A's. Growing up together, we were the closest of friends
and intimates, especially Agnes and I, for Allen spent his
winters at school in Boston, while Agnes and I went to
Farmington.

As we grew into our teens, games gave way to long walks
or sessions up in a big apple tree or on the rafters of the carriage house, with talks about everything, from theology to
our plans for life. For some years my plans for the future were
definite. I meant to be a medical missionary to Teheran, having been fascinated by the description of Persia in O'Donovan's
The Merv Oasis. I doubted if I could ever be good enough
to be a real missionary; but if I could care for the sick, that
would do instead, and it would enable me to explore far
countries and meet strange people. Later Agnes and I read
Charles Kingsley and Frederick Denison Maurice and became
interested in the English social question, and though we knew

nothing about American social evils, life in a big city, exploring the slums, began to seem to me as tempting as Persia.

Fort Wayne, outside our own yard, touched us chiefly
through the church which played a large part in our lives —
not so much socially, for we were fairly self-contained socially,
but as a pervading background, as something that came next to
home and family. My father's family was Presbyterian and
we all went to the First Presbyterian Church, a lovely Christo-
pher Wren building of red brick with wide steps up to a
white-pillared portico. I saw one exactly like it in Athens,
Georgia, years later, when the one in Fort Wayne had burned
down and been replaced by a rough-stone, pseudo-Richardson
monstrosity. Sermons were long, services scrupulously plain,
but I do not remember being bored. Indeed our "puritanical"
Sunday was distinctly pleasant, probably because it was so
different from all other days and followed so strict a tradition. Breakfast, dinner, supper, on Sunday were unvarying
but different from the meals on other days, the books we read
were "Sunday" books, and church and Sunday school were
interesting partly because they constituted our rare excursions
into the outside world.

The religion we were taught was sober, not colored with the
fervent evangelism which was so prevalent in those days. My
father, Montgomery Hamilton, had a passion for theology. There was a time when I knew more about Arianism,
Socinianism, Gnosticism, and the other heresies than I knew
about the history of my own country. He insisted that my sister Edith and I learn the Westminster Catechism, and many a
struggle we had over that heathenish production. It was only
a struggle to memorize the words — we never bothered with
the meaning. My mother, Episcopalian as she was, sometimes

protested against giving such strong meat to babes, but apparently one can shovel very tough particles into a child's mind without causing indigestion. I can still remember some of the worst answers: for instance, "All mankind by Adam's fall lost communion with God, are under His wrath and curse and so made liable to all the ills of this life, to death and to the pains of Hell forever." I suppose a sensitive child should have been profoundly affected by such horrible teaching, but it made not a dent on us. Luckily for Margaret and Norah, my father was tired of the Catechism when they came along, and they escaped it.

To offset the Catechism we learned Psalms for my mother and the Sermon on the Mount and the first chapter of St. John. And in summer we went to her church, the little Episcopal Church in Mackinac Island, where we were steeped in the collects and the Litany and the *Te Deum* until they became a part of us. We learned to love the service better than we had ever loved the Presbyterian. The Bible was more familiar to us than any other book, and, as is true of everything we learn in childhood, it is so deeply imprinted in my memory that more often than not when I hear it read in church I can keep just a little ahead of the minister. Such training would be preposterous nowadays, but I wonder whether we have not gone too far in the other direction, whether children brought up with no knowledge of the Bible are not robbed of part of their heritage. For it permeates our great literature and our great art, much of which must be incomprehensible to young people educated in modern schools. Quite apart from one's faith or lack of faith in the teachings of the Bible it seems to me that an education which leaves it out is thin and poor. I think of the young Americans I have seen in Mexican churches gazing at the devout worshipers before some holy image as they would gaze at animals in a menagerie, with as little realization of what it is all about. To them *Paradise Lost* and Chartres must always be things written in a foreign language.

Religion, as it was taught to us, had little authoritarianism; certainly credulousness was not encouraged. The first piece of "research" I ever undertook was when I was about twelve years old. My father set me the task of finding proof of the doctrine of the Trinity in the Bible. His own belief was that this doctrine was a later addition to the Gospels, and he had no hesitation in setting me on an inquiry which might bring me to the same conviction. But in those days there was no pragmatism to shake a child's belief in Christian ethics. We never questioned the rightfulness of truth-telling, honorable dealing, unselfishness, self-control. To base them on practical advantage to oneself or even to society would have been to shake the foundations of our moral world. Actions were right or they were wrong, and when they were wrong we knew that the eyes of the Lord are in every place beholding the evil and the good. This unquestioning acceptance of a moral code, together with a strong family background, made us more "rooted and grounded," but not, I think, so dependent on our elders as are the children of today.

Our education was very uneven, with serious omissions. Fort Wayne had only public schools, and my mother objected to the long hours from nine in the morning to four in the afternoon. My father objected to the curriculum — too much arithmetic and American history, neither a subject which interested him. So we did not go to school and we could be out of doors during the sunny hours. We had a smattering of mathematics, taught by a day governess, but I never got beyond the beginning of algebra. We learned what our parents thought important: languages, literature, history. We had formal teaching only in languages; the other subjects we had to learn ourselves by reading, and we did. Most of the hours we spent indoors were spent over books. My father taught us Latin; my mother talked French with us when we were little and saw to it that we had French lessons later on; our German came first from the servants, who were always German, then from a Lutheran schoolteacher.

Of science we had not even a smattering, beyond what we could gather from my father's favorite Max Müller. Yet in a way we were trained in habits of scientific approach. We were not allowed to make a statement which could be challenged unless we were prepared to defend it. One of my father's favorite quotations was, "Be ready always to give a reason of the hope that is in you." When he could not answer a question he would send us to the *Encyclopedia Britannica*, to look it up. Of course the articles were often beyond our comprehension. When I told him that my cousin Allen was studying physics in his Boston school and I wanted to study it too, he said, "It is all in the encyclopedia." And it was, but not in a shape for a girl of fourteen.

The habit of doing one's own searching for the knowledge one wanted was valuable, but the field that attracted me was too limited. As I reached my teens, instead of turning to the natural sciences, of which I was completely ignorant, I taught myself Greek and Italian and read the French classics. Of American literature I knew little. My father had a great impatience with what he considered the woolgathering of the New England school and I knew nothing of Emerson, little of Hawthorne. Poe was the only American poet he respected. He liked clarity and definiteness — Macaulay and Froude, Addison, Pope. He read us Macaulay's *Lays* and

Scott's poems, and he made Edith and me learn the whole of *The Lady of the Lake*, reciting a few lines every evening, to "train our memory." Later on he would give us a page of Addison which we must read over three times and must then write out in Addison's words. He hated sentimentality, and though that term to him sometimes covered my mother's generous enthusiasms and indignations, it was probably a wholesome factor in a household of women.

My mother, Gertrude Pond, was of a quite different temperament. She was less intellectual but more original and independent in her approach to life; indeed she was an extraordinary woman for her day and generation. Perhaps it was because she had spent much of her young womanhood in Germany and France that she was free from the Victorian prudery which was considered essential to a lady. My mother could speak of such subjects as pregnancy, childbirth, suckling, quite unconscious of the taboo in Fort Wayne. Even more, she faced sex problems with courage and originality. I remember a discussion she had with the women of my father's family, in which she took the stand Browning takes in "The Statue and the Bust," that the woman who is virtuous because she fears public opinion is not virtuous at all.

I remember also a friend's coming to her in great distress over her brother who was living with a mistress and who must be persuaded to marry her, to make the relation moral. My mother insisted that the woman was the seducer; that such a marriage would be degrading, not moral; that he should be persuaded to break up the relation. But her attitude seemed shocking to her friend, as indeed it would have to almost all women in those days.

She had been the oldest daughter in a family of eleven, and though my grandfather was well-to-do and there were servants enough in the big household, she had to play mother to the younger children because my grandmother was usually absorbed in having another baby. She had a passionate love of freedom, of going her own way undisturbed by the demands and compulsions of family life. This spirit she carried into her own home, so far as she could. Never was there a mother less possessive. The motto she chose was that of the monks of Thelema, "Fay ce que vouldras," and she taught us that personal liberty was the most precious thing in life.

Some seventy years before Virginia Woolf wrote *A Room of One's Own,* my mother believed in the right of every woman to privacy, even if she were the mother of a family. Another of her traits was equally rare — her capacity for enthusiasms and for indignations over events and causes which had no personal bearing whatever. She could blaze out, even in her old age, over tales of police brutality, of the lynching of Negroes, over child labor and cruelty to prisoners. She made us feel that whatever went wrong in our society was a personal concern for her and for us. But her indignation was not so much against the individual policeman or prison warden; it was against the whole class and especially the system which made such cruelty possible. Something she said once gives a picture of her quality and of the atmosphere in which we girls grew up: —

"There are two kinds of people, the ones who say 'Somebody ought to do something about it, but why should it be I?' and those who say 'Somebody must do something about it, then why not I?' "

She was no lover of Scott or Macaulay. For her I learned Gray's *Elegy* by heart and with her we read aloud *The Mill on the Floss* and *Adam Bede.*

The German Lutheran Church was opposite the Old House

and was to us children second in importance only to the First Presbyterian Church, for our maids all attended it. So did the hired men. (We all had hired men, not gardeners or coachmen or housemen, but plain hired men.) Then at Christmas it was the Lutheran Church to which we went, for our church ignored completely that Popish holiday. The maids would call us at half-past five on Christmas morning and after a hasty glass of milk in the kitchen we would steal out into the dark winter morning over to the church, which was brilliantly lighted, and had great Christmas trees on either side of the altar. We heard a simple, naïve sermon in German addressed to the children and then the classes from the Lutheran Schools up in the gallery sang their Christmas hymns, "*Vom Himmel hoch da komm ich her,*" "*Uns ist ein Kind geboren,*" "*Ihr Kinderlein kommet,*" and many more. As the congregation streamed out we followed them, up one German street and back on another, to see the little lighted Christmas trees in every window. The memory of those Christmas mornings, and of an old hired man and a very lovely nursemaid, are enough in themselves to keep me from ever lumping all Germans together in a general condemnation.

Our summers were spent for some years at the Old Sweet Springs in West Virginia, where we were among the few Northern children. It is a lovely spot and when I saw it not long ago, deserted and silent, I was impressed by the excellence of the architecture, reminiscent of Thomas Jefferson's University of Virginia. Mostly one's childhood memories of buildings are much too big and imposing; it is a disillusionment to see them in later life, but the Old Sweet is as stately and spacious as I remember it. But I did not carry any picture in my memory of the mountains, though I could picture clearly a little pebbly brook. I wonder if children ever do see distant views — if they pay any attention except to what is near and tangible.

When I was ten we began to go to Mackinac Island, which became our summer home for many years — the years when impressions of the outside world are keenest and deepest. It is a beautiful island, lying in the Straits, with Lake Huron to the east and Lake Michigan to the west, their horizons as wide as the ocean, but north and south faced with the Michigan shores and with low-lying islands. There is a legend that it rose from the waters in the days when only Indians were there. It is much higher than the land all about it, and it has imposing cliffs of limestone rock. In my childhood it was still untouched by modern progress, by the hideous architecture of the eighties and nineties. The old Mission House and Mission Church had set the standard, and the village might have been in New England except for the picturesque bark cabins of the Indians on the Point. On the hill above stood the whitewashed stone buildings of Fort Mackinac, which are still there but are no longer used by the Army. And behind it the woods began with all the beauty of Northern woods: white birch and silver birch, beech, hemlock, and those pines which one sees only in the North, tall and straight-stemmed, with bark that has a rosy hue and forms great irregular scales.

We came to love it passionately, almost painfully it seems to me now as I look back on the tragic eagerness with which we returned each year. We would scan the shore as the boat came near and break our hearts over any change in the beloved view. The changes came thick and fast in the nineties, as the place became a resort, and indeed we helped to spoil Mission Hill by building a homely cottage there. But woods and shore remained much as they had been in my grandmother's time when she took her babies there, and our life was spent in the woods and on the water. As I look back on our education it seems, as I have said, incomplete and scrappy, but it gave us two precious things: a love of out-of-doors and a love of reading, and with those one is protected against any possible kind of boredom.

Poetry belonged to Mackinac, or perhaps it was interpreted and made real there. At any rate when I used to read "Tintern Abbey," or bits from the "Hymn before Sunrise," or "The Heavens declare the glory of God, the firmament showeth His handiwork," or even Byron's "Colosseum by Moonlight," it was all Mackinac to me — the pine cliffs on the west, the moonrise over Lake Huron, the deep, deep woods near Scott's Cave, the tremendous sweep of sky and straits and wide horizons during an equinoctial storm. Wind in pine trees, water lapping on a pebbly beach — I have heard them in Switzerland and in Bavaria and in Sicily, and always Mackinac has come sweeping back to me and I think it always will. Among the most vivid memories are the nights spent in an open boat, or on the shore of the mainland, when my father would take us with him on one of his fishing trips. There would be no sound but the lapping of the water in that vast solemn night, or now and then the loon's long cry, so musical and so deeply mournful.

Miss Porter's School in Farmington was a tradition for Hamilton girls. My father's three sisters had been sent there; and, one after another, as we of the next generation reached the age of seventeen, we were sent for the two years — which also was traditional. In all, there were ten of us at Farmington, ending with my youngest sister, Norah. It is hard to make anyone who is not an old Farmington girl understand the love and loyalty we hold for Miss Porter's School, for some of the teaching we received was the world's worst.

The system was purely elective, so that I was allowed to shirk my two weak subjects, mathematics and natural science, and we certainly were not made to study so hard or so many hours as we should have done.

I elected Latin, Greek, German, and mental and moral philosophy. These last we studied with the aid of Noah Porter's textbooks, but studying meant simply committing so many paragraphs to memory and reciting them to an elderly German who kept his eyes fixed on the ceiling, for he claimed that he knew both books by heart and need never look at the text. There was no discussion, and no explanation. The only one in the class who rebelled against this mode of instruction was Theodate Pope (Mrs. John Riddle of Farmington). She had an idea that mental philosophy really meant something, and she would mull over Noah Porter and try to puzzle out some ideas instead of just memorizing it. We told her that was a silly waste of time. "Why do you bother?" we said. "It doesn't mean anything. All you need do is to learn the words." That was all we had to do in German literature also, which was taught by the same gentleman, only this time the words were in German. I spent days reciting stuff about somebody called Klopstock but I never read anything he wrote and certainly never wished to.

On the other hand, Latin and Greek were very well taught; so was German conversation; so were drawing and music. Even those of us who did not "take music" had the benefit of wonderful recitals by famous pianists. And in the spring term old Professor Seymour, grandfather of Charles Seymour of Yale, came to stay at Miss Porter's and to lecture on Shakespeare and take over the classes in Greek and Latin. He was a delightful scholar, to whom the beauty and loftiness of the classics were everything — not the second aorist or the uses of the subjunctive. I read Tacitus, Horace, and Lucretius with him, and Aeschylus and Sophocles — not Euripides, for to Mr. Seymour that was only "silver Greek." As a special privilege I was allowed to read Dante with him too, going down to Miss Porter's house after supper in the long spring twilight. Neither of us had ever heard Italian spoken, so we pronounced it as if it were Latin, and with the old-fashioned English pronunciation at that.

So much for Farmington's educational system. But that was, of course, only a small part of our life there, as I suppose it is in any school, no matter how excellent. Personal relations are the important factors in adolescent life. For my cousin Agnes and me the school meant a sudden and thrilling entrance into the outside world; it meant meeting, and passionately admiring, girls who had had an upbringing quite different from our own — an astonishing experience to our narrow little minds. The school was completely free from any kind of snobbishness; girls stood on their own feet and were liked or disliked for their own qualities only. That lifelong friendships were founded there every old Farmington girl knows. A great encouragement to such friendships was the requirement of a two-hour walk every afternoon, for luckily we had no gymnasium. The long talks against the background of New England's beautiful winters gave us something calisthenics could not.

Miss Porter's personality was a pervasive influence, though I find it impossible to tell how she got it across to us. She gave us somehow the best of the New England tradition — integrity, self-control, no weakness or sentimentality, love of beauty, respect for the intellectual, clear thinking, no nonsense; but she conveyed it more by the atmosphere she created than by any formal teaching.

III

I Chose Medicine

AFTER I came back from Farmington, Edith and I decided that we must train ourselves to earn our living, for the family finances were rapidly diminishing and our only hope of a wide and full life, of going out into the big world, lay in our own efforts. There seemed only a few careers open to us — teaching, nursing, the practice of medicine. Edith chose teaching and began to prepare herself for Bryn Mawr College by studying mathematics and botany. I chose medicine, not because I was scientifically-minded, for I was deeply ignorant of science. I chose it because as a doctor I could go anywhere I pleased — to far-off lands or to city slums — and be quite sure that I could be of use anywhere. I should meet all sorts and conditions of men, I should not be tied down to a school or a college as a teacher is, or have to work under a superior, as a nurse must do. So I studied physics and chemistry with a high-school teacher, then entered one of those little third-rate medical schools which flourished in the days before the American Medical Association reformed medical teaching. It was in Fort Wayne and I spent a year studying anatomy chiefly; then, since that year convinced my father that I was in earnest, I went on to Ann Arbor for a real course.

Those were very happy and exciting years. The Medical School of the University of Michigan was then one of the few schools with courses in physiology, biochemistry, bacteriology, and pharmacology which were taught by men with German training, and in laboratories more than in the lecture hall. The training fostered a spirit of inquiry, a habit of following a problem to its solution if possible, of accepting only what could be proved. My teachers were John J. Abel in pharmacology and W. H. Howell in physiology — both of whom went the next year to the newly established Medical School at Johns Hopkins — F. H. Novy in bacteriology, Victor Vaughan in biochemistry, and George Dock in medicine. They were a remarkable group of men.

Lectures were given in one of two huge amphitheaters, filled with students, most of them men. We women sat in a little group of about fifteen at one side. At first I watched with excited apprehension the antics of the men, but soon they palled; and like the rest of the women students I found I could study my notebook undisturbed by the wildest din. The lectures on theoretical subjects were attended by the homeopaths, the dentists, and the pharmacists as well as the regular medical students. The rule was that the lower seats belonged to the regulars, the others sitting higher but in a strict order with pharmacists at the top. While we waited for a lecturer it often happened that a homeopath or a dental student would be discovered in the seats of the mighty, and then he would be seized by the regulars and "passed up" over the backs of the benches to the top, while his classmates fought to free him. Some of the lecturers had a hard time restoring order when they entered on such a scene, but Dr. Howell never. He would pause a moment, looking at the class, a small slight figure, then speak with his soft Southern accent, and at his first word the confusion would cease, the men would slip back to their seats and fumble for their pencils. It was not discipline at all;

it was simply the eagerness of his students not to miss a word of what he had to give them.

The school was coeducational and had been so for some twenty years, so we women were taken for granted and there was none of the sex antagonism which I saw later in Eastern schools. A man student would step aside and let the woman pass through the door first, the women had the chairs if there were not enough to go round, but when it came to microscopes or laboratory apparatus it was first come, first served.

This was really my introduction to the world of science. I shall never forget the revelation that came to me when I saw through the microscope the cells which make up the human body, and realized that later on I should be looking at these cells changed by disease — that the actual processes of disease could be viewed by the human eye. In physiology it was the same. We were not told of the processes of digestion, of nerve reflexes, of blood circulation; we reproduced them in the laboratory. We followed Pasteur's law in Novy's laboratory, isolating the anthrax bacillus, cultivating it, injecting it into an animal and recovering it again. When I reached clinical work, under Dr. Dock, it was the same method, modified because it dealt with human patients instead of guinea pigs, but following the same principles.

Dr. Dock put me on his staff for my last year, which meant that I took histories, made the routine rounds with him as well as the formal ones, and did as much of the clinical laboratory work as I could, snatching the time for it from surgery, obstetrics, and gynecology — subjects which interested me not at all. Dr. Dock belonged to the new school of clinicians — he had been one of Sir William Osler's assistants — who utilized the microscope and chemical analysis as well as physical examination in the diagnosis of a case. My spare time was spent chiefly over the microscope. Then, best of all, would come the discussion, summing up all the findings, from history, present condition, laboratory tests; and if one part of the picture puzzle was lacking, Dr. Dock would never fail to pounce upon it. The hospital was small; we saw few patients and we worked up their cases with great thoroughness. Most of them were rather obscure ones, for the hospital was a consultation center for the whole state.

Ann Arbor also gave me my first taste of emancipation, and I loved it. I loved to feel that nobody was worrying about me when I came back late from the library, nobody even knew when I came. At home, if I went in the evening across the yard to the Red House, either my father or my mother would stand in the door to hear me call back that I was safe.

My vacations were spent in Mackinac where we four sisters had happy reunions every summer. Edith and Margaret brought from Bryn Mawr Ruskin, Matthew Arnold, Pater, D'Annunzio, Flaubert, Huysmans, Maupassant, the Goncourts. Norah, who was at the Art Students' League in New York, taught me to sketch, for which I have been grateful, lo these many years. Those days remain in my mind as full of outdoor beauty and of intense enjoyment in talk, especially over a campfire on the shore of British Landing, where our Chicago friends, George and Caroline Packard, had their summer home.

Our first introduction to the literature of revolt had come in Mackinac when another Chicago friend, Judge Edward Osgood Brown, who used to join us often in our long walks, had started us reading Bernard Shaw and Henry George's *Progress and Poverty*, for he was an ardent Single-Taxer. Even more exciting was his espousal of the cause of the anarchists who were hanged for the Haymarket bombing. To us girls that episode had been one of criminal violence threatening the whole country and Judge Gary's conduct of the trial we had never thought of criticizing. Our talks with Judge Brown were eye openers in a field quite new to us, but we never thought of rejecting his ideas because they were new and upsetting. If they were true we had to accept them, and therefore they must be carefully thought out.

It was natural that a graduate from Ann Arbor in those days should turn to the laboratory branches. I soon decided that I would go into bacteriology and pathology instead of medical practice, but Dr. Dock urged me to take a year in a hospital first, saying that my training would be too one-sided otherwise. There were few internships then open to women; I had two months in the Hospital for Women and Children in Minneapolis, then nine months in the New England Hospital for Women and Children outside Boston. The first is just a blur in my memory, a blur of fear and bewilderment and fatigue, for the resident physician went off on her vacation and so did the majority of the staff, and I was left largely alone to cope with cases of typhoid fever (we had never seen typhoid in Ann Arbor) and with obstetrical cases, which were the most terrifying of all, since my training in that field had been very scanty. It was an utterly lonely life and I rejoiced when the call to Boston came, to a hospital with six internes and a resident physician and a dispensary in a poor section of the city where part of our service was passed.

This was my first experience of life in a big city. All I had known up to then was New York for brief visits, shopping and theater and the Metropolitan Museum. Boston had much to offer and I took it all eagerly. But what interested me most was the life down in the Pleasant Street Dispensary where I worked with people of thirteen different nationalities and where each new call was an adventure. The first evening I was there I was called to a case over a saloon some distance away. It seems absurd, but really I had never been on a city street alone at night before. The case lasted till midnight, and coming back I lost my way. I dared not ask help of any of the men who passed me but presently a little woman came hurrying along and I stopped her. She was very kind. She led me back to my street and laughed at my fears. She was a chorus girl, she told me, and she never had any trouble. "Just walk along fast with your bag in your hand, not looking at anybody, and nobody will speak to you. Men don't want to be snubbed; they are looking for a woman who is willing." It was good advice and it worked. I never had one unpleasant experience, though my night work took me into notoriously tough quarters of the city, and several times into houses of prostitution.

Among my fellow internes was a Russian girl who had been a revolutionist in Russia and who used to hold me enthralled by the stories of her life. She was Rachelle Slobodinskaya, afterwards Dr. R. S. Yarros, a specialist in obstetrics and one of the early founders of the birth control and of the social hygiene movements. She seemed to me the most exciting person I had ever met and I marveled as she told of joining the Russian revolutionists when she was thirteen years old, fleeing to this country when she was seventeen, and working in sweatshops in New York to earn her living. At seventeen I was starting for Farmington and in all my life I had never had to think where my next meal was coming from. Being so sheltered and so ignorant seemed contemptible. Years after, Dr. Rachelle and her husband, Victor Yarros, came to Hull-House to live, and the friendship begun in Boston still continues.

My year of European study came soon after. Edith had won

a European fellowship at Bryn Mawr and my Ann Arbor professors had told me that if I hoped to devote myself to bacteriology and pathology I must study in Germany, otherwise I should never be accepted as an expert. Such was the status of American scientific training in the nineties. (As a matter of fact, I found that in bacteriology Leipzig had nothing to give me that I had not already had from Dr. Novy, but neither Germans nor Americans would have believed it.)

In the fall of 1895 Edith and I sailed on what seemed to us a great adventure. Even gaining permission to study in one of the German universities was a long and difficult enterprise, for of course women were not admitted to any of them. But if an individual professor were liberal-minded, he could give permission to attend his classes, though a degree of any kind was out of the question. Sometimes the classical faculty where Edith wished to work would be willing to accept her but the scientific faculty would refuse me, or vice versa.

We did succeed in gaining entrance to the University of Leipzig, where they told us we should be considered "invisible," and to Munich, though there the negotiations were prolonged and elaborate. The trouble lay in the classical faculty, for Munich University was Roman Catholic and the seminarians attended the courses in Greek and Latin. They might have to sit next a woman, perhaps even share a manuscript with her, if there were not enough to go round. Fortunately for Edith there was enough antagonism between the Catholics and Protestants on the faculty to make the latter espouse her cause. We heard that several compromises were suggested — one that a little "loge" be built in the lecture hall where she could sit hidden by a green curtain. Finally she was given a chair up on the platform beside the lecturer, facing the audience, so that nobody would be contaminated by contact with her. It was very trying for a girl who had not even gone through the mild ordeal of a coeducational college. Most trying of all was her experience on the opening day. One of her professors, a kindly old man, told her he would meet her at the entrance to the University Place and escort her to the classroom. She assured him it was not necessary, but was thankful indeed for his protection when she found the Place crowded with students waiting to see a woman enter.

My work in Munich was very pleasant. The atmosphere in the laboratory was quite different from that in Leipzig; it was gay and easy and friendly. Bavarians are like our Southerners in many ways. Professor Buchner was a dear. When he appeared at the door each morning with his gentle "Grüss Gott," we all felt a surge of affection for him. He liked to have a woman working under him and gave me a great deal of attention — but he could never forget that I was a woman. I wanted to work on a problem he was studying, the part played by the white cells of the blood in combating infection, but that would have meant animal experiments. Professor Buchner told me gently that he knew such experiments would be impossible for me. So he set me to studying a thick-capsuled bacillus from India which he hoped would turn out to be a companion and aid to the cholera bacillus, perhaps neutralizing the acid in the gastric juice which inhibits the cholera bacillus. It turned out to be nothing but a big, fat nonentity.

In Leipzig there had been a fair number of foreign women students; in Munich we two and an Englishwoman, a student of archeology, were the only ones. Six German women who applied were refused. The authorities said that the only reason women wanted to study was to prepare themselves for subversive political activity; if foreign governments wished to run that risk, all right, but the German government had too much sense. My lot in both Leipzig and Munich was easier than Edith's because I wanted laboratory work, which nobody objected to, and lectures were of secondary importance. In Leipzig two professors permitted me to attend their lectures, but in Munich all were closed to a woman. When I heard that Professor Buchner was to give an exposition of his work on immunity to a class of graduate physicians, I begged him to let me hear it. He hated to refuse me, but it was a most revolutionary request. Finally he arranged it. I must be in the laboratory ten minutes before lecture time when the oldest research student, a grandfather, would escort me to the empty classroom and seat me in a separate chair in a corner. Then, when the lecture was over, before the students left their seats, Professor Buchner would hastily escort me out. And those dangerous men from whom I was being protected were all graduated physicians, doubtless settled and staid heads of families.

However, it is not for a woman who has been on the faculty at Harvard to be too derisive about German universities in the nineties. It is still true that though women work in Harvard museums and are permitted to read in Widener Library, they are always obliged to leave at six o'clock. They are assured that this rule is for their own protection, against the undergraduates! And when the Germans did admit women, they went the whole way — no dormitories, no rules, no Dean of Women, the same freedom for women students as for men. In 1912 when I was in Germany, one of my friends told me about her daughter, a student in the University of Munich. She and a girl friend lived in a furnished room and took their meals wherever they pleased. Carnival time was just over and the girl had written her mother that she had *bummelte* all night in the streets with the crowd of students. "It seems shocking," said my friend, "but really no harm seems to come of it." It is true that those were girls who went to the university with a serious purpose, to work for a career; fun was only an incident, and none of them would have dreamed of regarding the university as a place in which to pick up a husband.

Life in Germany in those days was very pleasant, though sometimes exasperating for an American. I had to learn to accept the thinly veiled contempt of many of my teachers and fellow students because I was at once a woman and an American, therefore uneducated and incapable of real study. The Bavarians were much pleasanter than the Saxons. I hardly minded being a woman in Munich. In Frankfurt am Main, where we went for the long spring vacation, I was treated quite as an equal in Weigert's laboratory. There I did a bit of research for Professor Edinger and formed a friendship with him and his wife which lasted while they lived and now goes on with their daughter Ottilie.

But everywhere, not only in Saxony, one was continually reminded that one was a woman and inferior. Students would march along the sidewalk, four abreast with arms locked, and if one did not step quickly into the gutter one would be pushed there. Officers would stride by in their gorgeous uniforms, with perhaps a drab peahen of a wife trotting along carrying the parcels which no officer might carry. If one was in a crowd, rushing for the cheap seats for the opera, one must expect to be pushed and shoved by the men; indeed once when I, being light and quick, had dashed up the steps to the gallery and secured a front seat, a great blond Siegfried of a student caught me under my arms from behind, lifted me out and took my seat. It was a man's world in every sense, and at the top was the army, living in a world of its own, adored and feared by the common man.

There was a professor in the University of Munich who had nine daughters, a frightful misfortune, for he could provide dowries for only three; the other six had nothing to look forward to in life except spinsterhood in a crowded home, for a professor's daughter might not earn her own living. So it did not seem surprising that one of the condemned girls should run away with a young lieutenant. What was surprising to us Americans was the universal assumption that she was hopelessly ruined. "Can't her family make him marry her?" we asked. "But he cannot marry her if he would," we were told. "The Kaiser has forbidden an officer to marry unless the girl has the necessary dowry. Otherwise they cannot keep up the state which the Kaiser insists on as proper for officers."

Although we were often exasperated by these German attitudes, we were much oftener charmed by the warmth and kindliness of the people and the easy, simple way they took the enjoyable things in life. At home, if we wanted music we must go to a concert; in Germany we could step out into the park, sit under the trees with a glass of beer or a cup of coffee, and listen to lovely music. The opera there was not a social function to be attended rarely because of the cost of tickets and the lateness of the hour; it was something one could enjoy four or five times a week, for a few marks; and since it was over at ten o'clock, it did not interfere with the next day's work. It was the easiest thing to get off into the country (what a contrast to Chicago!), only a short ride in a fourth-class coach and then fields and mountains and lakes, and, at every lovely view, a tempting beer garden with perhaps a group of students singing as Anglo-Saxon students do not sing.

Even the scientific meetings to which Professor Buchner took me were informal and pleasant as ours seldom are. Not long ago I was impressed by the contrast, by the way our passion for mechanized efficiency can ruin all *Gemütlichkeit*. I was asked to speak to the Medical Society of Pittsburgh and was escorted to the Mellon Institute, where, I was told, the meeting would be held in the most up-to-date auditorium. "I must get there early," said my host, "so that I can have a front seat, because the acoustics are bad and the air-conditioning machine (of course the room is air-conditioned) makes so much noise that one cannot hear well at the back of the room." I was taken up to a high platform, placed in front of a microphone, and warned not to move away from it or I should not be heard. After I had spoken, not to the audience, but to the machine, the chairman announced that if there were any comments or questions he must ask the questioner to come up on the platform and speak into the microphone. Of course nobody wanted to do that. The three papers were read, there was no discussion, the meeting closed efficiently.

And I thought back to a meeting in Munich where Dr. Buchner had demonstrated some of his observations on phagocytic action. It was in a delightful Old World restaurant and we all sat around informally, some drinking beer or coffee or even having supper. In the middle of the room was a long table with microscopes. As the Professor talked we could, if we wished, step up and look at the slides he was describing. The discussion that followed was really a conversation, absolutely informal and easy. One wonders when we Americans will get over our childish love for mechanical gadgets and sweep some of them away.

Work in a German laboratory was novel enough to keep me amused and interested, not only in the actual study but also in the men around me. Leipzig, where I did pathology, had as chief of that department old Birch-Hirschfeld, who really gave us nothing at all. He would pass through the laboratory occasionally and we would all stand up, face around, and bow profoundly, but that was all we saw of him. The men in Leipzig worked hard, but long hours were never the rule. In the middle of the morning the *Diener* would come in with *Frühschoppen* — beer, rye bread, Swiss cheese — and at once the room would be full of gayety. One of the men could make music with a comb and the others would dance to it. The same thing would happen at *Dämmerschoppen* in the afternoon. I could never get used to the mixture of profound learning and childlike clowning in these men. In Munich the atmosphere was still gayer, for Professor Buchner was not a wet blanket like Birch-Hirschfeld. There in the month of June we had no fewer than thirteen holidays, five Sundays and eight Church feast days, which Protestants celebrated quite as much as Catholics. And yet these Germans produced more first-class scientific studies than did the hard-working Americans I knew at home. Professor Edinger commented on that fact once. He said, "You Americans are in too much of a hurry to succeed, you push yourselves too hard. Now look at me. Never have I worked longer than eight hours in a day, but I shall keep that up till I die. Your American scientists are finished at fifty. After that they produce no more original work."

I saw Germany again in 1910 and 1912, when I visited her excellent lead smelters and white- and red-lead works and potteries; again in 1915 when I went with Jane Addams to place before the Chancellor, Bethmann-Hollweg, and the Foreign Affairs Minister, von Jagow, a proposal for a neutral commission of mediation to end the war; then in 1919, again with Jane Addams, this time to make a survey of the effects of starvation under the food blockade for Herbert Hoover and the Quakers; in 1924 on my way to Russia, when life under the Republic seemed drab and poverty-poor; and finally two visits to Hitler's Germany, the first in the early months of his regime, the last during "Munich week," when so great and so terrible a change had come over that land of great learning and of easy gayety that I could hardly believe it was Germany.

By the autumn of 1896 our year in Europe was over and we came home. Edith had a position waiting for her. She became headmistress of the Bryn Mawr School in Baltimore. Because no position awaited me I went with her for a winter's work in the Johns Hopkins Medical School. In spite of my year in Germany, nobody seemed to want my services. The demand for trained bacteriologists and pathologists did not begin till some years later, and the only thing to do was to keep on fitting myself for a career and hoping that some day an opening would come.

Those were the great days of the Johns Hopkins Medical School. I met there not only my former teachers, W. H. Howell and J. J. Abel, but William Welch, Simon Flexner, William Osler, Howard Kelly, John Finney, Franklin Mall, Lewellys Barker. Exciting as it is to work in a foreign laboratory there is something satisfying in returning to one's own country and one's own language, in every sense of that phrase. Baltimore was not gay and colorful as were Munich and Frankfurt, but the men I worked with accepted me without amusement or contempt or even wonder, and I slipped into place with a pleasant sense of belonging.

Dr. William Welch used to stop by my table now and then and exchange German experiences with me, and that was always a red-letter day. I saw him for the last time some three months before his death in Johns Hopkins Hospital. He was deeply absorbed in a description he had just read of the anti-tuberculosis work which Soviet Russia was carrying on and which John Kingsbury and Sir Arthur Newsholme had just written up. There was not a trace of anti-Bolshevist prejudice and skepticism in his attitude — only warm admiration and even envy.

My regular work, which was pathological anatomy, was done under Simon Flexner. It was really pure enjoyment. He gave me two cases to work up and helped me to have them published. It was Dr. Flexner who first taught me that important part of research, the thorough and critical review of all that has been written on one's problem and the scrupulous care one must use to give credit where credit is due.

The Johns Hopkins was one of the few schools in the country which gave one a chance actually to see the malarial organisms; patients from the deep South came there, and seamen from the tropics. I went often to the dispensary to study malarial blood, and sometimes I would drop work for an afternoon and attend Dr. Osler's clinic, just for the pleasure of seeing how admirably he conducted it. He was freer from what the English call swank than almost any other great man I have known. His manner with the students was that of an equal, and he always fretted against the hospital etiquette which required a nurse to stand in the presence of a doctor. That was, of course, the absolute rule in Johns Hopkins Hospital, and it was with real trepidation that the clinic nurse would sit down when he bade her. He told me with much irritation that he had once had to pass repeatedly by a nurse who was rolling bandages, and each time he did so she rose to her feet. "Such a silly waste of time and strength." He used to bring in out-of-the-way references in his talks with the students which would lead them far afield from their narrow medical path. Once it was "What is the best way to stop a hiccough?" And after an array of approved, scientific methods had been offered him, "Well, how about making the victim sneeze? Don't you remember — the physician in Plato's *Symposium* cures Aristophanes that way?" Another time it was "Why do we call lead poisoning 'saturnism'? That goes back to the days when the ancients knew only eight elements, and they believed that the eight great heavenly bodies were each composed of one of these — the sun of gold, the moon of silver, Jupiter of copper, Mars of iron, Venus of tin, Mercury of quicksilver, Saturn of lead, Vulcan of sulphur. That is why we call quicksilver mercury and silver nitrate lunar caustic. And when we treat rubber with sulphur we call it vulcanizing."

Dr. Osler was adored by his assistants and all his students, so that many of them could not help trying to imitate him, his walk, his gestures, his accent, his expression. Often I would find myself watching a little crowd of semi- and semi-demi Oslers. I liked it; I knew that the copying was not merely superficial, but that the young men had taken as their ideal a great leader.

That was the last year of student life for me — the delightful life at once free from responsibility and full of varied interests. Although I dipped into it again for short periods, at the University of Chicago and the Institut Pasteur in Paris, it was not the same, for it was only an interlude in my real work. My first job was offered to me that summer, to teach pathology in the Woman's Medical School of Northwestern University in Chicago. I accepted it with thankfulness, not only because it meant employment in my own field, but because it was in Chicago. At last I could realize the dream I had had for years, of going to live in Hull-House.

Agnes put this idea in my mind. Neither of us had heard

much about social reform in our sheltered youth. Free trade and civil service reform were the only movements we heard discussed at home. My father took Godkin's *Nation;* its program of reform, which meant integrity and expert knowledge in civil office, taxation for revenue only, no tariff protection for special interests, satisfied him completely. Fort Wayne had no slums, there was no unemployment; the problem of poverty was individual in each case: it was due either to misfortune, which called for charity, or to shiftlessness, which called for stern measures. The first appeal we ever heard for the righting of a wrong outside our own country was in a speech at school in Farmington on the Hindu child widows.

During the two years in Fort Wayne, however, between Farmington and Ann Arbor, Agnes came across Richard Ely's books. She was fired with enthusiasm for his program of Socialism and won me over to it easily. We began then to read about the settlement movement. Now it happened that in the spring before I went to Germany, Jane Addams came to Fort Wayne to speak in the Methodist Church. She was already famous, though Hull-House was not more than six years old. Norah brought the exciting news to Agnes and me, and we three went to hear her in the evening. I cannot remember my first impressions; they blend into the crowd of impressions that came in later years. I only know that it was then that Agnes and I definitely chose settlement life. Years later we carried out our resolve: Agnes went to the Lighthouse in Philadelphia and I found myself a resident of Hull-House.

This was not so easy as it sounds. It was difficult to gain entrance to Hull-House as a resident, even in 1897, for already it had attracted many young men and women. No salaries were paid. The residents either had incomes of their own and so could afford to give all their time, or they gave their evenings and Sundays apart from their regular occupations. Everyone paid his own way, as Miss Addams always did, and there was never any difficulty in filling the available bedrooms. The rooms were all filled when I went there in the spring of that year. I can remember how the place charmed me as I sat waiting for Miss Addams in the high-ceilinged, old-fashioned reception room, and how my heart beat when she came in. She had won me over already in the church in Fort Wayne, but now, face to face, I felt even more attracted to her — to the mixture of sweetness and aloofness, of sympathetic understanding and impersonality, and the total absence of that would-be charm and false intimacy which school and college had made me dislike heartily in older women.

Mrs. Kelley passed through the room as we sat there, and Miss Addams introduced me to that vivid, colorful, rather frightening personality whom I came later to adore. But though my desire to live at Hull-House increased with every minute of that interview, my hopes died, for Miss Addams made it clear, gently but firmly, that all the rooms for the coming fall were taken. But I could not at once give up my long-cherished dream of settlement work, so I went up to the Commons, Graham Taylor's settlement, a couple of miles to the north of Hull-House. It was in much the same sort of neighborhood and almost as old as Hull-House. Unluckily for me, neither Mr. nor Mrs. Taylor was at home and the resident I spoke to said I should be of little use if I could give only my evenings. That seemed to settle it, and I could do nothing but look for a place to live — which I found in a studio building on Ohio Street. But I was still resolved that in some way, somehow, I would make my way into a settlement. I had a conviction that professional work, teaching pathology, and carrying on research would never satisfy me. I must make for myself a life full of human interest.

So it was a matter of great rejoicing when during that summer Miss Addams wrote me, up in Mackinac, that there was a vacant room. I might come in September.

IV

Hull-House Within

THE LAST DECADE of the nineteenth century (how amusing now to recall that the phrase *fin de siècle* used to connote extreme modernism, sophistication) was simpler in many ways than any period which followed it. Perhaps Edith Wharton was right when she called it the Age of Innocence. We had more uncertainty then, but on the other hand we had more faith. We were far less certain of what was needed to make society over; we were groping and seeking. We, ordinary Americans, had no ready-made system into which we could fit, which we could accept in its entirety, as a Communist accepts Marxian dialectics, with an end after that to all questioning. But on the other hand we had more faith in human nature, we really believed in a steady progress of mankind, we never dreamed that the pendulum would swing back and an age of barbarism would return.

Hull-House was founded in 1889, three years after the terrible Haymarket riot and the trial and executing of the anarchists which had stirred Chicago to its depths and implanted in the minds of ordinary people a horror of radicalism (then called anarchism), a horror which every now and then broke out in blind panic and cruelty.

It is hard for a Chicagoan to realize that most Americans now living have never heard of the Haymarket bombing, which affected Chicago so deeply for decades after its occurrence. But since I am assured that this is true, I must describe as briefly as possible that shattering event which happened in the spring of 1886. For some time there had been a growing movement among Chicago's trade-unionists in favor of the eight-hour day. This had been taken up by radicals, anarchists, who, though a small group, made a great noise. They openly advocated "direct action," the "propaganda of the deed." Then there came a strike and a lockout in the great McCormick Harvester works, in the course of which several workmen were shot by the police. This led to a protest meeting in Haymarket Square, a big market place on the West Side about a mile north of Hull-House where a great crowd of strikers and sympathizers assembled one evening. Toward the close of the meeting a group of policemen suddenly marched into the Square as if to disperse the crowd and at that moment someone threw a bomb. It killed one policeman and wounded seventy. A wave of terror and anger swept over Chicago. Nobody knew who had made or who had thrown the bomb, but the anarchists who had advocated violence were promptly arrested, seven of them. One of the group, Parsons, felt so confident of acquittal that he came back to Chicago and gave himself up to share trial with his comrades.

But so intense was the feeling against these men that all the usual rules about selection of jurymen and about court procedure were abrogated. The demand for conviction spread over the whole country, and though none of the eight men could be shown to have had any part in the crime, all were found guilty. Four were hanged, one committed suicide, three went to the penitentiary. Six years later Governor John P. Altgeld pardoned those three, in the face of bitter denunciation, not only by the conservative press but by such men as Lyman Abbott and Theodore Roosevelt. Sigmund Zeisler, a young lawyer then, set back his professional career for many years, I was told, because he espoused the cause of the anarchists. The Haymarket riot cast its sinister shadow on all of us working at Hull-House in the late nineties.

Miss Addams has given so fully the history of Hull-House, of the birth of an idea and of its fulfillment, that I can make only a modest addition to the picture. As one reads her earlier writings one sees that she was moved not only by the greater inequalities and injustices of society but perhaps even more by less evident, more intangible and rarely voiced evils from which men and women suffer but which sociologists often miss. She knew, because she understood people, that political equality meant little in comparison with social equality; she knew that the social exclusiveness of the well-to-do, the social ostracism of the "Dago," "Polack," "Hunky," "Greaser," Negro, was harder to bear than political corruption and rotten city government. Bad government led to wretched conditions, but it did not degrade the poor man in his own eyes; on the contrary, the clever political boss flattered the voter's self-respect, made him feel himself of importance. Contempt, she said, is the greatest crime against one's fellow man.

So she looked upon Hull-House as a bridge between the classes, and she always held that this bridge was as much of a help to the well-to-do as to the poor. We talk much nowadays of the frustrated idealism of our young people, of their longing for leadership, for a dedication of themselves to a great cause, for courage and hardship, for such blazing devotion as we see in the Nazis and the Fascists. Miss Addams felt that need strongly and she made an inspiration of a life among the city poor, the bewildered and exploited immigrants. She offered young people of education and culture and gentle ways a place where they could live as neighbors and give as much as they could of what they had. They were not to live in sordid tenements — that sacrifice was not asked of them — but they were to suffer with the rest from the squalor and discomforts of the slums so far as outer things were concerned, and in the knowledge they acquired they would be better equipped to fight against these evils. It is true that Hull-House gave them both beauty and comfort, but so far as was possible they welcomed their neighbors in to share.

When I look back on the Chicago of 1897 I can see why life in a settlement seemed so great an adventure. It was all so new, this exploring of the poor quarters of a big city. The thirst to know how the other half lives had just begun to send people pioneering in the unknown parts of American life. Now, when we have floods of books and plays on every aspect of that life, from Southern share-croppers to Pennsylvania coal miners, from Scandinavian farmers in the Northwest to the Cajun fisher folk of Louisiana, it is hard to believe that when Miss Addams came to Chicago the first book of that kind was still to be written. Jacob Riis brought out his *How the Other Half Lives* in 1891. It was in the early nineties that Walter Wyckoff, a Princeton graduate, did what was then unheard of: he took to the road as a casual laborer and wrote of his hopeless quest for jobs. So to settle down to live in the slums of a great city was a piece of daring as great as trekking across the prairie in a covered wagon.

My first evening at Hull-House is still clear in my memory. There was a rather large company at dinner that night and ex-Governor Altgeld was the guest of honor. I saw the admiration and appreciation with which he, the defender of the Pullman strikers and the pardoner of the imprisoned anarchists, was greeted by Miss Addams, Mrs. Kelley, and Miss Lathrop. I listened while Mrs. Kelley talked with him about her experience as Chief State Inspector of Factories under his administration, when for the first time such inspection was enforced, and of the working of the short-lived eight-hour law for women (which was declared unconstitutional two years later). I heard them discuss also his attack on the Supreme Court for declaring a Federal income tax unconstitutional and I listened to his denunciation of the Carnegie Company's actions in the bloody Homestead strike in 1892.

In those early days at Hull-House the group of residents was rather small and we had a fairly intimate life, if one can use such a word to describe a relation which was almost entirely devoid of personal intimacy. We knew each others' opinions and interests and work and we discussed them often and freely, but the atmosphere was impersonal, rather astonishingly so for a group composed chiefly of women. Miss Addams was warm and magnetic, but she never tolerated the sort of protecting, interfering affection which is so lavishly offered to a woman of leadership and prominence. Nobody ever ventured to refuse her to visitors, or even to take her telephone calls unless authorized to do so. She was impatient of solicitude, and her attitude brought about a wholesome, rather Spartan atmosphere.

Mrs. Florence Kelley, Julia Lathrop, and Alzina Parsons Stevens were all there when I came. Mrs. Kelley was one of the most vivid personalities I have ever met. She used to make me think of two verses in the Old Testament: the one in Job about the war horse who scents the battle from afar and says among the trumpets, "Ha, ha"; and the one where the Psalmist says, "The zeal of thine house hath eaten me up." It was impossible for the most sluggish to be with her and not catch fire. A little group of us residents used to wait for her return from the Crerar Library, where she was in charge evenings, and bribe her with hot chocolate to talk to us. We had to be careful; foolish questions, half-baked opinions, sentimental attitudes, met with no mercy at her hands. We loved to hear her and the Scotch lawyer, Andrew Alexander Bruce, discuss the cases they had had under the Altgeld administration. Mr. Bruce won an important judgeship later on and I am sure he deserved it.

Mrs. Stevens came of a good Maine family, a Parsons of Parsonsville, but her father's death in the Civil War reduced the family to poverty and she had had to go to work in a textile mill at the age of thirteen, where she lost one of her fingers in the machinery. She had gone into the labor movement from the bottom and had thrown all her energy and intelligence into it. I remember her as intolerant equally of opposition to the labor movement and of sentimentality about it. Once when one of the residents stood up for a notoriously crooked labor leader Mrs. Stevens turned on her fiercely. "That is the worst kind of snobbishness," she said, "to assume that you must not have the same standards of honor for working people as you have for the well-to-do."

It was Mrs. Stevens who introduced me to Eugene Debs, that lovable, warm, vivid personality whom I remember as I do few men. She was a close personal friend of his, one of the little group who used to stand by him during the hours of dark discouragement in the Pullman strike, keeping him from drowning his depression in drink, or when he could bear it no longer shielding him till he came back to himself. She did not live to see him sentenced to prison for opposition to the war, but those of us who admired him felt deep indignation over this act of intolerance and over Wilson's refusal to release him when he was nominated for the Presidency, although by then the war was over. I voted for him, partly as a protest against this unjust attitude, partly because to me Debs seemed head and shoulders above Harding and Cox. One of the most ironical happenings I have ever known concerned Debs during Harding's administration when Harry Daugherty was Harding's Attorney General of unsavory fame. In response to many petitions, Daugherty sent for Debs to come from Atlanta Penitentiary to Washington for an interview and then announced that he could not recommend Debs for pardon because he found that he had not yet repented his sins nor even seen the error of his ways.

When I try to describe Julia Lathrop the word that comes first to my mind is "disinterested." This is a rare quality, even in philanthropists, in people who are devoting their lives to others, for sacrifice and devotion can go with a certain kind of self-centeredness, and frequently do. Julia Lathrop did not see herself as the center of what she was doing; she really was not thinking at all of her relation to it. Florence Kelley was more stimulating; Julia Lathrop never roused one to a fighting pitch, but then fighting was not her method. (Nor was it mine. I have always hated conflict of any kind, but with me this led to cowardice, to shirking unpleasantness. Never with her.) She taught me a much-needed lesson, that harmony and peaceful relations with one's adversary were not in themselves of value, only if they went with a steady pushing of what one was trying to achieve. So often, when I have succeeded in breaking down the hostility of an employer and in establishing a friendly relation with him, I have been tempted to let it go at that, to depart without risking unpleasantness. Then I have remembered Julia Lathrop and have forced myself to say the unpleasant things which had to be said.

It was during my early days at Hull-House that I went with

her to visit one of the large insane asylums of Illinois. The superintendent was at first distinctly hostile, but Julia's tact gradually softened him until at last he was pouring out all his many grievances and difficulties. She listened with sympathy and I thought that would be the end, that we should depart feeling we had conquered his hostility and left him friendly and well-disposed. But to Julia that was only the preparatory spade work. She then proceeded to tell him gently, but with devastating clarity, what was wrong with his administration of the asylum, for which he, after all, was the only one responsible. He took it, with startled meekness, and I learned a lesson I never forgot.

She was the most companionable person, with a sense of the absurd and a way of telling absurd stories that was unique, and she had a large store of them, gathered as she journeyed back and forth over Illinois during the many years she was on the State Board of Charities. Later, when she was made the first Chief of the Children's Bureau, Hull-House felt the loss deeply. (But by that time I was working in Washington, so it was my gain.) Julia Lathrop had more than her share of human wisdom. I think women have more of this than men — at least, I know that when I have wanted a solution to an intellectual problem, I have taken it to a man, but when it was a problem concerning myself, or others, I have gone to a woman for wisdom, most often to Julia Lathrop or Jane Addams, or Mary Rozet Smith.

I cannot describe Jane Addams. Perhaps I am too close to the trees to see the forest. When I try, I seem to get only bits of her, pieces which should be fitted together in a pattern of great beauty, but I am not capable of producing that pattern. Some day it must be done by a mind great enough to

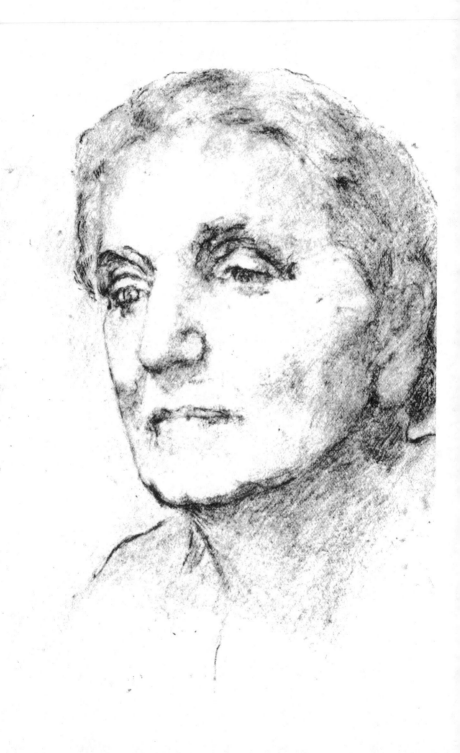

deal with so great a woman. All I can do is to give something
of the impressions made upon me.

She had intellectual integrity; there was nothing of what
George Meredith has called "merciful muddle" about her.
She never sentimentalized over the poor, or labor, or the half-
baked young radicals, or the conscientious objectors, and so,
having no illusions to start with, she could never be disillusioned or disappointed. She never shrank from painful facts.
She never refused to listen to damaging evidence. I well remember how indignant I was when she told me that she had
invited a grief-stricken young couple to come for a visit, and
I knew that those very people had treated her with a contemptible injustice born of panic and fear. When I reminded
her of it she said vaguely, "Why yes, that is true, they did.
Strange, wasn't it?" And then she dropped the subject. She
did not excuse them, for there was no excuse, but her pity
was just as tender as if she had shut her eyes to the facts.

She was a pragmatist in the best sense before that word
was invented, holding that anything one had learned in college and from travel must be tried out in actual life. "Truth
must be put to the ultimate test, the test of the conduct it
dictates and inspires." Her young womanhood was passed
largely in study, reading, travel, for she was a semi-invalid for
years, and she had had more than her fill of theoretical knowledge; it made her rather impatient. She turned from it eagerly
to practical application, in the field of action. As was natural,
John Dewey, then at the University of Chicago, became one
of her closest friends and counselors. This practical approach,
together with her complete absence of personal pride, made
her ready to try out a new scheme and equally ready to drop
it if it proved a failure. Always she held that a settlement
should be a place for experiment. When a new enterprise

had proved its worth the settlement ought to try to make the city take it over and go on, itself, to new fields. This happened again and again, with our playground, our public baths, our kindergarten, our volunteer probation officers and truant officers; all were taken over by the city. And though sometimes it seemed to us that we had managed these services better and more disinterestedly than the city did, Miss Addams insisted that the move from private charity to public responsibility was a step forward, even when poorly handled.

She never took a stand for the sake of consistency; she was no slave of her own theories. When we were in Paris just after the war, she shocked the Frenchwomen of the pacifist group by accepting an invitation to a reception given her by a group of American doughboys waiting to be demobilized. The women begged me to remonstrate with her, to make her see that this would be a public abandonment of her principles. I labored in vain to convince them that she had no principles against conscripted men, whatever she thought of conscription, and that to hold herself aloof from them would require a sort of fanatic belief in her own rightness which she never possessed.

She had two conflicting traits which sometimes brought her great unhappiness: she was very dependent on a sense of warm comradeship and harmony with the mass of her fellow men, but at the same time her clear-sighted integrity made it impossible for her to keep in step with the crowd in many a crisis. Most reformers I have known have enjoyed, more or less, the sense of being in advance of their times, of belonging to a persecuted minority. That was never true of Jane Addams. The Pullman strike, the rise of the I.W.W., the war fever of 1914–1918, the sudden, panicky persecution of the radicals after the war, to mention only a few instances, were for her the most painful of experiences, because then she was forced by conviction to work against the stream, to separate herself from the great mass of her fellow country-men. Nor did she ever fall into the mire of self-pity or take refuge in a sense of self-righteousness. She simply suffered from the spiritual loneliness which her farsighted vision had imposed on her.

There is one supremely lovely figure which rises to one's mind whenever one thinks of Hull-House in the years from its founding to 1934, and that is the figure of Mary Rozet Smith, Jane Addams's closest friend and the most universally beloved person I have ever known. She left no mark on history but she left a deep mark on all who knew her, even slightly, for she had a genius for personal relations. I suppose that means quick insight, warmth, and a "heart at leisure from itself." She was one of those persons whose biographies are never written but who have a deep and abiding influence on their time. Her large, gracious home on Walton Place was a refuge for Miss Addams, who could hardly have carried on had she not been able to slip away to it from the West Side now and then. It was also a place of refreshment for many of the rest of us. And to Hull-House her coming was not only a joy but a sustaining help in time of trouble and perplexity for all the years up to her death in 1934. Miss Addams survived her by only one year.

I did not know Mrs. Bowen in those early days. My intimacy with her began in 1912 in connection with the Pullman incident which I shall relate in due course. Louise de Koven Bowen was one of the earliest friends of Hull-House and is now its oldest friend, for she still guides its destinies when all the others are gone. She was always a prop and a stay to Miss Addams, even when, as in 1917, she did not agree with Jane

Addams's anti-war stand, for her generosity is of the spirit as well as of the purse.

Hull-House in 1893 was a very attractive place. It still is, though I shall always feel that the great changes which came in the following years took away some of the early charm. Changes always do that. The house had been built in 1846 on much the same plan as my grandfather's Fort Wayne house, which was five years older. There were the same hall and stairway, the same long drawing room with carved white marble mantelpieces, the same French windows at both ends, and the same lofty ceilings with elaborate cornices. This was the original house which Mr. Hull had built on unfashionable Halsted Street, hoping thereby to attract other well-to-do people to that part of the West Side, for he was a large land-owner. He never succeeded in this, however; the neighborhood, when Miss Addams and Miss Starr came exploring for a home for their new scheme, was one of small tenements, mostly of wood, and only two stories high, inhabited by newly arrived European immigrants. The house itself had gone through various vicissitudes; it had been a lodging house for workmen, a temporary home for the Little Sisters of the Poor, and Miss Addams and Miss Starr found it housing some Polish immigrants. But they saw at once that it was still solid and beautiful, just what they needed.

Life at Hull-House was very simple so far as luxuries went, but it was full of beauty. Miss Addams and Miss Starr brought with them many charming furnishings and whatever they bought had the two qualities of durability and beauty. Our food was inexpensive but dinner was served to us in a long, paneled dining room, lighted with chandeliers of Spanish wrought iron; breakfast in a charming little Coffeehouse built in imitation of an English inn. To me, the life there satisfied every longing, for companionship, for the excitement of new experiences, for constant intellectual stimulation, and for the sense of being caught up in a big movement which enlisted my enthusiastic loyalty.

My part in it was humble enough. At that time there were few of the social services which now we take as a matter of course. Hull-House had to have its own day nursery, kindergarten, public baths, playground, as well as all the other activities which settlements still carry on. There were no baby clinics, and, though I did not feel at all competent to treat sick babies, I did venture to open a well-baby clinic which very soon was taking in all the older brothers and sisters, up to eight years of age. Miss Addams let me use the shower-bath room in the basement of the gymnasium and provided a dozen little bathtubs, with soap and bathing towels, for most of the work of the "clinic" was bathing the children. Some of them came all sewed into their clothes for the winter, but I found I could get past the Italian mothers' dread of water if I followed the bath with an alcohol rub and anointing with olive oil. Then I gave what I had been taught was the best advice about feeding babies — nothing but milk till their teeth came. When I see the varied diet modern mothers give their babies, anything apparently from bacon to bananas, I realize that those Italian women knew what a baby needed far better than my Ann Arbor professor did. I cannot feel I did any harm, however, for my teachings had no effect. I remember a young mother who had brought her baby to me, showing me her fine specimen of a three-year-old son, and telling me of his difficulties when he was a baby. "I gave him the breast and there was plenty of milk, but he cried all the time. Then one day I was frying eggs and just to make him stop I gave him one and it went fine. The next day I was making cup cakes and as soon as they were cool I gave him one, and after that I gave him just whatever we had and he got fat and didn't cry any more."

So now when I see an Italian baby sucking a slice of salami I feel quite serene. Garlic, we are told, is full of most valuable vitamins and salami is full of garlic. Evidently long before vitamins were discovered men decided that garlic was endowed with peculiarly beneficent properties. An elderly anarchist who used to come to Hull-House and talk to me about violent revolution and assassination (though I was sure he would not hurt a fly) underwent a radical conversion under a self-styled Hindu Mahatma, which led him to give up not only his revolutionary dreams but his way of life, so that he was changed to a shadow of his former self. He was instructed to plant his feet on the earth, lift his head to Heaven, say "I am divine," and eat nothing but garlic and popcorn. No better way could be devised for deflating a revolutionist.

Much more disquieting than the food habits was the recklessness of these Italian mothers toward contagious diseases. Perhaps fatalism is a better word. It was hard to argue with them because, after all, the results of exposure are so unpredictable and so many cases occur without any known exposure. Once I was remonstrating with a woman who had deliberately taken her year-old baby into a room where there was a child with diphtheria, but instead of impressing her I shocked her sense of right and wrong.

"Do you think," she said, "that God would punish me for going in to help Maria with her sick child? No, He would rather punish me if I did not." I might have known her baby would not catch diphtheria. They never did when I said they would.

This woman was a worker of "white magic," which is the

kind that cures sickness and brings good luck. It is valued
among the Italians but not nearly so much as is "black
magic," the kind practised by witchmen and witchwomen
who, in Italian, are called *il mago* or *la maga* — the same term
that we use for the Three Wise Men. That sort of magic is
always very secret; it is sought by unsuccessful lovers who
pay as much as ten dollars for a love philter, by jealous lovers
who want to cast a spell over a rival and make him or her
waste away in a "consumption." Sometimes a woman will
ask for a spell to be cast over a girl who has ensnared her son
and whom she is willing to kill rather than accept as a daughter-
in-law. One malignant old woman, who herself was a *maga*,
sent a curse way over from her Calabrian village to West Polk
Street, Chicago, which made her son's first-born baby pine
away and die, just because he had married a girl who had no
dowry. It was the young mother herself who told me about
it, a girl born and brought up in Chicago, a product of the
public school, but as firm in her belief as if she lived in
Calabria. All the old woman had had to do, Cristina said,
was to take a lemon and call it by the baby's name and stick
a pin in it every day; then, as the lemon slowly shriveled, the
baby pined away.

Mostly, one needed more than a lemon — a doll was surer.
A grief-stricken mother told me how she had lost her only
son from what the doctors called consumption, but what
was really black magic. A girl he had jilted bought a doll at
the ten-cent store and stuck it full of pins, and when there
was room for no more she threw it into Lake Michigan. The
poor mother knew nothing of this till she visited a *mago* who
told her that the only way to save her son was to find the
doll and pull out the pins. Of course she could not find a doll
in the Lake and so her son died.

I asked another woman how one told a sickness that was

just ordinary from one caused by black magic. "It's easy," she said. "If the doctor can cure you, it's a natural sickness, but if he can't do nothing for you, and the more medicine you take the worster you are, it's witching." Her husband and her oldest son had been "witched" by a malignant stepsister who was the daughter of a witch and had learned the art. Mike's blood was turned to water and he had strong fits, while Pasquale shook all over, "even his teeth shook on him." "How did she do it?" I asked. "For Mike, it was for death, so she put it in his wine, but for Pasquale it was only for sickness all his life long, so she put three hairs on his coat. He was lucky. He picked them off with his left hand. The *maga* said if he'd done it with his right hand, she couldn't have done nothing to save him." "What did she do to unwitch them?" I asked, full of curiosity. Feluccia hesitated. "It's prayers," she said — "only not Christian prayers." Then, feeling my skepticism, she got up, folding her shawl about her. "Everybody believes it," she said. "Only Protestants don't, because Protestants don't know how to witch and they don't know how to unwitch."

Life in a settlement does several things to you. Among others, it teaches you that education and culture have little to do with real wisdom, the wisdom that comes from life experience. You can never, thereafter, hear people speak of the "masses," the "ignorant voters," without feeling that if it were put up to you whether you would trust the fate of the country to "the classes" or to "the masses," you would decide for the latter. But it also makes you distrust the sharp division which young radicals are always making between "proletariat" and "petty bourgeoisie." (Why always "petty"? Is the *haute bourgeoisie* more enlightened than the *petite*?) I have found plenty of typical, petty-bourgeois mentality in the same families that produced ardent Communists. If one's contact with the poor is only through their organizations, their clubs and trade-unions, one gets a very one-sided, distorted impression of the working class, which contains not only rebel youth but conservative middle age, not only the radical leader but his wife, who cares more for a nice flat and an electric refrigerator than for the emancipation of the workers. And if you follow for years the career of an ardent young radical you may find him slowly changing into a steady, conservative head of a family.

When I heard my wealthy friends speak of the spread of Bolshevism and the imminent danger of revolution, I would think of the families I knew, their devotion to their hard-won little properties, their reverence for property rights, their instinctive fear of change, their absorption in everyday life, and revolution seemed pretty remote. One evening young Upton Sinclair, who was living in Mary McDowell's Stockyards Settlement, and writing *The Jungle*, told me with quiet conviction that the next President would be a Socialist. As I remember it, he proved to be McKinley.

I think it is the undying hope of better times coming which keeps our poor from the desperation that drives men to revolt. A German immigrant once said to me: "In the Old Country you know you are just what your father was and your grandfather, and your son will be the same; here you can go higher and he can go higher still." In the winter of 1914 when unemployment was very great and Chicago was full of drifting men from all over the Middle West, the French dramatist, Brieux, came to Hull-House and I happened to be the one to "tote" him. (In Hull-House that is the convenient term for showing people over the House, and we speak also of "toters" and "totees.") M. Brieux said he wanted to see poor people, the really, abjectly poor. So I took him over to Bowen Hall, our largest auditorium, which we had thrown open to the unemployed and which was full of men, some in groups talking and smoking, some making coffee in a big boiler in the kitchen. "Here you have our very poorest," I said — "men from all over the country who have had to leave their wives and children to the charities while they travel off in desperate search for work." He looked around the room, then he said, "This is not poverty. This is a sudden, temporary disaster. It is not what we French call *la misère*. These men are normal and they will go back to normal life again. In France we have people who for generations have not had enough to eat."

In settlement life, as one comes to know simple people intimately, one loses one's contempt for the banal, the bromide, the cliché, because one hears them used with such complete sincerity. You cannot laugh at "There's nothing like a mother's love" when you hear it said by a widow who has made up her mind to turn scrubwoman in a downtown office rather than send her child to an orphanage. When a young Irish girl said to me, "It would be selling my soul. I'd rather starve," the words did not sound melodramatic, for I knew that she was making the choice between working for eight dollars a week at the Fair and following one of her friends into the luxury and idleness of a prostitute's life.

I used to go to the Friday-evening meetings of Mrs. Pelham's Friendly Club, made up of scrubwomen chiefly, and I would listen with real emotion when they sang "Thou wilt still be adored, as this moment thou art, Let thy loveliness fade as it will. And around the dear ruin each wish of my heart, Shall entwine itself verdantly still." I could see the dreamy look in the "dear ruin's" eyes as she thought back to the days when "himself" was not an old drunken brute, but a gallant Irish lad whispering sweet promises. That a sense for fact was not lost in the sweetness of memory I realized when I heard one of them say, "My sister's got it good. Her old man's dead."

This sort of outspoken frankness sometimes startled me, but I came to see that it was only complete sincerity quite free from self-consciousness. A young Italian mother came to see me at the end of one of Chicago's most unendurable summers. Her baby had been sick for weeks, and night after night she had been up with him until she was exhausted. She said, "I'd look at him and think, 'My God, if you're going to die why don't you die?'" It was not hardhearted, it was only frank. The same thought might surely flash into the mind of any mother who was at the end of her strength, but she would push it back in horror. Antonia faced it without any shame; to her it was natural, but it did not make her stop pacing the floor with the baby.

In settlement life it is impossible not to see how deep and fundamental are the inequalities in our democratic country. That belief, so dear to Americans, that opportunity is open to all, that the exceptional child can rise to the highest position in the community if he will, may be true in politics, in business, even in the learned professions, but certainly not in the arts. One of the saddest things in the lot of the poor is the crushing down of artistic talent. My sister Norah, who had art classes in Hull-House for several years, used to suffer again and again the grief of seeing some promising young artist, Italian or Mexican, or Bohemian, leave school for the barren monotony of factory work, too tired after hours of it to do anything creative, his gift wasted. Yet no one can deny the need in our country for those gifts which the immigrants from countries with a more highly developed artistic life could bring us.

V

Hull-House Without

THERE WERE two things I acquired from my life at Hull-House which were certainly undesirable, and which, at long last, I have rid myself of: a deep suspicion and fear of the police and a hostility toward newspaper reporters. Both feelings had plenty of foundation in experience. Chicago's police were Tories in their political thinking and they treated those they considered rebels against the social order with little consideration for the Bill of Rights. Also, though many were foreign-born, they despised the foreign-born of other nations. My first experience with the Chicago police came during my first year at Hull-House. At that time our neighborhood streets were lined with big, wooden garbage boxes, very convenient seats on a pleasant day. At the noon hour two Italian workmen were sitting talking on the one in front of their tenement when a Polish-born policeman told them to move on. The command was senseless; it was their garbage box, and they refused, whereupon he drew his revolver and shot them both. I came by a few moments later to find an angry mob of Italians storming our little playground house where the policeman had taken refuge (he was soon rescued by a patrol wagon), and the wounded men with their weeping wives waiting for the ambulance. One of them died in the County Hospital from a wound in the lungs.

This was so shocking a deed that we felt we could not let it be passed over in silence, as the Chief of Police had decided was best. When a delegation of Italians came to us to appeal for some sort of action we asked Clarence Darrow, then living not far from Hull-House, to bring charges against the Polish policeman, and we collected, in nickels and dimes, some four hundred dollars for a retaining fee. But nothing came of it. Darrow never pushed it: he explained that his role was that of defender, not prosecutor, and the policeman was not even suspended.

In our mass meetings the sight of an officer in uniform, instead of bringing a sense of security, would fill us with dread of some violent deed, not on the part of the audience, but of the police. There was a big meeting of Russians one evening, Mensheviks and Bolsheviks, gesticulating furiously and shouting at each other, but I knew nothing worse would happen if the police would let them alone. But a panicky resident had called up the Maxwell Street station and a group of burly Irish policemen gathered in a corner muttering to each other. I went up to them and said that it was only a discussion of two theories of government and I was sure it would end peacefully. "Lady," said one of them, "you people oughtn't to let bums like these come here. If I had my way they'd all be lined up against a wall at sunrise and shot." I lived through an hour of wretched suspense but luckily there was no chance for the use of police clubs and the meeting broke up without any incident.

But almost as much did I fear the newspaper reporter and my fear was shared by all the residents of Hull-House. We knew that anything that went wrong at the House was a "story," and that ingenious twisting might turn the most innocent answer into a ridiculous or a damaging statement. And, of course, there was no redress. To write a protest only made matters worse by giving added publicity to the story.

It was an unwritten rule that these gentry were not to be handled by anyone but Miss Addams or Miss Lathrop, a rule we were all thankful to follow. One of our worst experiences was over the Averbuch murder, a story that Miss Addams has told in her *Twenty Years*. Averbuch was a young Russian Jew, an anarchist, who had been in this country only a short time. He went, on some errand never explained, to call upon the Chief of Police, who, when he saw a swarthy foreigner facing him, lost his head and emptied his revolver into the lad's body, most of the bullets entering from the back. Averbuch had no connection with Hull-House; he was studying English at another settlement, but Hull-House had more news value. The reporters came in swarms to interview us and to prove that Hull-House was a nest of anarchism.

I learned then the deadly use the papers can make of the word "admit." Clara Landsberg, who was in charge of our adult education department, insisted that Averbuch was not among the students. "Would you have accepted him if he had applied and you knew he was an anarchist?" "Certainly," she said, "we do not ask anyone what his political theories are." But the reporter's words read: "Miss Landsberg admits that there are anarchists in the classes at Hull-House." Miss Addams was in bed with tonsillitis just then and Julia Lathrop was away. I struggled in vain with a relentless young man and finally in despair took him up to Miss Addams. He listened to her in silence and then, blinking his colorless eyes behind his thick spectacles, he remarked, "I may as well tell you, Miss Addams, that I have orders from my paper to link Averbuch up with Hull-House and that is what I'm going to do."

It was the Averbuch case, by the way, which started a long friendship between Miss Addams and a young Chicago lawyer, Harold Ickes. When she sought for a lawyer to take up the case, vindicate the young victim and bring to light the methods the police had made use of, she was refused by all the established, eminent lawyers. But one of them suggested that she try a young fellow who was known to have radical sympathies; she did, and Harold Ickes took the case. His effort was of value only as it served to show our terrified immigrant neighbors that there were still people in Chicago who believed in justice and freedom, and it did rescue from the hands of the police poor Olga Averbuch, the lad's elder sister, whom the police had tried to "third degree" into a confession of an anarchist plot.

Life at Hull-House did not leave us much free time, for most of us were working people who were away all day and could give only evenings to the work of the House, but there was plenty of interesting activity to fill our Sundays and the evenings when we had neither a club nor a class. There was a Yiddish theater not far from us where we saw excellent plays, acted so well that we needed little help from interpreters in the audience to follow them. The English-speaking theaters had delightful old-fashioned melodrama, *Way Down East, No Child to Call Her Mother, East Lynn, Uncle Tom's Cabin*, all acted just as they should be, with hero and villain, heroine and villainess, recognizable the moment they stepped before the footlights. It was inconceivable that the heroine should ever be a brunette, or the villain wear a flannel shirt open at the neck — that was the mark of the hero; the villain must be in slick clothes and a bowler hat. Sundays we spent bicycling whenever the weather allowed, sometimes along the North Shore, which then was open to all from Rogers' Park north, sometimes to the western suburbs, or south to Palos Park. Usually the party consisted of Gerard Swope, then in the Western Electric Company, and Mary Hill, who is now

Mrs. Swope, and young Nicholas Kelley, whom we called Ko. We would stop in a roadhouse for ham and eggs and beer and come home late at night, slipping through the dark alleys, tired and deeply refreshed.

At Hull-House one got into the labor movement as a matter of course, without realizing how or when. As I look back I can remember a few startling experiences which must have pushed me farther along the way, but I cannot remember when I began to see the working world through the workers' eyes. One of these experiences came to me through an Italian girl whom I was helping with her English. Filomena was the eldest of a large family and, as used to happen fairly often, she was sent over to this country to pave the way for the rest, to earn money for the family's passage. It was hard to understand an Italian family sending a young girl out into the world alone, especially when one saw how strictly she would be guarded as soon as her family arrived. Only a complete ignorance of what such a journey meant and of the difference between Chicago and a Calabrian village could explain it.

Filomena had but one purpose in life, to earn money. She worked in one of the great men's clothing factories and soon rose to the skilled job of making buttonholes on the lapels of men's dress suits. This was shortly before the great strike of 1910, Sidney Hillman's strike, and the work in the factories was let to subcontractors who acted as foremen and whose one idea was to push the work as much as possible. There was much talk of revolt among the girls in Filomena's department but she told me she paid no attention to it, she stuck to her buttonholes and the girls called her a mean pace-maker.

Then one day the boss said to her, "How many needles of thread do you use in a day, Filomena?"

"About three hundred," she answered. "Why don't you take your needles home with you and thread them evenings?" he suggested. "You'd make a lot more if you did." Filomena was much impressed, she followed the suggestion, and that week she made more buttonholes than she had ever dreamed of. The foreman let all the other girls know what Filomena had drawn in her pay envelope and one after another the girls began threading their needles at night. Then, when nearly all were doing this, he cut the pay so that they would make just what they had before. That was at last too much for Filomena; when the strike broke she went out with the others.

Another happening which is stamped on my memory concerns a young Irish girl of sixteen, gentle and shy, with the natural good breeding which one finds often among the poorest Irish and which makes one believe that they are right in saying that theirs was an old civilization when we Anglo-Saxons were still savages. Celia was a waitress in an all-night restaurant, for at that time a girl might work twelve hours a night seven nights in the week in Illinois. For her own protection I had her join the waitresses' union and when her place went on strike she took her turn picketing. Chicago police have never felt it part of their duty to observe the law toward strikers; violence, often needless and unprovoked, has been the rule. I felt personally responsible for Celia and made my way through the crowd outside the restaurant just in time to see her dragged along, unresisting, by a huge policeman and hustled with abusive words into a police van. We did get her off without a jail sentence but not till the next day.

Nobody who has not had to look on helplessly while servants of one's own government treat humble people with brutality can realize what rage it arouses, how all one's love and pride of country vanishes for the time being. Another time when this anger came over me was in the Kuppenheimer strike in Chicago. I do not remember the year but it must have been after 1915 for I know that I told Miss Addams I had seen nothing in occupied Belgium that so enraged me. Brutality in Belgium was the Germans' responsibility, brutality in Chicago was partly mine. I had undertaken to picket in that strike and had just reached a factory on the far West Side when I saw a little group of men running wildly in all directions. They were the pickets, thin, stoop-shouldered young Jews and Italians, and they were pursued by big thugs hired by the company, who struck and kicked them as they ran. A little knot of uniformed policemen, sent there to "keep law and order," looked on idly.

In the great Hart, Schaffner and Marx strike of 1910 I did not picket but went on a citizens' committee formed by Miss Addams, which met at Hull-House. She has told the story of that strike and how wisely it was settled, with a Joint Board of Arbitration composed of employers and employed with an impartial chairman, a method which has averted strikes ever since. Sidney Hillman emerged as leader of the new union. I met him in the course of the strike when Julia Lathrop and I called on him in his tiny hotel bedroom (I remember there was only one chair in it), a slender, very youthful-looking man, quiet and a bit shy, but very wise and steady.

Picketing in different strikes was no unusual job in those days. I used to volunteer for the early morning picket usually, because the police were much less in evidence then and I was in mortal fear of having one of them seize me and drag me about. The fact of arrest was not as bad as the way it was done. But late one winter afternoon I found myself marching up and down in perfect safety because I was with Professor Hale, head of the Latin Department of the University of Chicago.

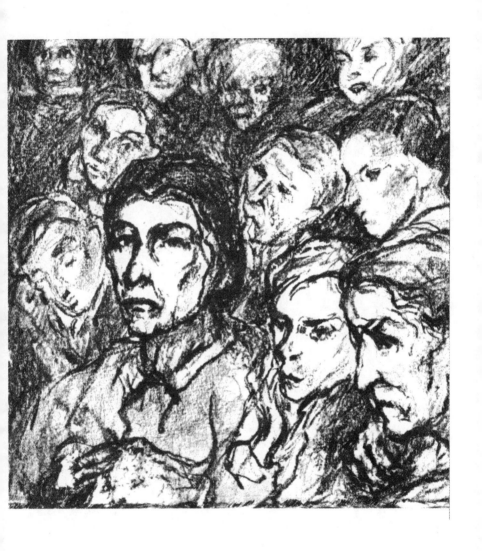

We were discussing the poems of Catullus, his favorite Latin poet. He was tall and very impressive, every inch a scholar and a gentleman, yet he could not understand why the police would not arrest him. "I am doing exactly what those poor fellows are doing," he said, "but they pay no attention to me." Of course the police had too much sense to provide such headlines for the papers.

Hull-House was the Mecca for many who came to Chicago in those days, for its fame had spread over the world with astonishing speed. It was said that Chicago had three *Sehenswürdigkeiten* — the University, the stockyards, and Hull-House. Some who came were radicals, Russian revolutionists, ranging from Miliukoff, who worked for a parliamentary system based on the English, to Nikolai, who at his party's command had assassinated some high dignitary and then had escaped from his Siberian prison in an empty hogshead. There were Liberals and Socialists of the moderate English type — Patrick Geddes, John Morley, J. A. Hobson, Sidney and Beatrice Webb, H. G. Wells, John Burns. The last was impressive but a bit amusing, for when, after a long discussion on all the shortcomings of our political system, someone said helplessly, "Well, what ought we to do about it?" John Burns responded promptly, "What you need in this country is one hundred John Burnses." John Morley won my heart by the way in which he took our shamed acknowledgment of corruption in city politics. "We British are partly to blame," he said, "for a great many of your political bosses are Irish and we are responsible for the Irish attitude toward government — that it is a weapon to be used by the victor against the defeated."

I met him again in 1915 when Miss Addams and I lunched

with him at his home outside London. He had resigned from the Government on the declaration of war in 1914 and he was a tragic figure. He told us that he had lived to see everything he had worked for in England swept away by the war and "I cannot hope to live long enough to see it come back." He did not — he died before the great social reforms which took place in postwar Britain had had time to occur.

Aylmer Maude, the disciple and translator of Tolstoy, came to see us on his way back from Canada where he had settled that strange sect opposed to war and to civilization, the Dukhobors, using the royalties from Tolstoy's *Resurrection* to defray the expenses. Lord Robert Cecil came after the war, and so did Graham Wallas. I remember a conversation between him and George Mead, professor of philosophy at the University of Chicago, and a devoted friend of Hull-House. Mr. Wallas had been reading some theses submitted by students of sociology for the Ph.D. degree. "Now look at these," he said, "careful, meticulously detailed studies of Chicago, of overcrowding, of housing, of recreation, but never once a bird's-eye view of the whole. Not one man ever stops to ask, 'Why have so big a city, anyway?'" Professor Mead protested, "But what use would that be? A student's ideas on such a subject are of no value. His careful collection of data is a real contribution." "Only to statistics," retorted Graham Wallas, "and you Americans have enough already. What you need is a wider outlook, a vision."

Henry Nevinson paid us a visit at the time of the Republican Convention that nominated Harding. I sat with him for some of the long hours of waiting in the hot Coliseum, listening to nominating speeches for Hoover, Lowden, and Leonard Wood, which were warmly applauded by the galleries but received in silence by the delegates, who simply waited for word from the little group sitting in the Blackstone Hotel. I cannot even remember who nominated Harding and when I went back to Hull-House and reported the result to Miss Addams, she said, "Harding, but who is he?" At dinner that evening we, with William Hard and Robert Lovett, tried to explain the who and why of Harding to Mr. Nevinson, but we all felt that he had unfortunately happened in on a spectacle of American politics at their lowest ebb.

Our English visitors sometimes surprised us by combining social radicalism with a total lack of democratic feeling, which to our way of thinking was most inconsistent. I remember a famous English Socialist who disapproved of our attempt at universal education up through the secondary schools. He believed that, after the essential primary grades, only gifted children should be helped to go farther. Another Fabian Socialist amused me very much when one morning I took him out into our neighborhood. He was talking eagerly about the need of vacation schools for London slum children as we stepped out into our courtyard, which was crowded with children waiting to go on a picnic in the country. He never saw them, at least not as slum children like those he was eager to help; he saw them only as obstacles in his way and he pushed them aside impatiently as if they were so many chickens, all the time telling me about the pitiful children in London. I thought to myself, "You may love humanity but you certainly do not love your fellow man." We found we could not always trust English radicals and Socialists to be nice to their American "comrades," when the latter were from an inferior social level, as most of them were, and we had some painful and embarrassing experiences when what was supposed to be a joyful meeting of kindred souls proved to be a meeting of the snubbers and the snubbed.

A great contrast to such visitors was Prince Peter Kropotkin, one of the most lovable persons I have ever met. He was a typical revolutionist of the early Russian type, an aristocrat who threw himself into the movement for emancipation of the masses out of a passionate love for his fellow man, and a longing for justice. His book, *Mutual Aid, a Factor of Evolution,* expounds a doctrine very different from that which now inspires Russian leaders, and he would be held in contempt by them as a sentimentalist; indeed that was true in his last years, after the Bolshevist revolution. I think he was as bitterly disappointed in the outcome of that revolution as was our other Russian revolutionary friend, Catherine Breshkovsky, but he never denounced it, as she did; that was not his way. He stayed some time with us at Hull-House and we all came to love him, not only we who lived under the same roof but the crowds of Russian refugees who came to see him. No matter how down-and-out, how squalid even, a caller would be, Prince Kropotkin would give him a joyful welcome and kiss him on both cheeks.

It was most unfortunate that his visit to us came just a short time before the assassination of McKinley. That event woke up the dormant terror of anarchists which always lay close under the surface of Chicago's thinking and feeling, ever since the Haymarket riot. It was known that Czolgosz, the assassin, had been in Chicago at the time when both Emma Goldman and Kropotkin were there and a rumor started that he had met them and the plot had been of their making — Czolgosz had been their tool. Then the story came to involve Hull-House, which had been the scene of these secret, murderous meetings. We went through a bad time but chiefly at the hands of reporters; the police did not molest us. They did, however, make arrests right and left, of all who could be suspected of radical opinions.

It was at that moment, when the reputation of Hull-House was at its lowest point, that Raymond Robins, who was living at the Northwestern Settlement, came to beg Miss Addams to do something to help a group of Russian Jewish anarchists ("philosophical anarchists") who had been caught in the police dragnet and were being held in jail incommunicado, while the police sought for evidence that would link them to Czolgosz. Robins had been able to do nothing himself but he believed Miss Addams might persuade the mayor to let them have a lawyer and she might bring back some reassurance to their frightened families. Nobody who has not lived through one of Chicago's attacks of anti-radical hysteria can understand what courage it took to do this. It would have been easy to reason that her first duty was to Hull-House, that these anarchists had never been inside its doors, and that if she espoused their cause she would be injuring an institution which could succeed only if it had the confidence of the public. But that was never her way of thinking. She went to the mayor, Carter Harrison, who told her that if she was ready to take the responsibility on her own shoulders, she might visit the prisoners and carry out their requests. She did, and of course she lived down the antagonism; Chicago came back to its senses and gave her again the warm admiration and help it always gave her in the long intervals between panics.

Chicago had some picturesque radicals in those days. Mrs. Stevens took me to hear Bill Haywood speak in Hodcarriers' Hall near Hull-House. He was a great towering hulk of a man, with a truculent, defiant way of speaking, not at all impressive or convincing. To me he seemed more down on the Socialists, who made up most of his audience, than on the capitalists he was supposed to be denouncing, but I soon found that that was true of many radicals. The heretic is always more detested than the heathen. It was Mrs. Stevens who took me to hear Emma Goldman also, this time as an interpreter, for Miss Goldman spoke in German. It was in a small Bohemian hall on DeKoven Street and, because the speaker was an avowed anarchist, a large number of policemen had been detailed to see to it that if she said anything dangerous (we had not yet found the word "subversive") the meeting was to be closed at once. But they were all Irish, not one understood German, and since Miss Goldman spoke without more than ordinary vehemence and the audience was orderly, they did not interfere, while she denounced government, law, police, religion, moral codes, and everything civilized society has built up as dykes to hold back chaos. It seemed to me a strangely fantastic doctrine, yet I could see that "philosophical anarchism," as we called it then to distinguish it from the "anarchism of the deed," was based on a profound idealism, on the belief that human nature is intrinsically good, that wickedness, cruelty, dishonorable dealing, are the result of tyrannical government, and man, if left to himself, can be trusted to act rightly.

Madame Breshkovsky was another aristocrat turned revolutionist and she inspired in me almost as much admiration as did Kropotkin. Those devoted people — and they were not the only ones we received as guests — made me feel so unworthy, for I knew that, no matter what misery I might see around me, I never should be capable of going out into a world of poverty, hardships, and danger as they had done. Madame Breshkovsky was an excellent actress — she could change in the twinkling of an eye into a dull, heavy, unresponsive peasant woman. I saw her do it once when a reporter came to interview her and she was afraid she might say something imprudent which would injure her cause, something which could be twisted into approval of assassination, the one thing which then fascinated all the reporters. So she told me she would understand no English, I must repeat all the questions in French, she would answer in French and I could censor her answers as I chose. She sat there with an expression of utter stupidity, with no flicker of understanding all through the interview, and the reporter departed thinking her a harmless old thing.

Marie Sukloff was another interesting Russian refugee, who had escaped from a Siberian prison and reached America through Japan. As a young girl of nineteen she had joined a group of Nihilists, and when it was decided that an official, I remember him as the Governor of Kiev, must be assassinated, the lot fell to her and to a young man not much older than she. They were to stand side by side on the pavement as his carriage passed by, she was to throw her bomb first, then he was to follow with his. She threw her bomb but it failed to explode (apparently bombs were pretty uncertain in those days), then his was thrown, exploded and killed the governor. Both were arrested and the young man was hanged, but public feeling against hanging a young girl under twenty was so strong that her sentence was commuted to life imprisonment. She escaped, as did so many, for Russian prisons were not very efficient. While she was with us she went to Joliet to see the great penitentiary and came back full of horror. "It is worse than anything in Russia or Siberia," she said. "Russian prisons are dirty and the guards are often cruel, but they are human — they may hit you one minute but the next minute they talk to you as if you were their sister. In Joliet it is all whitewashed and still, it works like a machine, it is terrifying." Later on when I went to Russia I visited a prison and felt about it just as she did. It was untidy, dirty even, but it was amazingly human in its informality, its crowd of chattering prisoners who gathered around me, full of curiosity. Actually I could not distinguish the prisoners from the guards. But that belongs in the chapter on Russia.

Some years later we had as guests two or three members of the Moscow Art Theater who came to us during the twenties, when the Bolshevist regime was well established. I remember our amusement when one of the actresses told us how frightened her family in Moscow had been to hear that she was to go to Chicago, the city of gangsters and racketeers. They said she must promise never to go out alone at night into those dangerous streets. "But I reassured them," she said, "I told them I should not need to go on the street, I could call for a taxi-airplane which would light on the roof and carry me to the theater. I saw it in an American movie." She was deeply disappointed, both in the apparent safety of Chicago's streets and in the lack of taxi-airplanes.

We had German visitors too. I remember a prominent German, a Geheimrat and a specialist in education, who was shocked by a debate he had witnessed in one of the high schools. I sat next him at dinner that evening and he commented on it to me. Those girls and boys had debated some question of public policy, I think it was the recall of judges, then very much to the fore. "How can you allow young people to discuss such things, nay more, encourage them and lead them to think that their opinions matter? Those are questions for their fathers to decide. Young people should not even think about them." I thought of this very un-American point of view years later, when I was in Vienna in 1921 and was visiting the child clinic of von Pirquet, a famous child specialist who gave us the first test for latent tuberculosis. For a time he taught at Johns Hopkins but he went back to Vienna when the war broke out. He had done wonders with children during the terrible years of starvation in Vienna, chiefly with linden leaves and sunlight, so far as I could see. As we left one of his sanatoria he said to me, "I suppose in America those boys and girls would be made into a self-governing community, with their own laws and judges and police. Here in Austria we do not put such responsibilities on children, we let them be just children." That appealed to me a good deal, at first, and I wondered if we were right to treat our children as if they were grown-up, to make them decide their own problems. But when I saw the appalling ease with which Austrians and Germans could be brought to submission by a ruthless leader I decided that our way is best.

One year when Miss Addams was in Europe and I was in charge of her mail a letter came to her from a woman who said she had read Miss Addams's book on prostitution, *A New Conscience and an Ancient Evil*, and wished to correspond with her about it. She stated frankly that she was an inmate of a brothel, so she knew what she was talking about. I wrote back at once, telling her of Miss Addams's absence and offering myself as a correspondent in her place. The writer accepted my offer and thus began a long exchange of letters which to me were very exciting, though I was somewhat disconcerted to find that neither Miss Addams nor Miss Lathrop would take the writer seriously. To me it seemed a thrilling glimpse into a terrible, unknown world filled with the helpless victims of man's lust. The woman would write to me usually in the early hours of the morning when her client had left her and the excitement of the night was as ashes in her mouth. She would quote Marcus Aurelius and Epictetus and especially Henley, for her head was always "bloody, but unbowed." She pictured herself as a captive bird beating her wings against the bars, and I was full of pity and of eagerness to free her from the life she loathed.

So when my work called me to Cleveland I resolved to stop over for a day in Toledo and see her, feeling sure that some way could be planned to effect her rescue. Julia Lathrop was provokingly skeptical, she would not believe the woman wanted to escape, she thought it was all probably play-acting, but that I could not believe. My mother was frankly nervous at the thought of my actually visiting a brothel, but, as always, she would not interfere, only she made me promise to go to the Charity Organization Society, tell them where I would be, and ask them to inform the police if I did not telephone them by five in the afternoon.

It was a sadly disillusioning experience. I found a house, luxurious but vulgarly ugly, and a woman of mature years, handsome, dignified, entirely mistress of herself. The pitiful little bird in the cage was a ludicrous picture. This woman was at once passionate and cold, a frightening combination. "Adelaide" had come to the house of her own free will and I soon saw that she had no intention of leaving it if that meant earning her own living. "I might make a good saleswoman," she said, "for I spend my time persuading men to spend money on what they don't really want. Most of the men who come here are only in search of a bit of gayety, fun, they don't really plan anything serious, but of course it is up to us to get them to spend the night." However, what she really meant to do was to get so strong a hold on one man that he would take her out and set her up in her own flat with a servant. Incidentally, that is just what she did. My last letter from her came from an apartment house in Cleveland.

My prostitute correspondent was as deeply disappointed in me as I was in her. My youthfulness put her off. "Oh dear," she said, "I imagined you quite different. Lavender and Old Lace, that is what I thought." Toward the end of my stay she interrupted her flow of talk about herself to ask what I did, and when I told her of my work she was frankly disgusted. "That is not the sort of thing I could possibly do," she said. "What I dream of is a little white cottage with green blinds and climbing roses, and babies." It was in this vein that she talked to her clients evidently, for she showed me letters from men who, like me, had accepted the captive-bird picture. I found too that there is snobbishness among prostitutes as in every walk of life. Adelaide was deeply contemptuous of the street walker, the woman who had to go out and pick up her clients. An aristocrat like herself simply saw to it that hotel clerks and taxi drivers had her address, then the clients could seek her.

I saw many intimate details of the life of a high-priced prostitute that day as the girl inmates wandered in and out, looking at me curiously. Their day was one of complete idleness: it was spent in the cult of the body, but there was no need to go out for the massaging and beauty treatment, not even for shopping — everything came to them. Life for those women was devoted to one thing alone, but for the men who visited them this was not true. For the man, such a visit was an occasional dissipation which cost him money; for the woman it was her sole preoccupation and at the same time it brought her money. After that I could never feel that the men arrested in a raid on a brothel were just as guilty as the women inmates nor as much of a menace to society.

I left that place of sordid luxury wiser for the loss of my illusions. It came over me that the revolt of the early Christians against the Roman baths was understandable. All that eternal bathing and anointing and massaging suddenly seemed disgusting and I could see how neglect of the body could come to seem holy and excessive cleanliness actually impure.

VI

Lawyers and Doctors

THE FIRST five years of my life in Chicago I taught pathology to the women students of Northwestern University which then maintained a separate school for women. It was a lonely life and I was afraid I should lose the desire for research for its own sake which Ann Arbor, Germany, and Hopkins had given me, so I went out to the University of Chicago two or three days each week and did a bit of work on a study Dr. H. H. Donaldson was making. His specialty was the brain and he set me the task of discovering whether, in the lower animals, there is a regeneration of the cells of the gray matter of the brain after an injury, as there is not in man. I worked on the brain of the newborn rat and found, as a side issue, that the maternal instinct of the rat is in her olfactory nerves, for if I handled the baby rat with my bare hand, the mother rat would promptly devour it as soon as it was returned to her, while if I first slipped absorbent cotton around it, not touching its skin, she would let it come back and suckle with the others.

There was another proof of the importance of scent in animals which I saw in that laboratory. John Watson, of later "behaviorist" fame, one day brought his mice and kittens into our room and showed us how they acted when they could see but not smell each other. When the mice were under a bell jar and the kittens outside, they paid no attention to each other, but when he substituted a wire cage for the bell jar the kittens clawed at it fiercely while the mice cowered close together in the very center of the cage. Yet, laboratory-born, the kittens had never met a mouse before nor the mice a cat.

Rush Medical School opened her doors to women in 1902, Northwestern University closed its women's annex, and I went to the newly founded Memorial Institute for Infectious Diseases, to do research in bacteriology under Dr. Ludwig Hektoen. I had already come to know him, and also Dr. E. R. LeCount and Dr. George Weaver, for I had had to turn to them for help when I first reached Chicago. When I arrived at the Woman's Medical School it was to find that pathology had been taught there by lectures only, there was no material for microscopic study, and had not the men at Rush Medical School helped me with the gift of all essential material, I could not have begun my course. Later on I was able to gather my own specimens from the autopsies performed in the morgue of Cook County Hospital.

It has been my good fortune to work under very remarkable teachers but none of them did more for me than Dr. Hektoen and I look back on those years in the Memorial Institute [1] with warm gratitude. We were a small group and the atmosphere was as informal and companionable as it had been in Munich and Frankfurt. At that time Almroth Wright's work on opsonins was all to the fore. Opsonins are substances in the blood plasma that act on bacteria and make it possible for the phagocytic white blood cells to swallow and destroy the bacteria — in short, opsonins are part of the defensive system of the body against infection. You can increase the opsonin content of the blood by repeated injections of very small

---

[1] The Institute was founded by Mr. and Mrs. Harold McCormick for research into bacteriological problems, especially the cause of scarlet fever, from which their child, John Rockefeller McCormick, had died.

quantities of the infectious germ, and therefore it was hoped that this procedure might be used to increase the resistance of human beings against such infections as are caused by well-known germs. These hopes have been realized only in part and even where such immunization is successful, opsonins are not the only substances responsible. I suspect that the general public knows of Almroth Wright's work only through Shaw's *Doctor's Dilemma*, where the doctor has only enough opsonin for one patient while two need it. My work with opsonins was chiefly in connection with tuberculosis and with the long-drawn-out effort to find a method of immunization at once effective and devoid of danger. The results, so far as opsonins were concerned, were negative.

A few years after my arrival Ruth Tunnicliffe joined the group and proved herself a really eminent bacteriologist, with as brilliant success as a woman can have in that field. This means that she could be a member of any scientific society she chose, could read papers and publish them, and win the respect of her colleagues quite as well as if she were a man, but she could not hope to gain a position of any importance in a medical school. I remember taking her to see the head of a department of pathology in a medical school where the chair of bacteriology was vacant. The pathologist received her with cordiality and respect and together they discussed their work for some time, then he spoke of the vacancy in the medical school and went over with her the qualifications of the different candidates who were being considered. Had she been a man she would almost certainly have been chosen, but it never occurred to him even to consider her.

It was while I was working at the Memorial Institute that an opportunity came for me to bring my scientific training to bear on a problem at Hull-House. (My efforts in the baby clinic could not be called scientific.) This was in the fall of 1902, when I came back from Mackinac to find Chicago in the grip of one of her worst epidemics of typhoid fever. At that time the water, drawn from the Lake, was not chlorinated; the only precaution taken against dangerous pollution was to make daily cultures of samples from the different pumping stations and the next day, when the cultures had had time to develop, publish the results and tell the public whether or not to boil the water. It was assumed that housewives would look up these instructions every day and act accordingly, but the actual result was that typhoid was endemic in Chicago and periodically it reached epidemic proportions. On this particular occasion Hull-House was the center of the hardest-struck region of the city — why, nobody knew. Miss Addams said she thought a bacteriologist ought to be able to discover the reason.

It was certainly not a simple problem. The pumping station which sent water to the Nineteenth Ward sent it to a wide section of the West Side; the milk supply was the same as that for neighboring wards. There must be some local condition to account for the excessive number of cases. As I prowled about the streets and the ramshackle wooden tenement houses I saw the outdoor privies (forbidden by law but flourishing nevertheless), some of them in backyards below the level of the street and overflowing in heavy rains; the wretched water closets indoors, one for four or more families, filthy and with the plumbing out of order because nobody was responsible for cleaning or repairs; and swarms of flies everywhere. Here, I thought, was the solution of the problem. The flies were feeding on typhoid-infected excreta and then lighting on food and milk. During the Spanish-American War, when we lost more men from typhoid fever than from Spanish bullets, Vaughan,

Shakespeare, and Reed had made a study of conditions in camps — open latrines, unscreened food — which led them to attribute an important role in the spread of typhoid fever to the house fly. That was what started the "Swat the fly" campaign.

Naturally, my theory had to be put to the test, so, with two of the residents to help me, Maude Gernon and Gertrude Howe, I went forth to collect flies — from privies and kitchens and filthy water closets. We would drop the flies into tubes of broth and I would take them to the laboratory, incubate the tubes, and plate them out at varying intervals. It was a triumph to find the typhoid bacillus and I hastened to write up the discovery and its background for presentation before the Chicago Medical Society. This was just the sort of thing to catch public attention: it was simple and easily understood; it fitted in with the revelations made during the Spanish War of the deadly activities of house flies, and it explained why the slums had so much more typhoid than the well-screened and decently drained homes of the well-to-do.

I am sure I gained more kudos from my paper on flies and typhoid than from any other piece of work I ever did. Even today I sometimes hear an echo of it. In Chicago the effect was most gratifying: a public inquiry resulted in a complete re-organization of the Health Department under a chief loaned by the Public Health Service, and an expert was put in charge of tenement-house inspection. But unfortunately my gratification over my part in all this did not last long. After the tumult had died down I discovered a fact which never gained much publicity but was well-authenticated. My flies had had little or nothing to do with the cases of typhoid in the Nineteenth Ward. The cause was simpler but so much more discreditable that the Board of Health had not dared reveal it. It seems that in our local pumping station, on West Harrison Street, near Halsted, a break had occurred which resulted in an escape of sewage into the water pipes and for three days our neighborhood drank that water before the leak was discovered and stopped. This was after the epidemic had started. The truth was more shocking than my ingenious theory, and it never came to light, so far as the public was concerned. For years, although I did my best to lay the ghosts of those flies, they haunted me and mortified me, compelling me again and again to explain to deeply impressed audiences that the dramatic story their chairman had just rehearsed had little foundation in fact.

Because of my access to medical help of all kinds, I was drawn into the fight against the cocaine traffic which Hull-House was forced to take up early in this century. A young girl from Iowa, Jessie Binford, later of the Juvenile Protective Association, lived at Hull-House, and her work was with delinquent children, for there were no probation officers for children then. The Juvenile Court had yet to be born. Miss Binford discovered that cocaine, "happy dust," was being sold to our schoolboys by agents of drugstores, who would stop the boys on their way home from school, give them a pinch of the powder to snuff up, and ask them how they liked it. The stimulating effect comes quickly, the boys told us they felt delightfully queer, "as if I was going up in a flying machine," "as if I was a millionaire and could do anything I pleased." Cocaine is far more tempting than morphine to the young and healthy and it worked havoc among these boys, who would get so desperate for a dose that they would commit a crime to get it, hold up and rob, smash drugstore windows, intimidate drug clerks.

Miss Binford and our fine Irish policeman, George Murray,[2] would round up the victims, sometimes from a hang-out under the old wooden sidewalk on Canal Street, capture the little boxes of cocaine, and hand them over to me for analysis. Dr. Walter Haines, toxicologist on the faculty of Rush Medical School, taught me the tests, and, armed with these, I would go to the trial of the druggist who had sold the stuff. This was the first of a long series of experiences with our legal system, as carried out in our lower courts, which nearly converted me to anarchism and left me with a strong conviction that the American system which most needs reform is the system of criminal law.

Chicago had police courts then, in dark, squalid police stations; the justices, all Irish in our neighborhood, were quite decent, most of them, but the jurors and the lawyers seemed to us of a lower criminal type than most of the accused and their manners were far worse. The defendant druggists in our cocaine cases always demanded a jury trial and their lawyers always intimated that we from Hull-House were meddling, high-brow reformers, trying to keep an honest man from earning his living. We had to work under a very inadequate law. In the first place, it covered cocaine but not the closely allied synthetic alpha- and beta-eucaine, which give the same chemical reactions. So the defense soon began to claim that the stuff sold was one of the eucaines, not covered by the law. The only way to prove that it was cocaine was to test it on the eye, for cocaine dilates the pupil, the eucaines do not. At first I used to test the specimens on laboratory rabbits, but I found that the defense lawyers could produce a real effect on

[2] George Murray was a policeman detailed to us for many years by the Maxwell Street Police Station. He had all the fine qualities of the Irish with none of the shortcomings.

the jury by dwelling on the well-known cruelty of the scientist toward animals and insisting on knowing what else we did to the poor rabbits in the Memorial Institute, so I tested the powders on myself, for I knew it would not injure my eyes and other people were quite understandably reluctant to take the risk. I used to go around the laboratory with one wide and one narrow pupil till everyone was so used to it that they took no notice. But one day Dr. Hektoen came in much amused to tell me that a doctor who had been talking with me went to him in great agitation to say that I evidently had a tumor of the brain.

A weak point in the law was that it did not make the druggist responsible for his clerk's action, so he could plead innocence, discharge his clerk, and hire him back the next day. Even if we secured a conviction, there was only a fine, no jail sentence, and the druggist could easily afford a fine. All this was so unsatisfactory that we soon found we must work for a new law.

After about a year we succeeded in getting a measure passed which covered the eucaines and provided a severer penalty, and under it we won thirteen cases in the police courts, which seemed to us no mean achievement. But the druggists had a clever lawyer who had spotted a weakness in the new law, all the cases were appealed, and the appellate judge threw them all out. He was one of Chicago's most respected judges, but he felt that he had done his whole duty by pointing out the defects of the law. He did not think, nor did any of his profession think, that it was up to them to see that we got the sort of law we needed. When finally a proper law was passed it was owing to the efforts of a Catholic priest and the head of the Bridewell. Nor would the legal authorities even tell us in advance whether the new law was properly framed, and that is certainly a strange thing. The legal experts may not pronounce on the constitutionality of a proposed law. No, it must first be passed, then challenged, and then they will consent to consider it and pass on it. That seems to me as absurd as if the Health Department should refuse to test the water of a proposed reservoir, saying, "No, we cannot tell you if this water is contaminated or not. You must put in the system and let the people drink the water, then if they get sick we will tell you whether it is typhoid fever and whether you must look for another water supply."

All of these cases were tried in the old police courts. Later on we got a grand new Municipal Court with big, well-lighted rooms, and a more formal procedure, but my experience led me to think that, so far as the administration of justice goes, the more it changes, the more it is the same thing. We at Hull-House did not find that the grand new courthouse was any freer from political influence than the old police court, or that the judges were any more impartial, or that the character of the prosecuting attorneys and the lawyers for the defense had changed in the least. Yet in that same period the dispensaries to which I had to take our neighbors had improved enormously, overcrowding and hasty examination had given way to the best of diagnostic service, and the poor could get medical and surgical care quite as good as that given the rich. Reforms in medical schools and hospitals have been put through with great thoroughness in the last quarter century. They seem to lag strangely in the field of criminal law.

As an American, nothing mortified me as much as the system of criminal law in Chicago, for it was impossible to explain it or to defend it to the immigrants whom one wanted so much to inspire with confidence in our American form of government. Take this instance, as one of many: a young black sheep in one of my Italian families who was a member of a gang of young hoodlums was arrested with two others for an attempted holdup. His parents came to me and as we talked it over I was keenly struck with the fact that I, who belonged to the country to which they had come, could not tell them to have faith in American courts, to trust in the wisdom and fairness of an American judge, and to believe that if the lad was sentenced to a reformatory, as he should be, he would come out a reformed character. I could not say these things because I feared that none of them was true. I knew the judge in that court, and was sure that he was not free from the influence of a powerful Italian politician (indeed a few years later he marched in the funeral procession of this Italian). I could not tell the parents that they were mistaken when they said the other boys would get light sentences because their fathers stood in with the political leader, while they did not, and that the heavy sentence would be given their son to satisfy the newspapers.

That the lad should be taught a lesson somehow, that he should be pulled up short before he became a confirmed criminal, I knew, but I also knew that he would never receive such teaching in the Illinois Reformatory as it was then, he would come out worse than when he went in. I do not know what I should have done; all I know is that I stood passively by while a kindly neighbor pulled the right political strings and the lad got off with a sentence so short that I could hope he would not be much the worse for it.

As I got more deeply into industrial medicine, my experience with the legal profession changed its character, for I went up into the civil courts, being called on to testify as an expert in civil suits for damages brought by workmen in the dangerous trades. Here I had a most bewildering experience. The laws of evidence seem to me the strangest thing about the whole legal system, and I never have got used to them. A witness is in the stand, doing his best to give a clear, connected statement of the facts as he knows them, but the laws of evidence (which are, I believe, peculiar to the Anglo-Saxon countries) require that the simplest story be interrupted, parts of it prohibited, the telling of it so cabin'd, cribb'd, confined that both witness and jury are confused. What is essential to the story must be suppressed for mysterious reasons, and the whole thing messed up hopelessly. When I have appealed to my lawyer friends for an explanation of this deliberate clouding of the waters of truth the only explanation I have ever had is that our courts are still working under laws which were framed when men were tortured to make them confess, and merciful judges tried to protect them, not by overthrowing the system — lawyers never do that — but by clever shifts which would do something while seeming to do something else. To a lawyer this explanation is apparently valid, to a physician it is as if he should say, "Yes, I know it is all wrong to bleed a consumptive patient because he has fever, but you see that practice dates back to the time when we did not know the nature of fevers, and thought that they all belonged to the so-called sanguineous type of disease and must be treated by depletion."

Once when I was still young and brash I tried to break through this curious system with results that may be imagined. I was on the witness stand, testifying as an expert, in a case which was variously diagnosed as chronic lead poisoning and as pernicious anemia, a hard enough problem for medical men but one which our legal system puts up to a lay jury to decide. The lawyer for the other side was putting questions to me in such a way as to increase the puzzlement of the already bewildered jury. So, when there was a moment's pause in the proceedings, I turned to the jury and said, "Now, suppose you let me tell you just what all this scientific stuff means." Heavens! If you could have seen the lawyer. Had I called on the jury to go forth and wreck the Constitution of these United States with force and violence he could not have been more horrified. The lawyer on my side rushed to my defense, though I am sure he was equally shocked, but that is part of the game. When the tumult and the shouting died I found that the judge had ruled against me and there was nothing to do but to sink back in my chair and go on giving answers to muddling questions. If these cases came before a court of experts, the system might work, but before a jury of ordinary people, how can it be expected to?

Then there is the curious fact that the legal profession, with all its manifest imperfections, is the most arrogant profession in modern life. In early days it was the clergy that claimed unquestioned authority and homage from the public, but they have lost it almost completely, and physicians never had it. Nowadays it is the judges who form our sacred priesthood; they are the only ones against whom *lèse-majesté* is still a crime. It is perfectly safe to revile the President of the United States, and one can utter blasphemies without even attracting attention, but to protest against an abusive tirade by an ill-bred or drunken judge may mean a prison sentence. And we are asked to believe that by the mystic laying-on of hands a passionately partisan prosecuting attorney who has been for years demanding the death penalty for all and sundry, and resenting as a failure the acquittal of any of the accused, is transformed in the twinkling of an eye into a wise, impartial dispenser of justice as soon as he is made a judge.

As for legal ideas on human psychology, they are very strange.

Maybe it is different now, but in the days when I frequented police courts it was still true that a witness who was upset and stammering and confused was showing "consciousness of guilt," while the fluent, self-possessed witness, with a marvelous memory for every detail, was proving his innocence. I used to watch, in helpless misery, an inexperienced and timid witness make a fool of himself under the ruthless handling of the opposing lawyer (why the best of judges never would interfere I could not understand), while the witness who I knew was lying gave a smooth, consistent, unshakable story. And the jury was led to believe that truth is always calm and unafraid, and that guilt is panicky and confused. Often I should have liked to ask the gentlemen of the jury how they would act if they were suddenly challenged to say what they were doing at half-past eight o'clock Thursday evening, two weeks ago, knowing that a jail sentence might hang on their answer.

There was once a dramatic poster on Halsted Street, advertising a melodrama in one of our neighbor theaters. It showed two men at a table, one starting back in horror as a waiter placed before him a platter with the bloody head of a man on it, the other leaning forward watching him intently and saying, "I have always maintained that if a murderer were suddenly confronted with the severed head of his victim, he would be startled into betraying himself." Apparently if he were innocent he would view the bloody head with complete nonchalance. But that is good psychology in a police court.

Doctors are a faulty lot, as we are told by the public again and again. But at least we ourselves admit it and strive to improve our ways. Some think that the medical profession is actually too quick to grasp for new methods, but surely it is well that it does not wrap itself in infallibility and shut its eyes to what is new. No physician could possibly rise to a high place in his profession if he did that. But apparently a lawyer could and can. My lawyer friends assure me that it is possible, and has actually happened, that a man can attain to the highest legal position in the land without ever having changed his mental attitude on any important point since he left the law school. That seems to me a pretty severe indictment of a profession.

As the years went on — my life there covered twenty-two years — Hull-House grew till it covered more than a city block and its activities increased in variety as the little group of residents came to include many people of many interests. We had Gerard Swope and his wife, Frederick Deknatel, whose son now continues his father's devoted service, George M. R. Twose, Edward and Charles Yeomans, George Hooker, William L. Chenery, Edith and Grace Abbott, Sophonisba Breckinridge, the Robert Morss Lovetts, Harriet Monroe, and many others. Once I expressed to Mrs. Kelley my wonder that a group of people so individual and so different could be held together, and she answered, "We have a common cult." She meant the personality of Jane Addams, but there was something more than that and it still lives after her death.

Hull-House still goes on, still works along the lines Jane Addams laid down fifty years ago. New features have appeared, some of the old ones have vanished; the old order changeth, yielding place to new, but the spirit remains much the same. Miss Addams always said that if after she was gone we opposed changes because "Miss Addams never did that," it would mean that a dead hand was crushing out the life of what should be a growing plant, for each generation should approach the problems of its day with fresh ideas, perhaps building on the foundations of the past, but following the lines of its own inspiration.

It is still a place for experiment in new ways, still a place where problems are studied not theoretically but with first-hand, intimate observation, a place where no one political or religious creed is followed but all may be discussed under a hospitable and tolerant roof, where the rare gifts of musical and artistic talent which are hidden by poverty can be discovered and fostered, where the young can come for pleasure and the old for comfort.

One often hears it said that settlements have had their day, that they belong to the sentimental era of the nineties, there is no longer a place for them. I do not think that is true; I think that now, when the tendency is away from the individual to the mass, the intimate, personal touch is much needed. We have no longer the same sense of the supreme importance of every human being; rather our tendency is to absorb the individual in the state, or the class, or the movement. There were many evils in the old, unrestrained individualism, but the new collectivism is not without its dangers. After all, was not the great gift of Christianity just that — the declaration of the supreme importance and worth of every soul in the sight of God? If we lose that, we shall have lost greatly. In all the multitude of organizations which work for the betterment of society, the settlement movement has its place. And for the younger generation which is espousing eagerly the cause of the underdog, it is well to have a place where the underdogs can be really studied, not only in their union headquarters or their Communist cells, but in their tenement homes, with all the family background and influences which play so large a part in their psychology. For only by such experience can the young crusaders gain a true picture of the "proletariat."

It was my life at Hull-House that brought me into the birth-control movement not long after Margaret Sanger started it, and I joined the Chicago Birth Control Committee which Dr. Rachelle Yarros, a pioneer in this field, had formed. I might quote from a letter on the subject which I wrote to the League of Women Voters.

Whatever we may think of the truth of the tale of the Garden of Eden in the Book of Genesis we must agree that it is a valiant attempt to explain some of the dark riddles of life, the blessed ignorance and innocence of childhood and the disillusion and burdens of later life, which are the fruits of the Tree of the Knowledge of Good and Evil. There is no sentimentality in Genesis about the contentment which manual labor brings nor the joys of childbearing, on the contrary the first is the curse laid on man and the second the curse laid on woman. Through all the centuries man has put his best energies into escaping his curse and the manual laborer has come to occupy the lowest social scale. But women have seldom rebelled against their curse, and when they have, Society and the Church have quickly suppressed them. When a Tolstoy tries to call men back to the joys of primitive labor, he meets with indulgent contempt, but woman's curse is still sacred and even the attempt to make childbearing less painful met with opposition from the clergy for many years, because it was contrary to Scripture.

It must have been some ten or twelve years after I came to live in Hull-House that I was suddenly asked one day in public whether I believed in birth control. Without stopping to think I answered at once that I most certainly did and then realized that this was the first time the question had ever been put to me or I had ever formulated my belief even to myself. The answer had been almost automatic, prompted by my daily experiences in a poor community, where I came in close contact with the lives of Italian, Irish, Slavic, German and Russian and Polish Jewish families, and saw what unlimited childbearing meant to them. I had pictures flash into my mind of the gradual slipping down of home standards and the loss of comforts, even decencies, under the pressure of too many babies, coming too fast. I could think of promising boys and girls whose parents had proudly planned for high-school education and a rise in the world and who had been forced to leave school at fourteen and take any possible job because there were so many mouths to feed that the father's wages would not suffice. I could think of dull, weary women, incapable of taking the part of mother as we think of that part, to the brood of children always increasing, who had to bring up themselves and their younger brothers and sisters because the one who should have done it had degenerated into a lifeless drudge. And so I found myself of a sudden an ardent advocate of a cause which till then I had hardly heard of, and all my experience since has only confirmed and strengthened my adherence.

The reasons which are convincing to those of us who live among and know the poor are perhaps not the same as those which seem most urgent to others. We are not, for instance, moved much by the plea that the upper classes are being submerged by the lower and that the poor must be kept from breeding too fast. We know that ability and character are not a matter of class and that the difference comes from the unfair handicaps to which the children of the poor are subject, and we would remedy matters by working for equality of opportunity for all children, instead of trying to encourage the propagation of one class and not of the other. The arguments for birth control which appeal most to us are based on the welfare of the women of the poorer classes and the welfare of their children.

A woman who starts her married life with a tiny flat and her wedding furniture and practically nothing more has an enormous problem in budget making before her at the best, one which she usually handles with a skill that amazes me when I think of her almost total lack of training except what she has had from her equally untrained mother. She can often, perhaps more often than not, make a very fair success out of it for the first years of her married life, while she is strong and the pressure is not too unendurable. But if the babies come year after year, she cannot, unless she is a very wonderful person — there are such in the poorest tenements — bear up under the continually increasing burden.

She does not always submit without a struggle. Birth control is carried on in the tenements all the time, in a form far worse than the prevention of conception, which the poor do not understand. It is in the form of abortion, which every woman can learn about if she wishes. Not long ago I invited a group of Italian women to spend a Sunday afternoon with me at Hull-House, all of them married women with large families. The conversation turned very soon on abortions and the best method of producing them and I was in consternation to listen to the experiences of these women, who had themselves undergone frightful risks and much suffering rather than add another child to a house too full already. One woman said she had thrown herself down the cellar stairs twice, but it had done no good. Another answered, "Next time take a tub of water with you and throw yourself down after it. I did that and it worked." These women were all Catholics, but when I spoke of that, they simply shrugged their shoulders. What could a priest know about a woman's life?

Karl Pearson once made a study of the children of large and of small families and, as I remember, decided in favor of the large family because he found the younger children on the whole much more worth while than the older ones. I wonder whether there is not a very obvious explanation for such findings. His investigation was probably made largely among the poor, who cannot defend themselves against the investigator any more than they can against the other ills of life, and among them it is usually true that the youngest children of large families are distinctly superior to the older ones in education and therefore more successful in life. But this does not mean more native ability; it means that the older sisters and brothers have been sacrificed for the sake of the later comers, they have been put to work at the earliest moment the law allows, if not earlier, they have been robbed of their youth and given burdens to bear which should never have been theirs.

It is not a question of introducing among the poor an effort to prevent excessive childbearing. Such efforts are made all the time now. It is a question of introducing safe-and-sane methods, and of spreading among them the knowledge that limitation of the number of children is possible without the risk of death or invalidism. It is a question of offering to the poor, who need them most, the knowledge and the power which have long been the possession of those who need them least.

VII

The Illinois Survey

IT WAS also my experience at Hull-House that aroused my interest in industrial diseases. Living in a working-class quarter, coming in contact with laborers and their wives, I could not fail to hear tales of the dangers that workingmen faced, of cases of carbon-monoxide gassing in the great steel mills, of painters disabled by lead palsy, of pneumonia and rheumatism among the men in the stockyards. Illinois then had no legislation providing compensation for accident or disease caused by occupation. (There is something strange in speaking of "accident and sickness compensation." What could "compensate" anyone for an amputated leg or a paralyzed arm, or even an attack of lead colic, to say nothing of the loss of a husband or son?) There was a striking occurrence about this time in Chicago which brought vividly before me the unprotected, helpless state of workingmen who were held responsible for their own safety.

A group of men were sent out in a tug to one of Chicago's pumping stations in Lake Michigan and left there while the tug returned to shore. A fire broke out on the tiny island and could not be controlled, the men had the choice between burning to death and drowning, and before rescue could arrive most of them were drowned. The contracting company, which employed them, generously paid the funeral expenses, and nobody expected them to do more. Widows and orphans must turn to the County Agent or private charity — that was the accepted way, back in the dark ages of the early twentieth century. William Hard, then a young college graduate living at Northwestern Settlement, wrote of this incident with a fiery pen, contrasting the treatment of the wives and children of these men whose death was caused by negligence with the treatment they would have received in Germany. His article and a copy of Sir Thomas Oliver's *Dangerous Trades*, which came into my hands just then, sent me to the Crerar Library to read everything I could find on the dangers to industrial workers, and what could be done to protect them. But it was all German, or British, Austrian, Dutch, Swiss, even Italian or Spanish — everything but American. In those countries industrial medicine was a recognized branch of the medical sciences; in my own country it did not exist. When I talked to my medical friends about the strange silence on this subject in American medical magazines and textbooks, I gained the impression that here was a subject tainted with Socialism or with feminine sentimentality for the poor. The American Medical Association had never had a meeting devoted to this subject, and except for a few surgeons attached to large companies operating steel mills, or railways, or coal mines, there were no medical men in Illinois who specialized in the field of industrial medicine.

Everyone with whom I talked assured me that the foreign writings could not apply to American conditions, for our workmen were so much better paid, their standard of living was so much higher, and the factories they worked in so much finer in every way than the European, that they did not suffer from the evils to which the poor foreigner was subject. That sort of talk always left me skeptical. It was impossible for me to believe that conditions in Europe could be worse than they were in the Polish section of Chicago, and in many Italian and

Irish tenements, or that any workshops could be worse than some of those I had seen in our foreign quarters. And presently I had factual confirmation of my disbelief in the happy lot of the American worker through the reading of John Andrews's manuscript on "phossy jaw" in the match industry in the United States.

Phossy jaw is a very distressing form of industrial disease. It comes from breathing the fumes of white or yellow phosphorus, which gives off fumes at room temperature, or from putting into the mouth food or gum or fingers smeared with phosphorus. Even drinking from a glass which has stood on the workbench is dangerous. The phosphorus penetrates into a defective tooth and down through the roots to the jawbone, killing the tissue cells which then become the prey of suppurative germs from the mouth, and abscesses form. The jaw swells and the pain is intense, for the suppuration is held in by the tight covering of the bone and cannot escape, except through a surgical operation or through a fistula boring to the surface. Sometimes the abscess forms in the upper jaw and works up into the orbit, causing the loss of an eye. In severe cases one lower jawbone may have to be removed, or an upper jawbone — perhaps both. There are cases on record of men and women who had to live all the rest of their days on liquid food. The scars and contractures left after recovery were terribly disfiguring, and led some women to commit suicide. Here was an industrial disease which could be clearly demonstrated to the most skeptical. Miss Addams told me that when she was in London in the 1880's she went to a mass meeting of protest against phossy jaw and on the platform were a number of pitiful cases, showing their scars and deformities.

All this I had learned, but I had been assured by medical men, who claimed to know, that there was no phossy jaw in the United States because American match factories were so scrupulously clean. Then in 1908 John Andrews came to Hull-House and showed me the report of his investigation of American match factories and his discovery of more than 150 cases of phossy jaw. It seems that in the course of a study of wages of women and children made by the Bureau of Labor, under Carroll Wright, investigators came across cases of phossy jaw in women match workers in the South. This impelled Wright to institute an investigation in other match centers. Andrews was asked to carry it out and did so, with a result most disconcerting to American optimism. Some of the cases he discovered were quite as severe as the worst reported in European literature — the loss of jawbones, of an eye, sometimes death from blood poisoning.

This episode in the history of industrial disease is very characteristic of our American way of dealing with such matters. We learned about phossy jaw almost as soon as Europe did. The first recognized case was described by Lorinser of Vienna in 1845; the first American case was treated in the Massachusetts General Hospital only six years later, in 1851. But while all over continental Europe and England there was eager discussion of this new disease, many cases were reported and all sorts of preventive measures proposed, practically nothing was published in American medical journals from 1851 to 1909, both laymen and public health authorities contenting themselves with the assurance that all was well in our match industry. When, however, the facts were at last made public in 1909, action was prompt. A safe substitute for white phosphorus had been discovered by a French chemist, the sesquisulphide, the American patent rights for which had been bought by the Diamond Match Company. This company, with rare generosity, waived its patent rights and allowed the free use of sesquisulphide to the whole industry, and this made it possible for Congress to pass the Esch law, which imposed a tax on white-phosphorus matches high enough to cover the difference in cost between them and sesquisulphide matches. So phossy jaw disappeared from American match factories.

There were a few other voices in the wilderness. I remember a trip to Washington, to a medical meeting, when Frederick Hoffman of the Prudential Insurance Company gave us a demonstration, with statistics and charts, of the relation between occupation and tuberculosis. It was a startling eye-opener to me and I feel sure that I was not the only one who was hearing such facts for the first time. Dr. George M. Kober of Washington and Dr. William Gilman Thompson of New York were two other pioneers in this field, and only a few years later Josephine Goldmark published her famous brief on the employment of women in industry. So there were stirrings here and there, the flood was rising slowly.

At the time I am speaking of Professor Charles Henderson was teaching sociology in the University of Chicago. He had been much in Germany and had made a study of German sickness insurance for the working class (the *Krankenkassen*), a system which aroused his admiration and made him eager to have some such provisions made in behalf of American work‧ men. The first step must be, of course, an inquiry into the extent of our industrial sickness, and he determined to have such an inquiry made in Illinois. Governor Deneen was then in office and Henderson persuaded him to appoint an Occupational Disease Commission, the first time a state had ever undertaken such a survey. Dr. Henderson had some influence in selecting the members and, as he knew of my great interest in the subject, he included me in the group of five physicians who, together with himself, an employer, and two members of the State Labor Department, made up the commission. We had one year only for our work, the year 1910.

We were staggered by the complexity of the problem we faced and we soon decided to limit our field almost entirely to the occupational poisons, for at least we knew what their action was, while the action of the various kinds of dust, and of temperature extremes and heavy exertion, was only vaguely known at that time. Then we looked for an expert to guide and supervise the study, but none was to be found and so I was asked to do what I could as managing director of the survey, with the help of twenty young assistants, doctors, medical students, and social workers. As I look back on it now, our task was simple compared with the one that a state nowadays faces when it undertakes a similar study. The only poisons we had to cover were lead, arsenic, brass, carbon monoxide, the cyanides, and turpentine. Nowadays, the list involved in a survey of the painters' trade alone is many times as long as that.

But to us it seemed far from a simple task. We could not even discover what were the poisonous occupations in Illinois. The Factory Inspector's office was blissfully ignorant, yet that was the only governmental body concerned with working conditions. There was nothing to do but begin with trades we knew were dangerous and hope that, as we studied them, we would discover others less well known. My field was to be lead, Dr. Emery Hayhurst took brass, Drs. G. Apfelbach and M. Karasek, carbon monoxide in the steel mills. Caisson disease [1]

---

[1] This is a disease caused by work in compressed air when the return to normal air pressure is too quick. The air absorbed by the body under pressure expands if that pressure is released too suddenly and this causes damage, especially in the delicate tissues of the brain and the spinal cord. Violent pain in the limbs (known as "the bends") and brain disturbances (called "the

had appeared in the state, in connection chiefly with the construction of tunnels in Chicago, and Dr. Peter Bassoe undertook the study of the 161 cases of this disease which had occurred up to this date. Dr. George Shambaugh contributed a chapter on boiler makers' deafness and Drs. F. Lane and J. D. Ellis one on the rhythmic oscillation of the eyes of coal miners, known as nystagmus.

While we were visiting plants, we set our young assistants to reading hospital records, interviewing labor leaders and doctors and apothecaries in working-class quarters, for we must unearth actual instances of poisoning if our study was to be of any value. Thus I was put on the trail of new lead trades, some of which I had never thought of — for instance, making freight-car seals, coffin "trim," and decalcomania papers for pottery decoration; polishing cut glass; brass founding; wrapping cigars in so-called tinfoil, which is really lead. Hospital records yielded cases from these and from many other jobs which were not mentioned in foreign textbooks.

One case, of colic and double wristdrop, which was discovered in the Alexian Brothers' Hospital, took me on a pretty chase. The man, a Pole, said he had worked in a sanitary-ware factory, putting enamel on bathtubs. I had not come across this work in the English or the German authorities on lead poisoning, and had no idea it was a lead trade, but the factory was easy to reach on the near West Side and I stopped in to ask about the man's work. The management assured me that no lead was used in the coatings and invited me to inspect the workroom, where I found six Polish painters applying an enamel paint to metal bathtubs. So

blind staggers") result if the worker goes too quickly into the open air. He is protected now by being made to pass slowly through a series of decompression chambers.

ignorant was I that I accepted this as the work of enameling sanitary ware, and did not even notice that all the men were painting the outsides of the tubs. I did note the name of the paint and went to the factory which produced it, but there I was told that enamel paint is free from lead. Completely puzzled, I made a journey to the Polish quarter to see the palsied man and heard from him that I had not even been in the enameling works, only the one for final touching up. The real one was far out on the Northwest Side. I found it and discovered that enameling means sprinkling a finely ground enamel over a red-hot tub where it melts and flows over the surface. I learned that the air is thick with enamel dust and that this may be rich in red oxide of lead. A specimen of it which I secured from a workman, who said he often took some home to his wife for scouring pans and knives, proved to contain as much as 20 per cent soluble lead — that is, lead that will pass into solution in the human stomach. Thus I nailed down the fact that sanitary-ware enameling was a dangerous lead trade in the United States, whatever was true of England and Germany.

It was pioneering, exploration of an unknown field. No young doctor nowadays can hope for work as exciting and rewarding. Everything I discovered was new and most of it was really valuable. I knew nothing of manufacturing processes, but I learned them on the spot, and before long every detail of the Old Dutch Process and the Carter Process of white-lead production was familiar to me, also the roasting of red lead and litharge and the smelting of lead ore and refining of lead scrap. From the first I became convinced that what I must look for was lead dust and lead fumes, that men were poisoned by breathing poisoned air, not by handling their food with un-

washed hands. Nowadays that fact has been so strongly established by experimental proof that nobody would think of dis-
puting it. But in 1910 and for many years after, the firm (and
comforting) belief of foremen and employers was that if a
man was poisoned by lead it was because he did not wash his
hands and scrub his nails, although a little intelligent observation would have been enough to show its absurdity.

This fact, that lead poisoning is brought about far more
rapidly and intensely by the breathing of lead-laden air than
by the swallowing of lead, is of the greatest practical importance. There can be no intelligent control of the lead
danger in industry unless it is based on the principle of keeping
the air clear from dust and fumes. The English authority,
Sir Thomas Legge, after some thirty years' experience in the
prevention of industrial disease, reached the conclusion that
the air is the only important source of occupational lead poisoning and that the only efficient measures for its prevention are
those directed toward the prevention of dust and fumes. A
hundred years ago Tanquerel des Planches, who is called the
Columbus of lead poisoning, noted that severe plumbism
never followed the handling of solid lead but only exposure
to dust and "emanations."

Lead is the oldest of the industrial poisons except carbon
monoxide, which must have begun to take its toll soon after
Prometheus made the gift of fire to man. In Roman days,
lead poisoning was known, for Pliny the Elder includes it
among the "diseases of slaves," which were potters' and knife
grinders' phthisis, lead and mercurial poisoning. Throughout
all the centuries since then men have used this valuable metal
in many ways, and from time to time an observant physician
has seen the results and described them, notably Ramazzini
in the eighteenth century, and early in the nineteenth cen-

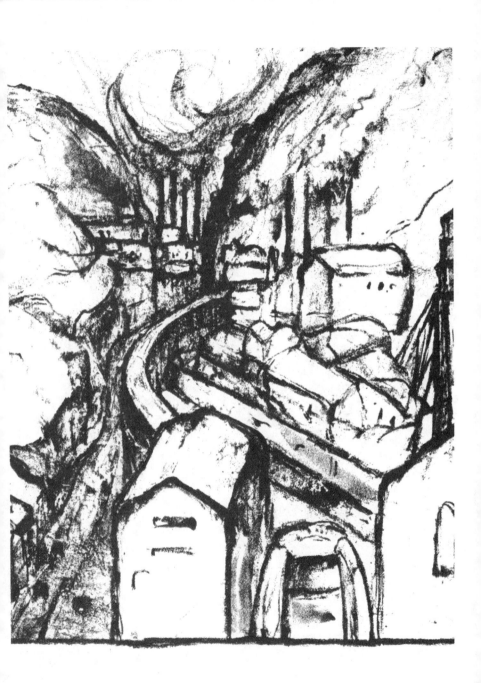

tury the great Frenchman, Tanquerel des Planches. It is a poison which can act in many different ways, some of them so unusual and outside the experience of the ordinary physician that he fails to recognize the cause. I could never feel that I had uncovered all the cases in any community, no matter how small, even after I had talked with all the doctors and gone through the hospital records, for some doctors would not pronounce a case to be due to lead poisoning unless there was either colic or palsy, which is as if he refused to recognize alcoholism unless there were an attack of delirium tremens.

It is true that a severe attack of colic is the most characteristic symptom of lead poisoning, and palsy — usually in the form of wristdrop — is the one most easily recognized, but there are many other manifestations of this protean malady, as every physician knows today. Thirty years ago it was not hard to find extremely severe forms, such as could come only from an exposure so great as to seem criminal to us now, but which then attracted no attention. Here are four histories, picked at random, from my notes of 1910.

A Bohemian, an enameler of bathtubs, had worked eighteen months at his trade, without apparently becoming poisoned, though his health had suffered. One day, while at the furnace, he fainted away and for four days he lay in coma, then passed into delirium during which it was found that both forearms and both ankles were palsied. He made a partial recovery during the following six months but when he left for his home in Bohemia he was still partly paralyzed.

A Hungarian, thirty-six years old, worked for seven years grinding lead paint. During this time he had three attacks of colic, with vomiting and headache. I saw him in the hospital, a skeleton of a man, looking almost twice his age, his limbs soft and flabby, his muscles wasted. He was extremely emaciated, his color was a dirty grayish yellow, his eyes dull and expressionless. He lay in an apathetic condition, rousing when spoken to and answering rationally but slowly, with often an appreciable delay, then sinking back into apathy.

A Polish laborer worked only three weeks in a very dusty white-lead plant at an unusually dusty emergency job, at the end of which he was sent to the hospital with severe lead colic and palsy of both wrists.

A young Italian, who spoke no English, worked for a month in a white-lead plant but without any idea that the harmless-looking stuff was poisonous. There was a great deal of dust in his work. One day he was seized with an agonizing pain in his head which came on him so suddenly that he fell to the ground. He was sent to the hospital, semiconscious, with convulsive attacks, and was there for two weeks; when he came home, he had a relapse and had to go back to the hospital. Three months later he was still in poor health and could not do a full day's work.

Every article I wrote in those days, every speech I made, is full of pleading for the recognition of lead poisoning as a real and serious medical problem. It was easy to present figures demonstrating the contrast between lead work in the United States under conditions of neglect and ignorance, and comparable work in England and Germany, under intelligent control. For instance, when I went to England in 1910 I found that a factory which produced white and red lead, employing ninety men, had not had a case of lead poisoning in five successive years. And I compared it with one in the United States, employing eighty-five men, where the doctor's records showed thirty-five men "leaded" in six months.

In 1912, I wrote this in the *Journal of the American Medical Association:* —

The contrast was brought vividly home to me by a description which I found in T. Weyl's *Handbuch der Arbeiter-Krankheiten.* He is drawing what he considers a shocking picture of "lead tabes" or "lead cachexia" as it used to be found years ago, but which is now almost never seen, thanks to prophylactic measures. He describes the striking pallor, the hanging head, bowed shoulders, hands that hang limply and can hardly be raised; the shambling gait, trembling movements of all the muscles of the body, the emaciation which is extreme.

From my own experiences I can unfortunately testify to the fact that, thanks to the lack of prophylactic measures, Weyl's lead tabes is far from being a rare condition in our country; that instances of it can be found in every town where there are lead industries of a dangerous character, and that it is not even a vanishing condition, for new instances of lead tabes are being added to the number every year. Surely there is every reason why we should devote to this disease the same intelligence and energy that we devote to other preventable diseases.

Life at Hull-House had accustomed me to going straight to the homes of people about whom I wished to learn something and talking to them in their own surroundings, where they have courage to speak out what is in their minds. They were almost always foreigners, Bulgarians, Serbs, Poles, Italians, Hungarians, who had come to this country in the search for a better life for themselves and their children. Sometimes they thought they had found it, then when sickness struck down the father things grew very black and there were no old friends and neighbors and cousins to fall back on as there had been in the old country. Often it was an agent of a steamship company who had coaxed them over with promises of a land flowing with jobs and high wages. Six hundred Bulgarians had been induced to leave their villages by these super-salesmen, and to come to Chicago. Of course they took the first job they could find and if it proved to be one that weakened and crippled them — well, that was their bad luck!

It sometimes seemed to me that industry was exploiting the finest and best in these men — their love of their children, their sense of family responsibility. I think of an enameler of bathtubs whom I traced to his squalid little cottage. He was a young Slav who used to be so strong he could run up the hill on which his cottage stood and spend all the evening digging in his garden. Now, he told me, he climbed up like an old man and sank exhausted in a chair, he was so weary, and if he tried to hoe or rake he had to give it up. His digestion had failed, he had a foul mouth, he couldn't eat, he had lost much weight. He had had many attacks of colic and the doctor told him if he did not quit he would soon be a wreck. "Why did you keep on," I asked, "when you knew the lead was getting you?" "Well, there were the payments on the house," he said, "and the two kids." The house was a bare, ugly, frame shack, the children were little, underfed things, badly in need of a handkerchief, but for them a man had sacrificed his health and his joy in life. When employers tell me they prefer married men, and encourage their men to have homes of their own, because it makes them so much steadier, I wonder if they have any idea of all that that implies.

VIII

The Federal Survey

WHILE the Illinois study was still in progress the commission decided to interrupt my part of the work by sending me over to Europe to attend the International Congress on Occupational Accidents and Diseases which was to hold its fourth meeting that summer in Brussels. Dr. Henderson suggested that I take time also to visit lead plants in England and on the Continent. This was an important journey for me, not only because it taught me much in the field of preventive hygiene but even more because it resulted in a definite break away from laboratory research and the taking up of this new specialty as my life's work.

The Brussels Congress was a very interesting experience for me, meeting and hearing the famous authorities I knew so well from their writings: chiefly German and English, but also French, Austrian, Dutch, Belgian, Italian. But for an American it was not an occasion for national pride. There were but two of us on the program, Major Bailey Ashford, with a paper on hookworm infestation in Puerto Rico, and myself, with one on the white-lead industry in the United States which revealed only too clearly the lack of such precautions as were a commonplace in the older countries. It was still more mortifying to be unable to answer any of the questions put to us: What was the rate of lead poisoning in such and such an industry? What legal regulations did we have for the dangerous trades?

What was our system of compensation? Finally Dr. Glibert, of the Belgian Labor Department, dismissed the subject: "It is well known that there is no industrial hygiene in the United States. *Ça n'existe pas.*"

There was one man in attendance at the Congress who felt as keenly as did Major Ashford and I the deplorable impression our country made and, being in a position to do something about it, he resolved that he would. This was Charles O'Neill, Commissioner of Labor in the Department of Commerce, for there was no Department of Labor till 1912, only a Bureau. Soon after I had come home and was again absorbed in the Illinois Survey, I received a letter from him asking me to undertake for the Federal government a similar survey, of the lead trades first, then perhaps other poisonous trades. The investigation was to cover all the states, taking one trade at a time, and it must be understood that I had, as a Federal agent, no right to enter any establishment — that must depend on the courtesy of the employer. I must discover for myself where the plants were, and the method of investigation to be followed. The time devoted to each survey, that and all else, was left to my discretion. Nobody would keep tabs on me, I should not even receive a salary; only when the report was ready for publication would the government buy it from me at a price to be decided on.

I accepted the offer, and never went back to the laboratory. Often I was homesick for the old life but I had long been convinced that it was not in me to be anything more than a fourth-rate bacteriologist. Interesting as I found the subject, and pleasant as I found the life, I was never absorbed in it. Hull-House was more vital to me by far, and I had no scientific imagination, one problem did not suggest another to my mind. I shall always be thankful for the training in scientific

method I had under Dr. Hektoen but I never have doubted
the wisdom of my decision to give it up and devote myself to
work which has been scientific only in part, but human and
practical in greater measure.

My service with the Federal government was thus quite free
from any red tape; it was really as pleasant and as independent
as was my position in the Memorial Institute, perhaps because
the chief under whom most of my work was done came to
Washington from the faculty of Princeton, with traditions of
university procedure. Dr. Royal Meeker was the Commissioner
of Labor Statistics in the new Department of Labor, appointed by President Wilson, and I look back to my service
under him with pleasure and gratitude. He gave me a free
hand, but was always ready to help in any difficulty; he never
edited my stuff and when nervous manufacturers asked to see
it before publication, he would arrange a conference with
them, call me in to defend my statements, and stand by me.
Also he refused to yield to requests for my dismissal during
the war because I was a pacifist.

This new job did not mean a break with Hull-House. I
could always go back to stay there when the time came for
getting my reports into shape and could stop over for a few
days whenever my travels took me from East to West and
back. It was not till 1919 that I finally gave it up as my home,
but even then, up to Miss Addams's death in 1935, I always
spent some months of the year there.

The first industry to be investigated under my new job was
one I had already studied in Illinois, the production of white
lead — "corroding lead," as it is often called — and of red lead
and litharge, or "roasting oxides." Both were then and are still
regarded as among the more dangerous of the lead trades.

The Old Dutch Process [1] was the one chiefly used at that time; it is still popular, though quicker ways of producing white lead have been in use for many years. It involves much handling of dry white lead, so that, unless elaborate dust-collecting systems are provided, the man must work in an atmosphere filled with poisonous dust. American methods produce far more dust than do the methods used in England and Germany.

In England, Sir Thomas Oliver had devoted himself for years to the task of cleaning up this industry, and when I visited the plants in East London, in Chester and in New-castle-on-Tyne, I found them a great contrast to ours. In some departments they were better than the German, in others the German surpassed the English, in none did I find conditions nearly as bad as I had found in our best plants. And the results were evident in the sickness records.

The form of lead poisoning I found in American hospital records was often very severe. Lead convulsions and lead insanity were rarities in England and Germany but there was a center of lead work in southwestern Illinois where everyone knew what "lead fits" were and it was easy to find histories of cases.

The study of the white-lead and lead-oxide industries for the Federal government took me from Omaha, through St. Louis, southern and northern Illinois, Cincinnati, Pittsburgh, to Philadelphia and New York and their environs. Here are a few of the notes I recorded at the time: First, a plant in

[1] This is a process that dates way back to the Middle Ages when the French discovered that if they put sour wine into lead pots a white powder was formed, which made the wine poisonous but was an excellent paint. We proceed in much the same way now, placing the sheets of lead in earthenware pots with a little acetic acid and then burying them in spent tanbark from the tanneries. The bark ferments, producing heat and carbon dioxide, and after some hundred days the pots are dug out and are found brimming over with a white powder which is the basic carbonate of lead.

St. Louis — "This is much the worst white-lead factory I have ever seen. It was built in 1843 and is crowded, dilapidated, dark, ill-ventilated. Dusty processes are carried on in the same room with dustless ones, so a needlessly large number of men are exposed. The dry corroded buckles and white lead from the separator and from the drying pans are wheeled in open barrows from building to building and even across the street. The enormous drying room is very dusty, but so is every department. There seems to be little concern for the health of the men and it is taken for granted that the majority will quit after a few months. As most of them are Negroes this is attributed, not to illness, but to their natural shiftlessness. Many of the men, especially the Negroes, wore no overalls and only two wore respirators. They were smeared with white-lead dust and their hair was full of it. I could not tell whether the grayish look of the Negro skin was due to pallor or dust. As I reached the plant, a Negro met me pushing a wheelbarrow of white buckles. He told me he had worked there a year and had had lead colic (he knew all about it) five times and that this was no unusual record. 'It is better paid than any other work a Negro can get, but it sure does break your health.' He gets $11.00 a week."

It is pleasant to find, in the same file with these notes, the copy of a letter I wrote in 1913 to an official of the big country-wide corporation which owned this plant. In it I congratulated him on the vast improvement which had been brought about in two years' time — new buildings, new devices for preventing dust, excellent housekeeping, a lavishly equipped "welfare house" with accommodations for Negroes as good as those for whites.

This was one of the many experiences which convinced me that the iniquitous conditions I so often found were not a proof of deliberate greed or even of actual indifference, but rather of ignorance and an indolent acceptance of things as they are. An alert and trained factory inspection service would have had little difficulty in righting these matters, for the employers were mostly very well-meaning, but throughout those early years I cannot remember ever seeing a single inspector or even hearing about one.

In those years, when I conjured up pictures of the cities I had visited, it was Pittsburgh which always appeared nearest to the infernal regions. Not that the white-lead and oxide works there were really worse than in other cities but there was something dark and menacing about that city, with its grime and soot, its flaming furnaces, its great somber granite Presbyterian Church which, from the center of the city, seemed to dominate it and to typify the religion that had inspired Pittsburgh's Scottish founders. I remember the official of a lead company who told me that he and his colleagues were spending large sums of money in an effort to "Christianize" their workmen, these last being Roman Catholic and Orthodox Slavs. I had been through their plant and had found a drying room with a ceiling so low that the men had to stoop way over while they emptied the top pan. The men had told me that room was known as "the morgue." A letter to my mother gives a picture of one of my days in Pittsburgh: —

April 1911

Today I went over to the West Penn Hospital to look through the records. It is an indescribably dingy place, smoke-begrimed and ugly. One of the great Carnegie Steel Mills is just below it and as I sat by the window I could watch the ambulances crawl up the hill to the accident entrance with a new victim inside. Three came while I was there. So many cases are sent from the mills that evidently the clerk got tired writing the name of the Company and had a rubber stamp made which, appropriately enough, he uses with red ink. All down the page came these red blotches, just like drops of blood. Andrew Carnegie himself is here today, making a speech out at the Institute. I went there Saturday afternoon and I saw the John Alexander murals of the steel mills, lovely pictures of clean, athletic youths, engaged in healthy sport against a background of Spotless Town. I suppose he was never allowed to look at the real thing. Did you know that the steel men still work twelve hours a day and seven days in the week? And that one of the fiercest defenders of the system is the minister of the most important Presbyterian church? It makes me ashamed to be a Presbyterian.

There are queer contrasts in life, aren't there? Sunday evening I was invited to the H——'s for supper. They are in steel and very wealthy, and I was all hot inside over the luxury of the house and the complacence of Mrs. H. And then their daughter came in. She has just returned from a year at school in Italy and she is the most exquisite young thing I have ever seen, beautiful, gentle, cultivated, modest. She is the product of this ill-gotten wealth; I suppose she couldn't be so exquisite had she not had it.

Philadelphia followed Pittsburgh, a far more attractive city but quite as full of dangerous trades. Pennsylvania has always been a strangely backward state in labor legislation, she still is, yet I suppose there is no state in the Union that has so many men employed in notoriously dangerous work. Accident compensation was not secured till 1915 and it was hedged about with many qualifications. As for occupational-disease compensation, Pennsylvania's workers never got that till 1938, under Governor Earle's administration, and the measure has since then had most of its teeth drawn. Under Governor Pinchot an effort was made to provide this form of protection, which was in force in all the other industrial states. John

Andrews of the Association for Labor Legislation and I were asked to come to Harrisburg and address a meeting on the desirability of a state survey to determine whether compensation for occupational disease was needed. This certainly did not seem a very radical procedure; Illinois had had such a survey more than ten years before and nobody had thought of protesting. But when Dr. Andrews and I faced our audience we found that we were looked on as meddling intruders, come to spread subversive doctrines, and we were not permitted to say a word. A big bull of a man, with a huge voice, stamped up and down the aisle demanding to know why they had been "gypped" into attending a meeting to hear outsiders tell the great Commonwealth of Pennsylvania what she ought to do. He called for immediate adjournment, the audience voted unanimously for it, and we foreigners departed, in helpless bewilderment. I asked who the champion of the employers was and they told me he was a very prominent coal-and-iron lawyer, so influential that when a boiler inspection measure came up before the Legislature he succeeded in getting exemption for the coal and iron people, so that even if all the other boilers in the state must be inspected, theirs were immune.

Harrisburg has always interested me more than other state capitals. The first time I visited the Capitol building it was with a company doctor. In the rotunda he made me pause before the statue of Matthew Stanley Quay in his marble niche. "Stand just here," he said, "and you can see the electric lights reflected over his head, just like a halo. And there, next to him, we shall have some day the statue of our Boies." "Boys?" I repeated, puzzled. "Boies Penrose," he said, "and the lights will make a halo for him too." It was this doctor who, at lunch, introduced me to a distinguished-looking, gray-haired man — "our Bayard, without fear and without reproach, Joe Grundy, who has taken on his own shoulders all the toil and the obloquy of our fight against the new Child Labor Law."

There were many white-lead and oxide plants along the Atlantic Coast in 1911. One of them provided me with a strange but very gratifying experience. It was a dreadful place, old, dusty with the dust of years, no attempt at any control of the obvious dangers, just hopelessly bad. The foreman who took me around was troubled to see the impression it made on me and as we stood in the yard watching the men from the dry-pan room eating their lunch on the steps, in their working clothes, with unwashed hands, he had a sudden inspiration. "I'll show you something you will like," he said, and he led me to a big stable where great dappled gray horses were standing on a clean brick floor, eating from clean mangers, and rubbed down till their coats shone. "Mr. B. is awful proud of his dray horses," he said. "He thinks nothing is too good for them."

That was the era of the muckraking article. McClure's Magazine was in full activity, and as I went back to my hotel I was strongly tempted to write an article for it describing Mr. B.'s horses and Mr. B.'s men in popular style. The contrast could have been made dramatic. But on soberer reflection I gave it up. The result would be only a temporary flurry, no lasting reform, and it would make any further work on my part impossible. A muckraking writer would not be permitted to visit other plants. So I went back instead and asked to see the head, old Mr. B., meaning to put the whole thing frankly to him as I had to Mr. Cornish in Chicago. I found him in an old-fashioned room, with horsehair furniture and an open grate, and I found him a gentle, genial soul, like Mr. Cheeryble in *Nicholas Nickleby*. He was very proud of his factory, he showed me photographs of its humble beginning under his grandfather and all the stages it had gone through to its proud present. I could no more have told him what his plant really was like than I could have told him his beloved child was a criminal. We parted without a word on my part of all I had planned to say.

I went back to the friendly foreman and put the case to him. "You must see Mr. Ed," he said. "He is really the one in charge now." I saw "Mr. Ed," a quiet, strong, efficient man, who listened without interruption to my long recital of the parlous conditions I had found. Finally, when I fell silent, he said, "May I have all that in writing, please. I have known for some time that things were not as they should be, but I did not know what should be done, nor whom to turn to for advice." He accepted my written report and at once began to follow its recommendations. That place was radically reformed, at the price of one single interview. If only there were more "Mr. Eds" in American industry.

Before I had completed my report for the Bureau of Labor I began to see the results of Mr. Cornish's conversion to the cause of industrial hygiene. The National Lead Company asked me to let them have copies of my notes on each of its plants as I visited them, and every now and then I would be invited to go back for a second visit and see what they had done by way of improvement. The results were really astonishing.

This does not mean that the production of white lead has been made quite safe. It will never be that. The mere fact that repairs must be made from time to time means that every lead industry has moments of danger, even in the best plants, and all our plants are not the best. But while the records of

Cook County Hospital in Chicago used to be full of cases of plumbism from the white-lead works, and the records of old Blockley in Philadelphia had so many that they did not bother to write the diagnosis — only the name of the particular plant the man came from — now one must search long for such cases. This is due not only to changes in manufacture but to that imperative reform which Mr. Hammar and Mr. Cornish introduced in 1911, the routine medical examination of all lead men, which is the only way to detect lead absorption and to prevent its going on to lead poisoning. Nowadays routine medical examination is accepted as an essential protection for all workers in poisonous trades, the examinations varying from once a week to once in three months, according to the degree of danger the man is exposed to.

The reforms begun back over twenty years ago have spread to practically the whole industry, certainly to all the branches belonging to the large companies. This was due in large part to the initiative of a few men, but also to the influence of insurance companies, which, since industrial diseases have come under the compensation laws, insist on preventive measures in the plants they insure. It is true, however, that a manufacturing company which has branches in many states often puts in the same reforms in all its plants, even those situated in backward states with no compensation laws.

My last visit to an Old Dutch Process [2] plant was in the spring of 1940 and I found little left of the risks which used to be universally present.

---

[2] I have described only the Old Dutch Process of corroding lead, because it was by far the most commonly used method and is still largely used, but there are quicker methods now, depending on the action of gases on atomized lead. The disadvantage here is that one is dealing from the start with a fine powder; the advantage is that the process is highly mechanized, needs few workmen and is easier to control.

IX

Smelting, Enameling, and Painting

WHAT WAS the prevalence of lead poisoning among enamel grinders and enamelers? That was a question I had the opportunity to explore before I left Chicago on my Federal survey. A strike was declared in a large sanitary-ware enameling works and it occurred to me that here was a chance to meet the usual working force, not only the invalided men, and to see if any of them were leaded. I went to A.F. of L. headquarters and there learned that the strikers were meeting in a Polish saloon and John Fitzpatrick was trying to organize them. He was willing to take me along, so while he harangued the men in the front room I interviewed them one by one in the back room.

Today the making of a diagnosis of lead poisoning is an elaborate affair, including examination of the blood, both chemical and microscopic, quantitative chemical tests of excreta, delicate tests for nerve response, as well as the usual physical examination. None of such aids were available to me, my methods were as crude as those of Tanquerel des Planches. I adopted a rigid standard. I would not accept a case as positive unless there were a clear "lead line" in addition to a typical history, or, if there were no line, a diagnosis of lead poisoning made by a doctor on the occasion of an acute attack.

The "lead line" nowadays is very rarely seen. It is a deposit of black lead sulphide in the cells of the lining of the mouth, usually clearest on the gum along the margin of the front teeth, and it is caused by the action of sulphureted hydrogen on the lead in these cells, the sulphureted hydrogen coming from decaying protein food in the mouth. Of course if a lead worker has a clean, healthy mouth, he will not have a lead line, and I am sure I have not seen one in over ten years, but in 1910 I looked on it as a common sign in lead workers.

Among the 148 men I examined — all Slavs, many of them powerfully built peasants — there were 54 whom I accepted as leaded but I refrained from adding 38 others who in these days would be classed as "probable cases." It would be simply impossible to find nowadays in this country a group of lead workers revealing such a condition, and after an exposure averaging less than six years. Fifty-four out of 148 is more than one third.

Because enameling tubs was notoriously hard, hot, and dangerous, most American men shunned it and I found in Pittsburgh and the surrounding towns, in Trenton and in Chicago, foreign-born workmen, Russians, Bohemians, Slovaks, Croatians, Poles. I remember a foreman saying to me, as we watched the enamelers at work, "They don't last long at it. Four years at the most, I should say, then they quit and go home to the Old Country." "To die?" I asked. "Well, I suppose that is about the size of it," he answered. It was not the lead, as I discovered then, that did the greatest harm, but the silica dust. Many of the doctors I talked to told me that there was where my attention should be turned, to the pulmonary consumption; lead poisoning was a minor evil. But lead dust was my job, not silica.

The lead dust was bad. In the enameling rooms of the

plants, this would be the picture. In front of the great furnaces stood the enameler and his helper. The door swung open and, with the aid of a mechanism which required strength to operate, a red-hot bathtub was lifted out. The enameler then dredged as quickly as possible powdered enamel over the hot surface, where it melted and flowed to form an even coating. His helper stood beside him working the turntable on which the tub stood so as to present all its inner surface to the enameler. The dredge was big and so heavy that part of its weight had to be taken by a chain from the roof. The men during this procedure were in a thick cloud of enamel dust, and were breathing rapidly and deeply because of the exertion and the extreme heat. I found that I could not stand the heat any nearer than twelve feet but the workmen had to come much closer. They protected their faces and eyes by various devices, a light tin pan with eyeholes and a hoop to go around the head, or a piece of wood with eyeholes and a stick nailed at a right angle so that it could be held between the teeth.

When the coat had been applied, the tub was swung back into the furnace and then usually there would be a few minutes of respite, for the man to relax, to go to the window for a breath of air or to take a bite of lunch. There was never any break in the eight- or six-hour shift, so the man had the choice between fasting (and an empty stomach favors lead poisoning) and eating his lunch with lead-covered hands in a lead-laden atmosphere. I saw plenty of sandwiches lying on dusty window sills and plenty of hasty lunches taken between two bouts at the furnace. Women told me of finding white powder in their husbands' lunch boxes.

I visited many of the homes of these workers. The enamelers are skilled men and the homes I saw were pleasant, the standard of living comfortable, yet they stayed only a few years in their well-paid jobs. I secured full histories of 186 cases of lead poisoning: 38 men had worked less than a year, 137 less than ten years. Lead poisoning and consumption both were notorious in those neighborhoods; I heard of them not only from the men but from doctors, priests, apothecaries, shopkeepers. And I found an unusually high proportion of severe forms among these cases, men who had had four, six, even eight attacks of colic. There were tragic stories of men who had gone back to their old homes in Austria-Hungary broken in health, paralyzed or dying. Sometimes the tales came from trustworthy sources but I could not add them to my records unless I had a doctor's diagnosis. I did, however, gain from doctors and from hospitals the details of 177 cases, and of these 28 had palsy, eight had the brain form of plumbism, and seven were fatal.

Seventeen years later, in 1929, I made a second survey of this industry, this time with special regard to the dust hazard. The risk of lead poisoning had been moderated; silicosis had by then become the most important of the industrial diseases and I knew that in making porcelain-enameled sanitary ware not only the enamelers but many other workmen were exposed to silica dust. I found the work of the enamelers not nearly so bad as it had been. In the first place no plant was using as much lead as it had in 1912 and three out of ten used none at all for ordinary enamel. Then there was far less dust both in the grinding room and in enameling. The enamelers' work was much less heavy, mechanical devices had been introduced for opening and closing furnaces, lifting ware, and controlling the turntable. The heat was still as great as ever, the workday still unbroken for lunch or rest, and now there are many double furnaces, which means that the men must work without even the few moments' break while the ware is heating. Even when the day is cut from eight to six hours, the work is more exhausting than on the single furnaces.

But the department that interested me most in this second study was the one where the ironware is prepared for coating with enamel. As the tubs come from the foundry their surface is smooth and enamel will not stick to it, so in order to roughen it a blast of fine sand is turned on and the million particles of sand make millions of tiny dents in the metal so that it is frosted all over. This, every industrial physician knew to be one of the most dangerous jobs in all industry and the National Safety Council had appointed a committee, of which I was a member, to study sandblasting and suggest how the danger might be controlled. So I had seen a good deal of this process in other industries but never anything approaching what I saw in sanitary-ware manufacture.

Imagine a great room filled with men cleaning mold sand off the tubs from the foundry. At one end through a thick fog of dust can dimly be seen eight lamplit little rooms open to the big room, in each of which a grotesque figure is manipulating a sandblast which, with a deafening roar, shoots sand at something, one cannot see what. Great clouds of sand come eddying out into the room and filling the air the cleaners must breathe. Some attempt is made to protect the sandblaster, none at all to protect the cleaner.

This was the worst plant I saw, but three others were almost as bad, all in states where no compensation law for occupational disease existed. The others were all much less dangerous and one was excellent in every respect. This was the Kohler plant in Sheboygan, Wisconsin, or rather in the charming village of Kohler. I remembered it from 1912, for Walter

Kohler was the only employer I met then who was seriously concerned with the problems of lead poisoning and of dust. In the intervening years he had done away with the lead and now he had brought the dust under control. In some of the other plants I saw excellent conditions, but Kohler's stood at the head in 1929. What Mr. Kohler had done was to make the sandblast chambers dust-proof, so that no man outside was endangered, and to provide the sandblaster with pure, dust-free air, fed to him through a pipe which led to his respirator. And of course a physician kept close watch of all these men.

Enameling sanitary ware is still a dangerous trade, for only the greatest precautions can prevent silicosis in sandblasters and enamelers, and even if there is no lead in the enamel the excessive heat is harmful. But compared with the situation in 1912 the trade has made enormous progress, aided, no doubt, by the passage in 1939 of a law in Pennsylvania awarding compensation for occupational disease.

There are several great lead smelters in southern Illinois and refineries in the northeast corner of the state, so I had been obliged during the Illinois survey to familiarize myself with the complicated processes of lead metallurgy so far as they were carried out in those plants. Other methods came to light as I journeyed from the Atlantic Coast to Montana for my Federal survey. Smelters are huge concerns, they require a large outlay of capital, and therefore their number is comparatively limited, but refineries can have a much simpler equipment — indeed they run all the way from little junk shops which undertake to recover lead from all kinds of scrap to huge plants which refine the products of smelting in Mexico.

In smelting, the danger comes from lead dust when the ore is ground and samples are prepared for the chemists, again when the charge is fed into the furnaces, and above all when the great flues and the baghouse must be cleaned out. Fumes from the furnaces travel along these flues depositing as they go very fine particles of lead oxides and sulphates, till they reach the end of the flue system, which is a high chamber with long, narrow cotton bags suspended from the ceiling, like organ pipes. Here the fumes cool completely and the last particles fall out. This is by all odds the most dangerous part of the smelter and cleaning out the flue system is a very ugly job, as everyone recognizes.

The second danger in lead smelting comes from lead fumes, and unless the equipment is excellent to begin with and kept so by constant vigilance, fumes will escape from the feed door of the furnace or from the discharge; indeed it is almost impossible to control them completely, although as long ago as 1912 I saw a German smelter, in Ems, which was as near perfection as one could wish. But the Germans did not use our most dangerous process, smelting on the open Scotch hearths. I have never seen this done in such a way as to protect the workman completely. On the whole, there is more danger from fumes than from dust in a smelter, except for the periodic flue cleaning, but in a refinery it is the dust especially that must be controlled. This is because refineries — and junk shops — handle all kinds of lead scrap, some of it very dusty. You may find in one plant a heap of old storage-battery plates, covered with brown lead oxide, near it a heap of white lead which corroded badly, one of red lead which went wrong in the roasting, and a quantity of lead dross, skimmings from the kettles in a printing plant. All these are often shoveled and tossed and swept up as carelessly as so much sand.

In the early days it was very hard to persuade men that wetting down was the only way to avoid trouble.

The great smelters were in Illinois, Missouri, Colorado, Utah, Montana, and along the Atlantic Coast. I went first out to southwestern Illinois for a second inspection of the great plants down there where the dangerous Scotch hearths are used, and then on to western Missouri, to what is called the Tri-State area, a region of zinc and lead mines, concentrating mills and smelters, situated where the three states, Missouri, Kansas, Oklahoma, come together. We think of it now as one of the chief centers of silicosis in the country but back in 1913 we knew only vaguely about that occupational disease and it was the smelting of lead that sent me to Joplin, the chief city of that region. A large smelter and oxide roasting plant not far from that city was being run by three young men who were in a desperate hurry to make money and down their competitors, but they had a great pride in their plant and had urged me to visit it. I got there on a bleak day in January, with a heavy, gray sky overhead, mud and slush underfoot. It struck me as a good plan to explore the village first, so I spent a day on Smelter Hill. It was the very dreariest, most hopeless community I had even seen, ramshackle, hastily built wooden houses, unpainted, sagging; and around the village not a tree, only great heaps of tailings, "chat" as the people called it, the refuse from the concentrating mills which formed huge pyramids of ground rock and wide stretches of fine sand as far as the eye could see. As I looked there came to mind that Old Testament verse: "And the heaven that is over thy head shall be brass, and the earth that is under thee shall be iron."

The villagers were quite as depressing. They were hill people from the Ozarks or western Kentucky, or farmers from Arkansas; they were full of malaria, hookworm, and silica dust from the chat heaps, to say nothing of lead. There was absolutely no touch of community life except a store which sold mostly patent medicines and liquor, and a water cart which creaked and slopped from door to door, peddling water by the gallon. It was easy enough to pick up cases of lead poisoning, of anemia and emaciation, of palsy, and plenty of histories of lead colic.

There was one amusing feature of that visit, however. I discovered that everybody in the village knew I was expected. The first woman who came to the door said, "Oh, you're the lady from Washington," and when I asked her how she knew about me, she said, "We all knew you was coming. They've been cleaning up for you something fierce. Why, in the room where my husband works they tore out the ceiling, because they couldn't cover up the red lead. And a doctor came and looked at all the men and them that's got lead, forty of them, has got to keep to home the day you're there." It was amusing, but irritating too. Of course, I knew that I had no power to cause the managers the slightest discomfort, but I was thankful they thought I had; on the other hand, I was provoked to know that I should not see the real state of things, but a hastily arranged special show. The most amusing part came when I had been over the plant and sat down in the office to face three pleased and proud young men who waited for me to give them the praise they thought they deserved. "I am sorry," I said, "that I cannot say anything about conditions here, because I have not really seen it as it is, only as it has been staged for me personally. You see, I spent yesterday on Smelter Hill and heard on all sides the story of the clean-up of the danger spots and the concealing of the cases of lead poisoning. So I simply do not know what I can say in my re-

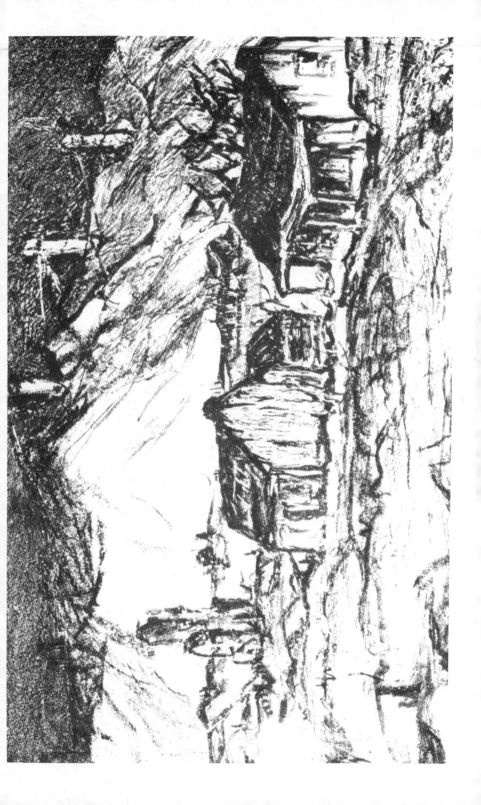

port to Washington." There was an appalled silence — the young managers looked like guilty schoolboys; it was so funny that I could not help bursting out laughing, and as they all joined in the situation lightened; they gaily admitted the fraud, and promised to let me see the doctor's report and to do everything they could to make the temporary reforms permanent, including a regular medical examination of the lead men.

That evening the doctor and one of the department heads came to see me in the hotel to tell me that they had had no share in the attempted deception and to assure me that their promises would be kept. Reforms were certainly needed. My notebook has records of 128 cases (none of them mild in character) in 1912, with three deaths, nine cases of cerebral plumbism, and ten of palsy. In the worst job, cleaning out·the flues, the rate of poisoning was 62.5 per cent.

Two years ago, in April 1940, I visited the Tri-State region again, this time on the invitation of Secretary Perkins, who called a conference in Joplin to consider the problem, not of lead poisoning, but of silicosis, far more widespread and important. Norah went with me to sketch that tragic mutilated country. There is still a lead smelter there, but the dangers have been better controlled; the rate of poisoning now must be far below that of 1912. But to my amazement I found the same abomination of desolation in the countryside as I had seen twenty-seven years before, not in the same place, but spreading out far more extensively, over parts of three states. Wherever new mines have been opened, there the great pyramids have risen and the flow of fine sand has spread around their bases and blown far and wide over the desolate villages huddled around them. One village we visited might have been Smelter Hill in 1913, except that the water peddler now drives a truck instead of a horse, and the people tell you about "miner's con" instead of lead colic. Of consumption there is plenty. Jasper County, Missouri, had a tuberculosis death rate of 130.5 per 100,000 in 1937, while that for the United States was 49; Ottawa County, Oklahoma, had a tuberculosis death rate in men of 379.9 in 1930, while the rate for the whole state was only 41.3. Oklahoma is now the chief center of zinc and lead mining — and of miner's silicosis.

I thought back over the years to a curious contrast I had noted when I made my first visit in 1913. The Colorado smelters were my next objective, after Joplin, but I made a side trip to Taos where my cousin, Dr. Allen Williams, was acting temporarily as government physician for three Indian pueblos. Taos was then untouched by tourists, artists, writers, and sellers of souvenirs, and the great pueblo was much the same as it was when the Spaniards discovered it. My cousin took me there on his rounds and I saw what seemed to me an astonishingly high development of community life, which struck me all the more strongly, coming as I had straight from Smelter Hill.

Here in the pueblo life was ordered, and wisely. The headwaters of the Rio Grande flow past the pueblo and the water served all possible purposes, but under regulation. Drinking water must be taken upstream, then came the pool for bathing, and below that the platforms for washing clothes. There was little organized recreation in the United States at that time, though Joseph Lee had started it, but here in Taos the dances and the excursions of the young people up the Canyon had always been arranged by the ruling elders. Allen told me that during an influenza epidemic he had said to one of the chiefs that he supposed the dance for the young men would be put off. "Not at all," said the chief. "Everyone is depressed and thinking only of sickness. We will have a dance to cheer them up and make them forget."

It was true, as Allen pointed out to me, that this well-ordered community had hardly changed at all since the Spaniards discovered it in the sixteenth century, there had been no progress beyond a few not very wise reforms our government had forced on them. But I had seen too much of the seamy side of our American enterprise, our passion for progress, to feel much enthusiasm for it. At least no class among the Indians had been sacrificed that society might progress. We have sacrificed the people of the Tri-State region for the sake of zinc and lead, the share-croppers for the sake of cotton, the migrants for the sake of beets and peas and fruits, and countless millions during the last century for the sake of "labor-saving" machinery. The Hammonds, in their study of the era of industrialization in England, say that it has taken the life of one generation to catch up with each great industrial change in that country. Perhaps we move faster than that but I am not sure.

Once I stood in a big iron foundry watching the men pouring molten metal into the molds. There was one man who caught my attention because he was so evidently straining at his work, using every ounce of strength to handle the heavy ladle. He was still in middle life, but nearly worked out. As I watched, the foreman said to me, "Come back in three years and you'll see none of this left. Let me show you what we'll be doing soon all through the plant." We went to another room and saw an automatic machine, ladles of molten metal filled at the furnace, traveling along a circular chain and needing only a guiding rod in the hands of a young lad to pour their charges into the row of molds on the floor. But my first feeling at the sight of this wonderful labor-saving device was not one of relief, it was dismay. What will become of the thousands of skilled iron and steel and brass and copper founders? "This will displace a good many men, won't it?" I asked. "I don't know how many thousands, in cast iron alone," he answered.

It came over me again how strange it is that our society should be so organized that an invention which does away with difficult, exhausting work and substitutes a job so easy that any untrained lad can handle it should be a cause for despair to the men in the trade, instead of relief and joy. There is little comfort in the assurance that though the foundrymen of today will be thrown on the scrap heap, the coming generation will profit and with it, since casting will be cheaper, the whole country.

I suppose any manufacturer would smile at the suggestion that the skilled founders be employed on the new machines at the same wage as before and that those displaced by the machines be pensioned, but really that seems the only fair way to manage such a situation if the benefits of progress are to be spread over all the classes of society. The introduction of machinery has always been met by labor with bitter if futile rebellion, and why not? Can we expect men to accept meekly a change which condemns them to poverty, on the plea that coming generations will be better off?

Leadville is high up in the Rockies, the highest incorporated town in the United States in 1913, so they told me. I knew it only from Bret Harte and from a story to'd me by the husband of Mary Hallock Foote. He was a mining engineer and he had taken his young bride, Quaker-bred and adorably innocent, to the camp to live. "I never let her know what went on there," he told me. "We had a house outside the camp and I remember One lovely evening we sat watching the sunset and she said how peaceful it all was, while I knew that right then down in the valley, they were hanging three horse thieves."

That time was over. Leadville as I saw it was an ordinary smelting and mining town but something of its history still clung around St. Vincent's Hospital when I went to study the records. The books go back to the eighties, and as I read the brief items — name, age, sex, diagnosis — a picture formed itself of a camp full of men, young men mostly, reckless, quick with knife or gun, working in lead without any protection, taking their sport in drinking and fighting. Case after case read, "Pneumonia, with alcoholism"; "Delirium tremens"; "Knife wounds"; "Gunshot wounds"; and, over and over again, "Lead poisoning." Rarely was there a woman's name in the list. Those nuns of St. Vincent de Paul, who had climbed the mountain passes on mule back, must have made the only center of gentleness, pity, order, and comfort in that wild and reckless place. I found them in other places, in Helena, Montana, for one. They were pioneers, they came in advance of the railroads and did a work of mercy that has never yet been chronicled.

From Leadville, Pueblo, Denver, Salida, I went on to Utah, where there were three large smelters. A letter I wrote my mother from Salt Lake City gives some of my impressions: —

I have seen only one smelter so far, one of the two large plants outside the City. I shall try for the second tomorrow. Yesterday I visited doctors and druggists and hospitals. I am amazed to see how lightly lead poisoning is taken here. One would almost think I was inquiring about mosquito bites. When I asked an apothecary about lead poisoning in the neighborhood of the smelter, he said he had never known a case. I exclaimed that that was incredible and he said: "Oh, maybe you are thinking of the Wops and Hunkies. I guess there's plenty among them. I thought you meant white men."

When I went through the records of the wards maintained in one of the hospitals by that smelting company, I realized why it seemed so unimportant, the accidents are so terrible and so numerous that a little thing like lead colic attracts no attention. My hair almost stood straight as I read of the burnings and crushings and laceratings, the amputation of both arms, the loss of eyes, the deaths from ruptured livers or intestines. And there is no system of workmen's compensation in Utah, the men themselves contribute all the money that their surgical and medical care costs.

At the medical meeting in Denver, I heard the head surgeon of the great —— Company describe the welfare work, hospital kindergarten, day nursery, domestic science school for foreign women, etc. Later on at lunch, I managed to ask most casually if the men's contribution covered all that program and he assured me it did.

It was much the same I found on my return to the East. On the Atlantic Coast, I visited a great smelter refinery where lead poisoning was rife among the immigrants who made up the poorly paid force. The wage scale was the lowest I had found, because the men could be hired as they landed, before they had a chance to learn American ways. There was no attempt to protect them from dust and fumes and so many sickened that the labor turnover was high. But that made little trouble — all the manager had to do was to go to the gates in the morning and pick out from the eagerly waiting crowd the number he needed. He took the company doctor with him to make sure of getting the healthiest men. This doctor, in charge of over 6000 men in several plants, was a hard-boiled man, a good servant to the company but with an attitude of contemptuous hostility toward his charges. When an accident occurred, a crushing or falling or burning, he was always ready to fend off a damage suit by certifying that the victim had heart disease and it was an attack of heart failure on his part, not negligence on the part of the company, that had injured or killed him. Yet the doctor's salary and the expenses of his dispensary were all paid by the men from whose wages a dollar seventy-five was deducted every month for medical care.

I found, as I talked with the men and their wives, that they did not trust him and resented his insolent ways, so those who could afford it went to other doctors and had to pay twice over for sickness. This system was very common then in the smelting industry, though I remember that the St. Joseph Lead Company of Missouri even then had an optional system, the men receiving care if they chose to pay a dollar a month. Nowadays the great smelters bear the cost themselves but the old system still survives in spots. I found it in force not long ago in one of the Mellon soft-coal mines in Pennsylvania.

It was somewhat dismaying, after I had had a painful interview with this old company doctor, to find that I was to dine with him that evening at the home of the works manager. What to talk about seemed a problem. But luckily I discovered that he was a Scotch Presbyterian and we ran a race with answers from the Westminster Catechism. I beat him on "Effectual Calling" but he beat me on "Reasons Annexed to the Fourth Commandment."

In smelting, as in white-lead production and pottery glazing and coating iron tubs with enamel, it was the pollution of the air with lead that one had to fight, that and the rooted prejudices of the employer who held firmly to the belief that poisoning was caused by the worker's own carelessness, by handling his food and his chewing tobacco without first washing his hands. I heard the head physician of one of the Colorado lead companies say in a medical meeting that it was not the lead a smelting worker encountered in the plant that poisoned him, only the lead he carried home on his body — certainly curious reasoning! I interviewed another doctor, a well-trained man, who was in charge of the employees of a great Utah smelter. He said to me, "I always tell the men that if they are careful to scrub their nails they need not fear lead poisoning." That morning I had been over the smelter in question and had watched the dumping of the Huntington-Heberlein pots. These are great round pre-roasters where the ore is made ready for the blast furnaces. I had seen the huge pot carried by a crane to the dump, a pit with an iron grating over it. The halves of the pot separated and the red-hot, fuming ore crashed down on the dump. Men came forward with long-handled bars to break up the big chunks and push them through the grating, working in such clouds of dust and fumes that I could hardly see them. These were the men who had been told to protect themselves by scrubbing their nails. Incidentally, the only provision for washing in this smelter was a cold-water hydrant out in the yard.

The painters' trade, the printing trades, and the making of storage batteries were next on my list; and then came rubber manufacture, the first trade I studied in which other poisons were more important than lead.

No industry has changed more radically in the years since 1913 than the painters' trade, especially certain branches, such as the painting of ships, automobiles, trucks, and railway cars. In those days there were only two poisons which threatened the majority of painters, lead and turpentine, and painters were perfectly familiar with the effects of both. But since in the painter's eyes the only good paint was lead paint with turpentine, and since he took pride in a good job, he never objected to the use of these two poisonous substances — indeed he preferred them. The new, cheap, quick-drying paints, with leadless pigment and naphtha, were beginning to come in, but the painter despised them and complained far more of the dopeyness and headache and nausea caused by naphtha fumes than he complained of lead poisoning.

The unwashed-hands theory of the causation of lead poisoning prevailed in full force in the painters' trade, and nobody had yet challenged its validity. Yet all painters knew that certain jobs were bad, mixing dry white lead or red lead with oil, sandpapering carriage wheels, rubbing down the painted ceilings of Pullman cars, chipping old red-lead paint from ships. These were, of course, all dusty jobs. We had been able to show the danger to painters of lead dust in our Illinois survey by examining the records of one hundred painters who had been treated in Chicago hospitals for lead poisoning. We found that most of them had worked many years at their trade before they knew they were leaded, but nineteen of them had had a severe form of intoxication after less than a year's work, and every one of the nineteen had worked inside and had had to rub down dry lead-painted surfaces.

The painters' trade was then, probably it still is, divided into two groups: first the independent house and sign painters, working now for one contractor, now for another, now on their own, skilled men and members of a strong trade-union; second, painters who work in manufacturing plants, some of them union members, many not. The house painter might work with lead paint on one job and with leadless paint on the next job; the factory painter was likely to use one or the other all the time. Consequently the men subjected to the greatest danger were those in manufacturing establishments where a paint rich in lead was used, and several coats applied, for one coat must be rubbed down after it dries before the next can be applied. It is this dry rubbing of a lead-painted surface, producing a fine lead powder to poison the air, which is the greatest evil connected with lead paint. That is why in European countries the use of white-lead paint in the interior of buildings was forbidden, though it was still permitted for the outside coating, where rubbing down is never used.

In those days automobiles were painted, and with many, many coats. Ford cars had some fourteen, Packards went up to nineteen. But not nearly all of these coats contained lead, nor was much rubbing down needed. Already steel and aluminum were replacing wood and lead-free color varnishes were replacing white lead except for a few coats. Carriage and wagon works — this was before the day of trucks — were much worse, for a great deal of lead was used and the coats sandpapered. White milk-delivery carts were especially bad. The same thing was true of the painting of wooden passenger cars and street cars, but worst of all was the job of painting the ceilings of Pullman cars. The paint used was rich in white lead and the painter who sandpapered it stood necessarily just in the right place to breathe in the fine dust he was producing. It was especially bad in the little lavatories.

The investigation of the Pullman works was by all odds the most interesting incident in my study of the painters' trade. During the Illinois survey I had been out there several times and had talked with many employees in their homes. It was the biggest and most varied industrial plant I had ever visited and I was deeply impressed by the hazardous processes which went on there — the many chances for serious injuries to the workmen. But my subject was lead poisoning and I stuck to it, particularly to the dusty job of painting and rubbing down the ceilings of Pullman cars. In the course of our searches through hospital records in Chicago, we had come across the histories of fifteen cases of severe acute lead poisoning in men who had done this work. They were not regular painters. It appeared that the risks were too well known in the trade; the job was left for recent immigrants. These men were peasants from Hungary, Serbia, Poland, and they had been so severely poisoned that the police had had to take them to the County Hospital, which must be twenty miles from Pullman.

After I had watched the men on that particular job I went to see the doctor, and my visit revealed an amazing state of affairs in a plant so huge. The medical department was of a primitive simplicity which seemed incredible. Its personnel consisted of one old doctor who had been a surgeon in the Civil War and who carried on all his work in the two front rooms of his private house. When an accident occurred, the first man summoned was always the company lawyer, who brought with him a diagram of the human body and noted upon it the parts apparently injured. Only then was the man carried to the doctor's office, where he was given the sort of treatment that can be given in a private house with a minimum of asepsis and of apparatus. There was no nurse and when I asked the old doctor how he managed when an anesthetic was needed, he said his wife was pretty handy. If the injury was serious, an ambulance was called from St. Luke's Hospital in Chicago, some eight or ten miles away (there was not even an emergency bed for a severely injured man). The long delay between accident and skilled surgical treatment must have affected seriously the outcome of many a case, especially a case of shock. But there was no compensation law in Illinois then. Needless to say, nobody paid any attention to such a trifle as lead poisoning.

I can remember how after that visit, as I would pass through Pullman on the train in the course of my journeyings, I would curse it in my soul, picturing what was going on there and realizing how powerless I was to do anything about it. But suddenly I found to my relief that there was a chance to bring about a change. I had poured out the story to Miss Addams and she made me repeat it to Mrs. Joseph T. Bowen, one of the first and staunchest friends of Hull-House, and a member of that all-too-small class of wealthy people who feel a direct responsibility toward the sources of their wealth. She was a large holder of Pullman stock and she told me she would see what she could do with a formal protest in her character as stockholder. It was not the first time she had done such a thing. Because she owned stock in United States Steel she wrote Judge Gary in 1911 protesting against the twelve-hour day, and again in 1921 she joined Charles Cabot of Boston in a protest not only against the twelve-hour shift, but also the seven-day week. They succeeded in abolishing the latter, but Charles Cabot did not live to see the former abolished. I can remember the interest with which Hull-House followed this effort and our dismay when we read the copies of letters from other stockholders, some of them clergymen, or philanthropists, defending the "right of steel workers to labor as long as they pleased."

The reforms in Pullman came far more quickly and easily. The matter was taken up at once and I was sent for to put the case myself before the officials, who were by now concerned. Changes took place with breath-taking speed, and by the end of 1912 there was a modern surgical department with surgeons in charge, an eye specialist, and a medical department to supervise the 500-odd painters. Moreover, a less dangerous form of lead was used in the paint and every effort was being made to protect the men against lead dust. The results were striking. When the physicians made their first examination of the painters in 1912, they discovered 109 cases of plumbism among 489 men during the first six months, but in 1913–1914 only three cases were found in a year among 639 men. Since then, lead paint has been almost entirely eliminated. The Pullman Company rose rapidly to the first rank of industrial corporations in its health and safety work and it still holds its place there.

During the last twenty-five years great changes have occurred in the make-up of coatings and in the method of applying them. The safest way of applying a coating is by dipping. I saw this done on a huge scale in the International Harvester Works in Chicago, the parts being lowered by machinery into great tanks of paint and swung out to one side to dry. Equally safe is flowing paint, from a hose, a method I have seen used to paint great electrical apparatus in the works of the General Electric Company. Brush work is not so safe; the man must be close to the surface he paints and if there are fumes, or if there is dust, he cannot help breathing them. But it is a skilled trade and the only kind of work the self-respecting painter believes in. Even in 1913 it was being displaced by "labor-saving machinery," this time the spray gun, which works with compressed air, sending a cloud of tiny droplets over the surface. This method is so quick and efficient that it enables one man to do the work of three or four and so simple that an unskilled hand can master it in a few weeks' time. At first the spray gun was used with harmful coatings and some serious cases of poisoning were reported, but during the 1920's changes for the better developed quickly, partly because by then a number of industrial states had workmen's compensation laws. Several careful studies of spray painting were made, by the National Safety Council and the Pennsylvania Labor Department and the Painters' Union, and soon lead and benzol disappeared to a large extent from coatings, and wood alcohol completely. Paints were thus rendered less poisonous and less paint was used, lacquers taking their place.

Today the house painter still uses the brush and still uses lead paint, on outside work, but not much on interiors. Ship painters use practically no lead at all (this reform we owe apparently to the Navy, which in its contracts calls for lead-free coatings) and though they still must work in small, enclosed spaces, the air they breathe is no longer full of lead or turpentine or anything more harmful than naphtha. Carriages and wagons belong to the past and so do wooden railway coaches and street cars. The painting of steel coaches and Pullmans is just as different from the method used twenty-five years ago as is their modern interior decoration from the ornamental orgies of that era. Now lead has been replaced by iron oxides and titanium oxide, which are quite harmless, and the liquid constituents are petroleum spirits with some turpentine, so although the spray-gun has replaced brush work and driven many men out of employment, the work itself has been made practically safe.

X

Europe in 1915

A MEETING of the International Congress for Occupational Diseases was planned for mid-August, 1914, to be held in Vienna, and the Department of Labor wished me to go as a delegate, a request I accepted with much alacrity. In one of my old notebooks there is a careful schedule of the places I planned to visit, centers of lead work of all kinds, in England and Germany, the model towns of Essen and Solingen, the rubber factories in Leipzig, and so on. My friend Katharine Ludington and I had taken passage on an Anchor Line steamer to sail from Montreal August second and, incredible as it now seems, we went up to Montreal the last day of July confident that nothing would interfere with our plans. Nobody who was not a mature person in the summer of 1914 can realize now how remote, how unbelievable, a European war then seemed.

To be sure there had been our war with Spain, but by 1914 we had come to regard that as a more than questionable exploit, one that could and should have been averted by good sense and good will. Almost nobody looked back on it with any pride and there was a strong party opposed to our holding the Philippines. There was much disapproval also of our interference in the Caribbean and in Central America and Mexico, while Bryan's peace treaties were held to be a move in the right direction. The Boer War was a great shock and aroused only indignation on this side of the water; indeed the first mass meeting I ever attended was one held in the old

Auditorium in Chicago to protest against that war. But the wise conduct of the British after the Boer defeat convinced us that they too realized the wrong they had done and were ready to forsake violence for peaceful methods. We read Norman Angell's *Great Illusion* with its irrefutable proof of the futility of war and, believing as we did then in the slow but sure progress of the human race, we looked forward to nothing worse than sporadic outbursts in such unknown regions as the Balkans or South America, never in the highly civilized countries of the Europe which we knew so well.

Perhaps this was especially true of those who lived in settlements for we saw emigrants from the countries in Europe which had bitter, centuries-old feuds living side by side in harmony. Croats and Austrians, Greeks and Bulgars, Poles and Germans seemed to leave their antagonism behind when they reached these shores and certainly their children felt none of it in school and in our social clubs. We could not help believing that in the old countries also these hatreds were dying down.

In Montreal we saw the incredible come true. The ship on which we had taken passage sailed for the war zone filled with Canadian volunteers. Belgium had been invaded, Britain had declared war, Montreal was full of marching crowds singing "God Save the King" and the "Marseillaise."

I returned to Mackinac to find my English uncle (by marriage) and his second wife, a Frenchwoman, staying with the family and by their intense personal feelings heightening the excitement, if that were possible. We are so inured to war now and we have had to see the destruction of so much irreplaceable beauty that it is strange for me to recall my horror over Belgium, over Louvain and Antwerp. Then for the first time war became real. The fighting in the Balkans, in South

Africa, in Cuba, was not real, I knew none of those countries, they were spots on a map. But Belgium's cities were vivid and to think of war actually reaching them was almost as impossible as to think of it reaching Chicago, or Mackinac.

We put all the blame on the Germans; we had no doubt as to their war guilt but I myself fastened it onto the Kaiser and the military caste. The Germans I had known, in my childhood in Fort Wayne, in my student life over there, could not be responsible for this ruthlessness and cruelty toward a small and helpless country; it must be laid to those arrogant, swaggering officers who had been so much in evidence in every German city. That the Germans would obey them meekly I was ready to believe, for never had I seen a sign of indignation, even of criticism, no matter how insolent an officer might be, but I was not ready to accuse the German people of anything worse than submissiveness to those on top. This affection for the Germans was, I believe, universal among Americans who had studied over there, and that means a goodly proportion of our university faculties. In almost every American university there was a German club of faculty members, who met to drink beer and sing German songs and reminisce tenderly about the golden days in Heidelberg, Bonn, Jena. There were no French clubs of that kind, nor, I believe, English. It was Germany that had taken us to her heart and given us a feeling of belonging.

Slowly, as the war went on, that feeling faded and the allegiance to Germany, the gratitude for what she had given us, disappeared under the horror of the destruction in France and the apparent ruthlessness of the German army. Also the attitude toward war changed and the demand grew strong and insistent that we throw our weight on the side of the Allies. As the pressure increased, the peace movement began to gather force and to take definite shape, to adopt a concrete program. As early as the fall of 1914 women [1] all over the country had begun to draw together for the study of possible steps toward a just peace, and, after a very dramatic lecture tour by two women from the warring countries, Mrs. Pethick Lawrence of England and Mme. Rosika Schwimmer of Hungary, the Women's Peace Party was formed with Jane Addams as chairman.

In March 1915 there came to Miss Addams a call, signed by British, Dutch, and Belgian women, to an international Congress of Women to protest against war. It was to be held in The Hague late in April and Miss Addams was asked to preside over a gathering of women from the warring countries as well as from the neutral. She accepted at once and I decided to go with her, as did some fifty American women. As I remember it, the only man in the group was Louis Lochner, who recently distinguished himself with the Associated Press in Berlin. We had a long journey over, on the *Noordam*, for we were held up from Friday to Monday off the coast of England near Dover, waiting for British permission to go on. What the reason for the delay was we did not know; it was easy to imagine a deliberate blocking of our peace move by the British War Office, though the cynical Dutch captain insisted it was only the English week end which, even in the war, tied up everything in government offices while the heads were off in the country. On the other hand, some support was given to the theory of deliberate obstruction by the fact, which we learned in The Hague, that the English delegation of eighty-

[1] Miss Lillian D. Wald, Mrs. Carrie Chapman Catt, Mrs. Anna Garlin Spencer, Mrs. Henry Villard, Mrs. Glendower Evans, Mrs. Lucia Ames Mead, Mrs. Louis F. Post, Mrs. Harriet Thomas, Miss Sophonisba Breckenridge, Mrs. Florence Kelley, Miss Grace Abbott, Mrs. Lucy Biddle Lewis, Mrs. Fannie Fern Andrews, Mrs. John J. White, Miss Emily Greene Balch.

seven women had not been permitted to leave Tilbury. Long as it was, the journey was far from tedious. There were interesting discussions while the American group formulated the concrete proposal which they intended to lay before the meeting in The Hague. This was the plan which came to be known as "continuous mediation," [2] and after the Hague Congress was over it was this plan which Jane Addams and Emily Balch carried to all the capitals of the warring countries and to several of the neutrals. It still seems to me the wisest and most practical scheme put forward by any group during the World War and I believe that had President Wilson (or Colonel House) been willing to try it, success might have followed, instead of failure, and the war brought to a close by a compromise peace without our having entered it.

The plan involved the formation under the initiative of the United States (simply because she was the only neutral who could be unafraid in that crisis) of a conference of men from the neutral nations, which should act as an agency of continuous mediation for the settlement of the war. We believed that while offers of mediation by a single nation might be rejected because one side might feel doubts of the impartiality of that nation, the same objection would not be felt toward a conference which would include nations of different sympathies, and that while a given offer at a given moment might be refused, repeated offers made by a continuous conference might in the end meet acceptance.

Colonel House's offer of Wilson as sole mediator was quite different, and one can understand the Central Powers feeling that he would be a prejudiced arbitrator. Had the women's plan been adopted, the Scandinavian countries, Switzerland, Holland, Spain, and the South American republics would have balanced the pro-Allies bias of the United States.

[2] It was first proposed by Julia G. Wales, of the University of Wisconsin.

We believed also that placing conditional proposals simultaneously before both sides would bring out into the open the real attitudes of governments and strengthen the hands of the pacifically inclined ministers who were struggling against the militarists and who, in the absence of any such strengthening, were destined, as the event showed, to go down before the bitter-enders. Governments at war cannot ask for negotiations, nor even express a willingness for them, lest this be at once construed by the enemy as a sign of weakness. But if neutral people commanding the respect of those ministers should study the situation and make proposals over and over again if necessary, something might be found upon which negotiations might start. I cannot see how anyone can read Lord Grey's book, *Twenty-five Years, 1892–1916*, without feeling that there were many moments during the war when such a neutral conference could have secured a hearing, would even have found a welcome in many chancelleries.

The Hague plan involved repeated offers. Can anyone believe that soldiers could have been held in the trenches through 1916 and 1917 if they had known that their governments were refusing peace terms which were fair and reasonable? For it would have been impossible to prevent all discussion of peace terms in the warring countries if such an international body had continually brought forward new propositions for the consideration of the belligerents. No government, we believed, could insist on gaining by bloodshed what might be obtained by negotiations, nor would it be possible to prolong the war for the sake of treaties among the Allies which could not be openly acknowledged.

The Congress of Women at The Hague was deeply impressive to us Americans. There were women from the neutral countries, and from Germany and Austria, from Belgium, from Russian Poland, and from England, for Mrs. Pethick Lawrence, Kathleen Courtney, and Chrystal MacMillan had luckily been on the Continent when the call came. Nothing we had read about the war had made us realize it as did a few talks with these women. I remember most clearly a lady from Vienna and one from Russian Warsaw. Miss Addams as always was the great figure at the Congress, the beloved leader, and the program she proposed for continuous mediation met with an enthusiastic acceptance. Indeed the reception went beyond what any of us had expected and we were startled to discover that the Congress was moving to appoint two delegations of neutrals to visit the capitals of the warring countries and of the principal neutrals and to place the plan before the Premier and the Foreign Minister of each, seeking endorsement of the plan if possible or, if not that, at least a pledge not to oppose it. Obviously Miss Addams was to head one delegation and, though rather dubious as to the wisdom of the scheme, she accepted. Emily Balch of Boston headed the second delegation, which was to visit the Scandinavian countries and Russia, while Miss Addams would go to England, France, Germany, Austria-Hungary, Italy, Holland, Switzerland, and the exiled Belgian government in France.

In my usual role of "confidante in white linen" I was to go with Miss Addams and with Dr. Aletta Jacobs of Holland, a famous suffrage leader, who also took a friend, Mevrow Palthe. But there was a delay of some eight days before we started and I took advantage of it to make a trip into Belgium with Mabel Kittredge, Grace Abbott, and Mrs. Lucy Biddle Lewis. I still have the long letter I wrote my family after I had returned to Holland and it pictures very vividly my first experience of life in an invaded country. "It is not a question of present horror, nor starvation, nor pillage, nor any kind of violence going on now, for all is decent and quiet and orderly; it is simply a conquered country under the heel of the conqueror and what that means is almost impossible to put into words."

Since then I have been in Soviet Russia and in Hitler's Germany and have learned to accept without surprise the atmosphere of suspicion and of underlying fear, the consciousness of being spied upon, the need for constant watchfulness, the heavy oppression of spirit, which belong to countries under the rule of tyrants. But then it was all so new as to be unbelievable: the search at the border when the German woman passed her hands all over my body and ran her fingers through my hair and cut the "Marshall Field" label from my hat and confiscated my Baedeker because it had maps; the strange atmosphere in the Hotel Britannique in Brussels where a voluble, English-speaking German woman tried to coax us to tell her our impressions and a Belgian headwaiter almost wept on our shoulders, then turned to wait on the German officers with the manner — I wrote my mother — of Epictetus serving his Roman masters; the visit to the Legation to talk with Brand Whitlock and to receive many warnings about spies and pitfalls which might mean confiscation of our passports and indefinite delays. And a surreptitious trip, for the Germans had our passports and we had no permits to leave Brussels, to ruined Louvain on the holiday of the Feast of the Ascension, when we could be lost in the crowd. A silent crowd, moving slowly past the wrecked houses, whispering, looking hastily over shoulders, to see if anyone was listening; a crowd so broken in spirit that even a sudden downpour of rain roused nothing but dull acceptance. To us it all seemed incredible, a horror that could not last, that civilized men must put an end to and soon. Strange to think that now the Belgian invasion in 1915 seems like a minor disaster of long ago, pale before the mass of horrors we have lived through since.

We got our passports back in time. It was my job to deal with the German officer in charge of that department, a gay young gentleman from Munich, and I found myself chatting with him about my student days in that city and receiving with equal gaiety his laughing assurances that all Germans were not heartless brutes. The others were shocked at my hypocrisy and I suddenly realized another of the effects of living under tyranny — it makes liars out of decently truthful people. For I wanted our passports more than I wanted to tell the truth.

Miss Addams met me in Amsterdam. She had gone on the first lap of her mission, to London, and had talked with Asquith and Grey, meeting with a courteous, almost sympathetic, but noncommittal reception. As she was leaving Asquith she said, "I suppose to you this seems a very foolish performance," and he said, "Not at all. It may be of some good. At any rate it is worth trying." She had also been able to discuss the plan for continuous mediation with a number of influential people — Lord Haldane, Morley, Bryce, Graham Wallas, Ramsay MacDonald, Charles Trevelyan, Bertrand Russell, the Bishop of London. This experience had given her a greater degree of confidence in facing the task put on her by the Congress, the task of penetrating the chancelleries of Europe and placing before the men in charge of their countries' policies a plan to shorten the war and to bring about a "peace without victory." She had of course no standing except that of an American citizen; nevertheless in each capital we visited our Ambassador or Minister secured interviews for her and Dr. Jacobs with the

Premier and the head of the Foreign Office. There were no difficulties on that score, nor did she meet with the slightest resentment from any of these statesmen.

As I look back on it now, that seems strange, but we have forgotten that in 1915 the war had not yet conquered people's souls. To talk of peace was then not nearly so impossible as it was two and three years later. Hatred had not yet congealed, atrocity tales had not yet accumulated to monstrous proportions, it was still possible for soldiers to fraternize together in the trenches at Christmas, the bitter-enders were not yet in complete control of the press. Miss Addams and Dr. Jacobs made a purely human appeal based on the cruelty and futility of war, protesting as women against the suffering, the waste of life, and urging that at least an attempt be made to bring about, through nonviolent discussion, adjustments of the quarrels which had given rise to the war.

They found often a surprisingly warm response to this appeal. One minister said that it was the only sensible thing that had crossed his threshold for months; another said that he had often wondered since the war began why women had remained so long silent, because since women cannot join in the fighting, they may make a protest against war which is denied to men. The only men who treated the suggestion with entire indifference were Delcassé, who of course was for war to the uttermost, and the Italians Salandra and Sonnino, who had just carried their country in triumphantly on the side of the Allies. Of course, we did meet with skepticism, even amused contempt, but, as I remember it, more from Americans in the legations and embassies than from Europeans, for our countrymen still idealized the war and many of them were openly ashamed of President Wilson for not joining in at once. I was often shocked to hear outspoken denunciations of the government from those who were supposed to represent our country's interests abroad, and from their wives.

Berlin was our first objective and there we met a number of interesting men: Prince Lichnowsky, Ambassador to Britain when war was declared; Hans Delbrueck, crusader for German colonies; Theodor Wolf of the *Tageblatt*.

One evening we went to see Maximilian Harden, editor of *Die Zukunft*, which Germans had told us was the most admired, feared, and detested paper in Germany, boldly attacking the Kaiser, the Junker class, and the army. Harden was antimilitarist till 1914, but then he went over completely to the war party. He even wrote this about the invasion of Belgium: —

Let us drop our attempt to excuse Germany's action. We willed it. Our victory will create a new order in Europe.

We found him in his study, standing behind a table, as was his habit in meeting people, for he was sensitive about his short, stocky body which made such an incongruous contrast to an enormous head with heavy, bushy hair. When he talked to us it was with defiance and truculence, with eagerness to repudiate his former pacifism. He poured contempt on German leaders for their hypocrisy in using the Sarajevo murders as an excuse for a war of conquest which had long been planned. We had heard of him as a champion of freedom, but we found that the only freedom he cared about was Germany's freedom to make herself supreme ruler of Europe. To my tentative mention of my visit to Belgium he replied gaily that Belgium would soon learn who her real friends were. "Belgium is like a little brother whom big brother has had to pull away roughly from bad playmates. Now little brother is in big brother's arms and he is pouting and his eyes are full of tears, but soon big brother will wipe away his tears and make him smile again."

We saw much of Sigmund-Schultze, an avowed pacifist but protected from harm by the personal affection of the Kaiser. We met also many of the women prominent in the *Frauenbewegung*. It was in talk with the latter that I gained insight into the attitude of Germans in general toward the war. They were absolutely sure that Germany was fighting in self-defense, they reverenced the military so deeply that to them the action of Belgian *francs-tireurs* was a horrible crime, and even the very best of them accepted the *Lusitania* incident without questioning. She was carrying munitions, the passengers had been warned, she was rightly doomed. One really lovely young married woman told us that the day the news came she declared a holiday and took her children on a picnic to the country to celebrate.

Miss Addams saw Bethmann-Hollweg alone at the chancellery, then she saw von Jagow with Dr. Jacobs. Both men gave her the impression that a peace offensive from the neutrals would not be unwelcome; certainly Germany would not take it as a hostile act. Von Jagow was insistent that Miss Addams must visit Belgium and carry back to America a true picture, but she refused very firmly. To me she said, "I always refuse to visit an industrial plant when there is a strike on, for I should see only what the employer wished me to, and I should be forced to say that I had seen nothing to criticize, which would of course be interpreted as a complete defense for the employer."

Vienna was sad, much sadder than Berlin, for even then in the spring of 1915 the Austrians were hungry. Our restaurant meals were made painful by the sight of pale, emaciated faces lurking just outside the window or behind the potted shrubs on the sidewalk, hoping for a crust to be slipped to them.

Already the official food ration was insufficient even for women. Everywhere we saw convalescent soldiers, on crutches or in wheeled chairs. The interviews, with Graf Sturgk and Count Burian, were easily secured by our Ambassador, Frederick Penfield, who was very kind to us. I was not allowed to take part in them but I did go with Miss Addams to see the former Minister of Foreign Affairs, Count von Berchtold, the man we all then held to be chiefly responsible for the war. He lived in a perfectly plain house in a little narrow street, but when the door opened it revealed a beautiful garden and a great hall and a lovely library opening on a terrace, where the Count received us. He struck me as the perfect type of diplomat, very high-bred, with easy, cordial manners, and an apparent frankness which covered absolute secretiveness. He was almost eagerly curious to hear all Miss Addams could tell him and plied her with questions, but when he had bowed us out and we looked back over the interview, we found he had said absolutely nothing.

Budapest was a very different experience. We went there because, though a part of Austria, Hungary had her own Prime Minister, the great Tisza, more important than either Sturgk or Burian, and the Hungarian women had insisted that Miss Addams see him. The atmosphere there was amazingly free. While in Berlin Miss Addams had been able to talk to the Women's Club only if she promised not to mention peace; in Budapest she spoke to a large audience of men and women who insisted on hearing all about the Hague Congress and her mission. The Hungarian aristocrats reminded me of our Southerners, both because of their warmly cordial manner and because of their pride and their fierce independence, which were apparently quite compatible with their subjugation of the despised Slovaks. We dined and lunched with a number of them, Telekys, Zichys, Palffys, and they spoke freely of their friendship with the English and their contempt for Austria. Count Tisza was very impressive, looking like a tall, broad-shouldered edition of General Grant. We had heard that he was a fire-eater but to us he spoke only of the senseless horrors of war, and he hoped the neutrals would step in with proposals for a compromise peace. "They would not find Austria-Hungary unreasonable in her demands," he said.

We went through Switzerland to Rome, to a country which had just entered the war and was triumphant, bewildered, jittery. On our way south, the conductor came and drew shades down over all the windows and when I protested against his shutting out the beauty of mountains and plain he answered that Italy was at war and in war nobody must look in or out of railway cars. In Rome, Miss Addams's formal interviews were purely perfunctory. Salandra and Sonnino would say no more than that Italy would not regard an offer of neutral mediation as a hostile act. But it was altogether different when we had our audience with Pope Benedict XV, for me the high spot of the whole trip.

Cardinal Gasparri arranged for the interview after a long and sympathetic talk with us. There was no question this time of my being left out, for His Holiness spoke only the Latin languages and I was needed to carry on the conversation in French. Our Italian friends were much excited when they heard we were to have a private interview and they saw to it that we were properly dressed, in long-sleeved and high-necked dresses — I remember much tucking of scarfs to hide the collarless state of our dresses — and veils of black Spanish lace on our heads. We were ushered in past the gorgeous Swiss guards one always sees when one visits the Vatican Galleries, to the inner part of the palace where they were replaced by still more impressive figures, men in beautiful suits of ecclesiastical red brocaded silk, or of black velvet faced with blue satin and trimmed with silver. As we sat waiting in the antechamber in a crowd of somber-clad women, I could not help speculating on this striking contrast between the sexes which was evidently planned deliberately. We women must so dress ourselves as to obscure all our charms — if any — lest we seduce the thoughts of the men, but they, on the contrary, might make themselves into figures so beautiful that we could not help being fascinated. It seemed to imply a much greater spiritual resistance on the part of the weaker sex, and it was certainly an indirect tribute to our charms — an undeserved one, I thought, for as I looked around the room I did not see one woman who could disturb the thoughts even of Saint Anthony the Hermit.

We had been told that when we were admitted we must kneel and kiss the Pope's ring and we were fully prepared to do it, but somehow it did not come off. Pope Benedict XV was a man of the world, he saw at once that we were Protestants and did not know how to behave, so he greeted us as any gentleman would and we found ourselves seated beside him without any awkward interlude. He was a little man, and very ugly, with a beaklike nose, sallow skin, and heavy-lidded eyes, but it was an ugliness that attracted, not repelled. He was dressed in a straight narrow gown of white (velvet, I think) with red buttons down the front and a red girdle, and his skullcap was also of white.

He had been given the outline of the plan for continuous mediation by Cardinal Gasparri and he put eager questions to us, as to the response of the statesmen Miss Addams had seen and as to the prospects of American backing. It seemed to him more promising than any effort he had heard of and he told us to convey to President Wilson his hearty wishes for its success. "I would offer myself as one of the mediators," he said, "did I not fear that it would be misunderstood and do more harm than good." Then he spoke to us of his deep grief over the war, with the Church split asunder, Catholics fighting Catholics and he himself accused by each side of partiality toward the other. Our interview lasted forty minutes, then he rose and dismissed us. We had been instructed to back out of the room and make a genuflexion when we reached the door, but again our host sensed our awkwardness and he himself led the way to the door, bowing us out as if he were simply a Marchese, not His Holiness the Pope, the Vicar of Christ on earth.

In Paris Miss Addams saw Viviani and Delcassé, the former approachable, even cordial, the latter absolutely hostile. He said that this time it must be war à l'outrance, there must be no possibility of a German revival, victory must be complete and final. If ghosts have any knowledge of our present world, Delcassé's must be an uneasy one.

Paris was full of Americans and some of them a queer lot. Dorothy Canfield has described them in one of her books, the Americans who were excited and fascinated by the horrors and whose one ambition was to get to the front. We met a wealthy lady whose gifts had entitled her to special consideration so that she could announce triumphantly to the lunch table that she was off to the front in two days. We met a trained nurse who collected gruesome war souvenirs and who always rushed out after a bombing to see the destruction before it was cleared up. She would not offer her services to nurse the wounded unless the authorities would send her to a base hospital just behind the lines. I am sure many Americans were doing useful work with refugees from Belgium and invaded France but some of

the well-meant efforts were queer, such as a traveling dispensary
with first-aid equipment and medicines, which some American girls drove through rural France. They were most courageous but not very successful. I could not help wondering what
sort of reception a similar enterprise by French girls would
receive in my native Indiana.

Jean Longuet and the Marquis de Chambrun, whose American wife was not in Paris at the time, were something of an
antidote to Delcassé. Longuet was a grandson of Karl Marx
and the leading Socialist, after Jaurès's death. "Not his suc-
cessor," he told us, "nobody living can fill his place." He told
us that he was sitting at the table in the café with Jaurès when
the young Royalist assassin killed him. Had he lived, Longuet
believed the anti-war party might have won out, in spite of
Poincaré's secret commitments to the Russians, but with
Jaurès lost the Socialists were like sheep without a leader. But
he was proud that the French Socialists had stood by their
principles when August Bebel and his German following
turned from international Socialism to join the war.

In Paris our Ambassador was William Graves Sharp, an
ironmaster from Ohio. We liked the Sharps very much; they
were the sort of family one likes to think is typical of America
— quiet, poised, sensible people, full of admiration for France
and intelligent enough to appreciate the best it had to offer
them, but not in the least carried off their feet by the charms
of their hosts no matter how aristocratic and titled. I used to
wonder if there were not some way in which our State Department could immunize the men (and their wives) who were
selected for service abroad against the seductions of the aristocrats they were bound to meet, men and women so much more
charming than any they had known at home, and such a contrast to the trouble-making radicals and Socialists. As it was,

the chief absorption of many of our representatives abroad seemed to be their personal relations with the nobility and gentry, and there was an inevitable, though doubtless unconscious, absorption of the mental outlook of those with whom they so gladly associated.

We sailed from England in a wretched little steamer, and when we reached home, Miss Addams faced the most difficult task of all, persuading President Wilson to put himself at the head of the neutral nations and with them to carry on continuing efforts for peace. She failed; Wilson preferred to work alone, through Colonel House, and secretly, not openly. And so the war went on; Colonel House was eventually persuaded that we must enter it, and, to judge from his *Intimate Papers*, he overbore Wilson's reluctance and triumphantly carried us in, thereby ensuring a smashing victory and a one-sided peace.

In Lord Grey's story of his part in the war, after telling of the resignation of the Asquith Coalition Government and his own departure from the Foreign Office, he allows himself to speculate on what would have happened if a peace which discredited militarism could have been made in 1916. "Two years of war in which expenditure of life and national strength and treasure at their maximum would have been avoided. European markets and trade might have recovered quickly, for the impoverishment and exhaustion would have been much less. The future peace of Europe, with the unreserved co-operation of the United States, might have been safer than it is today. Prosperity and security might be today more fair in prospect for us all than the victory of 1918 and the treaties of 1919 have made them; and there would have been a peace with no obnoxious, secret ideas of *revanche*. So disappointing have events been since 1919, so dark are the troubles still that we are tempted to find some relief in building castles in the air, and if the future is too clouded for this, we build them in the past."

Lord Grey's responsibility for the prolongation of the war is great, but he disarms his critics by his lack of arrogance, he has no faith in his own omniscience. To Colonel House no such doubts seem to have come, he seems never to have asked himself whether some other way might have been tried before the final step was taken. There are a few of us who believe that there was a better way and that if Wilson had been willing to follow it there might have been a shortened war, a peace brought about by negotiation before the war had done its worst, before militarism had entrenched itself everywhere and nationalism grown to monstrous proportions, a peace which would have saved America from war madness and its after-effects, and — who knows? — even a League of Nations growing out of this conference of neutrals instead of one formed by victors after years of bitterest conflict.

There was for Miss Addams a strange aftermath of this European venture. Soon after she reached New York she was asked to address a large audience there, in Carnegie Hall I think it was (I had been called to Mackinac by illness in the family), to tell about the Congress and what followed it. In the course of her speech she told of what we had heard repeatedly in England and on the Continent, that before a bayonet charge the English soldiers would have rations of rum served them, the Germans small doses of ether, to brace them up to this terrible ordeal. For some reason that simple statement of fact was taken as an insult to the brave Allies and, under the leadership of Richard Harding Davis, a newspaper campaign was launched against her which for bitterness cannot often have been exceeded. She was accused of insulting the heroic young men who were dying for their country, but nobody stopped to think that war does not mean only dying, it means killing; indeed no country wants its young men to die for it — that is most wasteful — but to kill for it. And surely it was no insult to say that decent young men, brought up in a Christian civilization, would not find it natural and easy to disembowel men like themselves whom they had never seen before. The English took it for granted that a stiff dose of rum was essential, but in 1915 — and for some years after — many Americans romanticized the war and resented fiercely anything that disturbed the picture they had created. She returned therefore to a very painful time of misunderstanding and growing bitterness and the disappointment of all her hopes.

War was declared on Good Friday, 1917. I was in Washington at that time and met Mary McDowell of the Stockyards Settlement who had come, with many others, to make a last protest against this step, to back up, so far as they could, the "little group of willful men" in the Senate who still stood out against it. After that, the temper of the country, at least in the Middle West, changed suddenly, became more militaristic and more intolerant of pacifistic dissent than the East, where the war feeling had prevailed for months. It seemed to me that the Middle West was like a gang of boys who, once they have decided on a plan, will brook no argument and will beat up any boy who opposes the majority will. Illinois and the neighbor states had opposed our entrance into the war, but once we were in there must be no more talk. Eugene Debs was arrested and spent some four years in Atlanta Penitentiary. Kate O'Hare was sent to Missouri State Penitentiary because at that time there was no Federal prison for women.

Debs and Mrs. O'Hare were the only victims whom I knew

personally but presently I met others, for the jail in Chicago began to fill up with the radicals and war resisters from the Middle and Far West, who, some hundred and twenty of them, came to trial, not singly but as a group, before Judge Kenesaw Mountain Landis and were given sentences up to twenty years. During the course of the trial some of the men developed tuberculosis and were released on bail. They used to come to Hull-House for companionship, and so did Elizabeth Gurley Flynn, who had been arrested with the others but promptly discharged by Judge Landis before the trial began, because, she thought, the presence of a woman (and a very attractive one) among the prisoners might arouse sympathy. There was no Civil Liberties Union to appeal to in those days, no possible way of rallying the liberally-minded remnant; there was simply nothing to do but to wait till the end of the war should bring about a lessening of fear and bitterness, which it did. Judge Landis's condemned were all pardoned not very long after the Armistice.

The intolerance which was invading the colleges and universities, especially Columbia and the state universities, was not nearly so evident in industrial life; indeed, the atmosphere there was wholesomely free from wartime hatreds. The employers frankly regretted having to dismiss their competent German and Austrian employees and the workers often spoke their sympathy for their former mates. Neither employers nor employed had time or attention to give to the campaign of hate which sometimes took childish forms, such as burning German toys and picture books, banning German music. I encountered it only now and then, as when a lady accosted me in the lobby of the Shoreham Hotel, requesting my signature to a pledge that never again would I listen to German music or look at a German painting or read a German book. I met it again in a small Illinois city when in the center of the town square there was erected a billboard, with the names of the German-American townspeople and farmers who had not bought as many liberty bonds as their patriotic neighbors thought they should. Those poor German Americans had a bitterly hard time — the men bullied into buying more bonds than they could afford, the women refused a share in Red Cross work, lest they sprinkle ground glass over the surgical dressings.

XI

War Industries

SOON after I returned from Europe in 1915 the war became my daily absorption, for Washington put me to work on the rapidly developing industry of high-explosive production for Britain, France, and Russia. Under the stimulus of an increasing pressure from the Allies, plants had sprung up, chiefly along the Atlantic seaboard, for the manufacture of shells and mines and of picric acid, dinitrobenzol, trinitrotoluol, smokeless powder, military guncotton, mixed powders, and fulminate of mercury. The French demanded picric acid, the British and Russians TNT and the "mixed powders" (which have nitrocellulose as their base), and all demanded fulminate of mercury, which is the "booster charge," the detonator to start the explosion. These are all nitrated compounds, made by the action of nitric acid on cellulose or glycerine or toluol or carbolic acid (phenol) or mercury, and therefore a great quantity of nitric acid was needed. Picric acid and TNT are made by nitration of coal-tar benzol and toluol, which are by-products of coke ovens.

Up to this time we Americans had had little or no experience in producing these wartime chemicals, we had bought what we needed from the Germans. Our coke ovens lined the tracks of the Pennsylvania Railroad, producing coke but letting those valuable light gases, benzol, toluol, xylol, escape into the air (later on I came to wonder whether this was not the best thing they could do). Once the blockade shut us off from Germany, we had to construct coke by-products plants to catch these gases, and to start production of nitric acid on a huge scale. These were new, unfamiliar procedures and brought new problems to our engineers. The blockade shut off German dyes also and aniline, which the dye and rubber industries depended on and which is another of the benzol derivatives. All the substances I have mentioned (except nitrocellulose) are poisonous to man, some producing their action through the breathing of fumes, some making their way into the body through the skin, all, with the exception of nitric acid and mercury fulminate, acting on the central nervous system, though in several cases this action is not so serious as the damage produced on blood and organs.

For me to enter this new field was again to embark on pioneer exploration. If there was anyone in Washington who knew where explosives were being produced and loaded (loading means filling shells and mines) he kept the secret. Neither Army nor Navy gave me any more information than I had been able to pick up myself. My chief in the Department of Labor, Dr. Meeker, could only tell me to follow my old procedure, visit the plants I knew and pick up gossip about the others. This method worked very well and I was helped also by the great clouds of yellow and orange fumes, nitrous gases, which in those days of crude procedure rose to the sky from picric-acid and nitrocellulose plants. It was like the pillar of cloud by day that guided the children of Israel. I would hear vaguely of a nitrating plant in the New Jersey marshes and I would spot the orange fumes and make my way to them. Sometimes it would be a group of "canaries" who would guide me to a plant. These were men so stained with yellow picric acid that they were dubbed canaries.

On one of my first trips in New Jersey, while I was waiting

in a small railway station, I noticed a Negro and a white man standing near, and the eyes of all who were waiting for the train were turned on them curiously. "Look at the canaries," somebody whispered. The white man was of a leaden hue, thin and weary-looking, but touched into incongruous comedy by smears of orange stain on his cheekbones and deeply dyed yellow eyebrows and hair. The Negro was frankly comic, nails of bright orange standing out from his black hands, hair and eyebrows orange-dyed, a golden burnish over the high spots on his face, the palms of his hands a deep yellow. I edged nearer and, being greeted with a friendly grin by the Negro, ventured a question: "Dyeing cotton goods?" "No, Miss, we're working over to the Canary Islands, making picric for the French." "Is it dangerous?" I asked. "Not this yellow stuff ain't, but there's a red smoke comes off when the yellow stuff is making and it like to knocks you out and if you don't run it gets you. You don't suspicion nothing much, you goes home and eats your supper and goes to bed, and then in the night you starts to choke up and by morning you're dead." I turned a questioning look toward the white man, but he nodded in confirmation and the Negro insisted: "Sure it's true, Miss. The man who had the bunk under me, he died that way. I ain't going to stay myself after next pay day."

I found the Canary Islands that same day off in the meadows with wide stretches of farmland about. It was not possible to visit the plant then, I needed a permit from the central office, but from the road I could see strange forms hurrying about — black men in motley garb with great stiff aprons, colored orange, woolen shirts eaten away to rags, high boots streaked with yellow, flaps of leather hanging down against their hands. As I was looking, orange smoke began to rise, rolling out in thick clouds that sank and spread over the ground and then sluggishly rose and rolled away, paling as they went, while a crowd of grotesque men came running out from a long shed and stood waiting for the fumes to scatter. A dog with his gray coat stained in absurd yellow spots came out from the guarded gate. Near the barrier to the east the land rose a little and the trees there were blackened and withered, for the west wind swept the gases in that direction and they blight whatever they touch. I wandered over to that side and suddenly I came on an old stone-flagged path with a decorous border of box on each side. There was a broken lilac bush, and near by a hearth and chimney, black with many fires, but the house it warmed had vanished. The rise in the land had saved the box and lilac, but all round them seeped a sluggish stream turning the earth into something poisonous and killing the roots of all green things. For wide stretches the lowlands were blackened and lay festering in the sunlight; only in one spot rose a tiny mound covered with wild rose and morning-glory. The poison had not reached it yet, but was creeping close.

A puff of wind from the west drove me, choking and gasping, before the angry fumes which were pouring out again and spreading over the spot where I stood. Escaped to clear air I found myself in a great field all grown up with weeds. Corn used to grow there but now ragweed and burdock. The men who tilled that land were in behind the barrier making the poisonous stuff for the French, and as they did it the kindly fruits of the earth perished and in their place were weeds and blackened stalks. It was better business to work for destruction than for life and so the farmers had left the fields for the acid sheds, and instead of yellow corn to feed men their harvest was heaps of picric to kill men.

I thought of the vision of Isaiah which for centuries men have cherished in their hearts. We have taken his words and

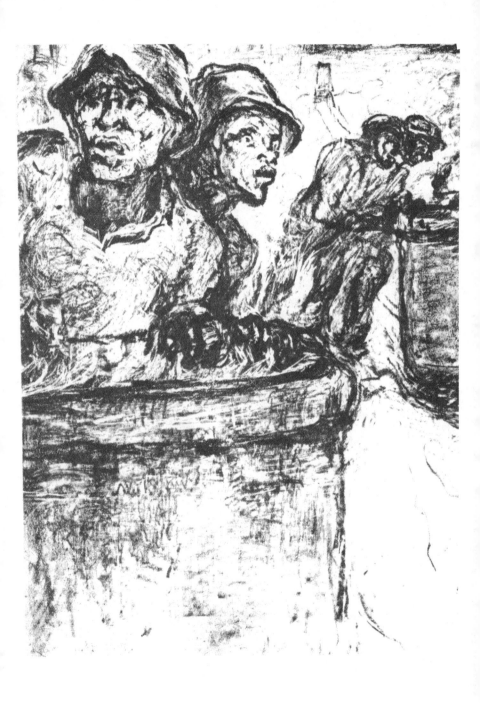

turned them about so that they read thus: "And they shall beat their plowshares into swords, and their pruninghooks into spears; nation shall lift up sword against nation, and they shall learn war."

Here were, as I have said, new engineering problems and they were being solved, not in advance of the actual production, but while it was going on. If anything went wrong it was not a laboratory accident, it involved the workmen on the job, men who knew little or nothing about what they were working with or how to protect themselves. Nitric acid is a very powerful caustic, it eats through metals and soldering materials, and when it encounters organic matter, such as cotton, or wood fiber, or glycerine, or coal tar (or even water), it gives off quantities of nitrous fumes which may exert enough pressure to blow off the lid of a machine or to burst it into fragments. This used to happen often in those days. During one day's visit to a great nitrocellulose plant I saw no less than eight such accidents, the orange fumes pouring out of doors and windows, the men fleeing before them. These fumes act on throat and lungs much as did the war gases used in Flanders, only they are not nearly so choking, but this is really an added danger, for while men will escape as quickly as possible from chlorine gas, which they simply cannot breathe, they may linger long enough in an atmosphere of nitrous fumes to get a fatal dose, when they do not realize the danger.

The picture of this form of industrial disease became very familiar to me as time went on. There were the very rapidly developing cases, probably rare, when the man died in a few hours after he was gassed, with little change in the body but with nitric acid in the blood, which apparently had acted on the respiratory center. There were only five of these that came to my knowledge, but nobody knows how many actually occurred, for most doctors knew nothing about nitrous fumes and would pronounce such a case heart failure or heat prostration. The typical picture of nitrous fume poisoning was as follows: The man was exposed a short time to heavy fumes or several hours to moderately heavy fumes, which made him choke and strangle, but in the open air this would pass over and he would go home thinking nothing serious had happened, eat his supper and go to bed, then awaken after some hours with a sense of tightness in his chest and an increasing difficulty in breathing. When the doctor arrived the man would be sitting up in bed, gasping and livid, using all his strength to pump air into his rapidly filling lungs. If the fumes had injured only part of the lungs then oxygen might pull him through till the exudate was absorbed, but if he had breathed deeply (and one's instinct is to hold the breath as long as possible, then gasp and hold it again) then he would have little chance, for all the lung tissue would be filled and he would "drown in his own fluids." In milder cases, as in gassing from chlorine during the war, pneumonia developed, sometimes quickly, sometimes after several days. And as was true also in the war, if the lungs were already tuberculous, the effect of the gas was to light up the trouble and turn it into a form of "galloping consumption." This happened more often with Negroes, for they are especially susceptible to tuberculosis, and therefore the largest munition company made it a rule not to employ Negroes on the "acid line." Unfortunately this was not true of some of the less responsible concerns.

The picric-acid plants were much the worst. Making the other explosives requires elaborate apparatus, but anybody can make picric acid by pouring carbolic acid into nitric acid and, if his mind is fixed only on profits, he can do it in a huge open shed, with nothing more elaborate than some big earthenware crocks. It was easy to hire Negro field hands from the deep South and, if the fumes were too heavy and some of the men choked and died, it was easy to convince the coroner that it was an advantage to the county to have this huge plant and that such deaths were due to "natural causes." That is exactly the history of the largest picric-acid works I used to visit, and from the spring of 1916 to the Armistice it grew steadily larger but nothing else was changed.

The first nitrocellulose works I visited was down in Hopewell, Virginia, where the du Pont Company had built an enormous plant on the James River, and also a model village for some 12,000 employees. Just over the line, however, across the railroad tracks, was a wide-open town of saloons, shooting galleries, gambling rooms, squalid barracks, and crowds of young men, most of them working in the plant but preferring the gay life outside the bounds of the model village, which was patrolled by du Pont police.

Mabel Kittredge went with me on this trip, out of curiosity over this new and exciting industrial development, and I was thankful to have her for, as we discovered at once, Hopewell was a strictly masculine community and a woman was a conspicuous and embarrassing intruder. When we asked for a hotel we were directed to a barbershop which had some rooms on the second floor. The barber was obliging but hesitant. He showed us a squalid room with a sagging bed, a tin wash basin, two chairs, and a floor so dirty that he was forced to apologize. "The room next to this is cleaner," he said, "but I'm afraid it might make you ladies nervous because of the bullet holes in the window. You see, we had a little shooting affair across the street last night." We could not help thinking that maybe the next shooting affair might send the bullets into that room, so we said we would think it over and we wandered down to the street letting him go back to his barbering.

As we stood there helplessly we were conscious of the close scrutiny of a mounted du Pont policeman, who evidently decided we were harmless and needed help. He kindly advised us to avoid Hopewell and go down to the river where we would find an abandoned steamer turned into a boardinghouse. The man in charge was respectable and had a Negress to see to the rooms. We were grateful for his advice but when we reached the riverbank we found the respectable man in the act of discharging his only female help. However we accepted his offer of two cabins, the walls of which, unfortunately, did not reach within eighteen inches of the ceiling, but except for the noise of the men coming and going when the shifts changed, we were unmolested.

That evening I had the somewhat flattering and quite unprecedented experience of being taken for a *fille de joie*. We went for dinner to a Greek restaurant where I recognized the proprietor as a Greek who had kept a saloon opposite Hull-House and sent his little daughter to our kindergarten. I waved to him and he came to greet me and talked to me for some time, attracting the attention of the whole room, but that seemed natural since we were the only women there. But the next noon when we came in he sat down at our table and whispered to me that a du Pont policeman had been there the evening before, and had reported to headquarters my bold-faced behavior. "You see," he said, "they've had an evangelist here and he's made the mayor clean out all the women and you're the first ones to turn up since then, so you see they're watching you." I meditated a while and then made another trip to the plant and explained the matter to the very polite and somewhat amused superintendent, who promised to set me straight with the police.

The tale of the evangelist interested us and when Sunday came we sought him out. He had a big tent, part church, part hospital, which latter had thirteen cots, all filled that day, mostly with victims of Saturday night's celebration. He was a tall yellow-haired Scandinavian with fierce blue eyes and a manner that was more than impressive. He told us he had been converted by Dr. Howard Kelly when he was serving a term in the Baltimore penitentiary, and when he was discharged he looked around for the wickedest place where he could go and do the Lord's work. Hopewell "across the tracks" seemed to offer what he sought and he had settled there. Since there was nobody to tend the lads who got shot or knifed in the drunken fights, he gathered them in, washed and bandaged and put them to bed, dealing all the time with their immortal souls as well as their bodies. For food he served coffee and soup, made in big iron kettles out in the yard.

But the achievement he was proudest of was his ridding the town of prostitutes. According to his story he could get no help from the mayor, since, as he discovered, the brothels were owned by the mayor, who collected big rents from them. "So," he said, "I went to see him one night and stopped him at his gate when he got home. It was a dark and windy night and he is a little runt of a fellow and I'm pretty tall. I said, 'Mr. Mayor, the Lord has sent me to you with a command — drive those women out. Now if you're reasonable and minded to obey quietly, the Lord tells me to treat you gentle, but if you're obstinate He has other methods. I'd like your promise here and now.' He was reasonable, the houses closed." I could certainly testify to his success.

Nitrocellulose is the stuff from which military guncotton

and smokeless powder are made. In the explosives industry everything that explodes is called "powder" even if it is a thick syrup (nitroglycerine) or looks like chunks of maple sugar (TNT) or blackish macaroni, spaghetti, vermicelli (smokeless powder). The first plant for the production of smokeless powder that I visited was Picatinny Arsenal and it was one of the very few places where I realized that I was studying explosives, not only poisons. We were in a small room on the third floor looking at a huge bin into which was rushing a stream of macaroni strips from a big pipe. My guide said, "How's the static today, Jim?" and flapped his hand over the bin. Jim flapped his and answered, "About as usual," and my guide went on to explain that what they had to look out for was a spark from the static electricity produced by the friction of the particles. "If that should happen," he said, "you dash for that window and slide down and when you hit the ground don't look behind you, keep right on running." I looked out of the window and saw a long chute going down to the ground. But no spark came there or anywhere and I soon grew as used to it as to TNT. Nitroglycerine always made me a bit nervous, though, that heavy syrup so scrupulously guarded, the plants often placed in narrow valleys to shut in the force of an explosion, the tanks of syrup poised over a reservoir of water into which the whole charge can be dumped at a moment's notice, if the temperature shoots up.

Washington was a strange place in those days. I went there often, staying with Julia Lathrop in her cool apartment in the Ontario and drinking in refreshment of spirit from her very presence. We were both pacifists but neither of us took a conspicuous anti-war stand, for the same reason — we were deeply attached to our jobs and feared to lose them. I have

never been sure I was right in this. Perhaps it would have
been better to make an open protest, but I knew I was not
influential enough to have that protest count for much, while
my work in the war industries counted for a good deal. As it
was, Dr. Meeker received more than one protest against
allowing a pacifist to enter munition plants, for I made no
secret of my views when challenged. Certainly my anti-war
feeling increased with every month of the war. It was not only
the sight of men sickening and dying in the effort to produce
something to wound or kill other men — that was bad enough
and certainly shook one's belief in the intelligence of the
human race — but it was also the strange spirit of exaltation
among the men and women who thronged Washington, engaged in all sorts of "war work" and loving it. I got an impression of joyful release in many of them, as if, after all their
lives repressing hatred as unchristian, they suddenly discovered
it to be a patriotic duty and let themselves go in for an orgy
of anti-German abuse. The industrial world seemed to be
given over to a sort of triumphant ruthlessness, with contempt
for any attitude save that of hard-boiled efficiency. It was perhaps not so much greed for profits as an intoxication of big-
ness, big plants, reckless spending (the "cost plus 10 per cent"
system made economy absurd), the sudden rise to importance
of mediocre people, who could be at one and the same time
patriots and profiteers. This does not mean that I met no fine
and disinterested people. I did, but they kept more in the
background.

With the Army I had very friendly relations and visited
arsenals as I did private plants, but the Navy was more difficult; every suggestion on my part that it would be well for
me to look into the mine-loading departments of Navy arsenals
met with a polite rejoinder that it was quite unnecessary, the

Navy had no cases of TNT poisoning. Since I knew this was impossible I decided to appeal to someone higher up and the young Assistant Secretary of the Navy, Franklin D. Roosevelt, was the one to whom I was referred. He received me very graciously and, what was far more important, he listened carefully to my plea. Then he sent for an Admiral, who came in, resplendent in white and gold and blue, a gorgeous creature who made me feel like a drab peahen. I cannot remember how Mr. Roosevelt did it but I know that in some way he secured from the Admiral the permission I needed and in such a way that the gorgeous gentleman never lost face. It was a remarkable performance.

The most carefully guarded branch of the explosives industry is the production of mercury fulminate and of percussion ("booster") charges made from it. This is more dangerous than even nitroglycerine for it is extremely explosive. Such a plant is built in small units, to lessen the damage done by an explosion, or there may be small cubicles for single workers, separated by a wall of concrete two or three feet thick. The floors are covered with rubber, but in spite of that the visitor must put on overshoes lest an exposed nail in a shoe heel strike against metal and produce a spark. The workers are given only tiny supplies of the stuff at a time, but even so the greatest care must be used. Fortunately handling mercury fulminate causes nothing worse than an itching eruption and even that can be avoided by careful washing. There were, I believe, no explosions of fulminate during the war; the accidents were most of them in plants handling harmless-looking TNT.

Mercury fulminate provided me with an experience I can never forget. We were in a large room where the fulminate was produced, by the action of alcohol on mercury nitrate, and the sublimed crystals had formed on the inside of great glass balloons. A workman picked up one and carried it across the room. I watched him, frozen with terror, for each crystal in that glass vessel would cause an explosion and there were thousands of them. Of course he did not stumble, nothing happened, but I still shiver when I think of it.

Much of this work was done in New Jersey and luckily the Department of Labor in that state had an excellent Commissioner, Colonel Bryant, who was ready to co-operate in every way with Washington. He assigned one of his inspectors, John Roach, to work with me and also a young chemist, Newell Gordon of Princeton, who was a great help, for chemistry plays a very important part in this industry. Before we entered the war there was very little interest anywhere in these new industrial developments, except with regard to the danger of explosions; poisons were not thought of, especially those unfamiliar ones, trinitrotoluol and picric acid. The former was the one that presented the most difficult problem although nitrous fumes did the greatest damage. In the list of 2432 cases of occupational poisoning which I published in May 1917, nitrous fumes accounted for 1389, and for 28 of the 53 deaths. But TNT came second, with 660 cases and 13 deaths, and while the prevention of nitrous fume poisoning was a problem for engineers and was dealt with more and more efficiently as the months went on, the prevention of TNT poisoning was much less simple.

The English told us to look out for absorption through the skin, much more important than breathing fumes. But this meant first-class housekeeping, scrupulous cleanliness; it meant also washable working clothes and shower baths. The English provided these as a matter of course, but our manufacturers did not. The discovery of cases of poisoning was very difficult, for no American physician knew what to look for, although we had plenty of information about it from England. Aside from the skin eruptions which are very common, victims of TNT poisoning suffer from injury to the liver and, more rarely, to the blood-forming tissues. The deaths in my list came from toxic jaundice or from aplastic anemia. But I knew my list was far from complete, for there were several company doctors who would give no information at all.

A welcome break in the strenuous program of wartime Washington was an invitation to dine at the House of Truth. This was the name given by Justice Holmes to a co-operative household of young men, all in some kind of government service, all bursting with ideas and eager to discuss them. There I would meet, either as permanent or as transient residents, Felix Frankfurter, Walter Lippmann, Eustace Percy, Robert Valentine, Loring Christie, Winfred Denison, and of course men from the diplomatic services, newspaper reporters, distinguished visitors from outside Washington.

The talk at the table must always be general, tête-à-tête conversation was frowned down, literally, and this made for a very lively conversation which could never degenerate into dullness because one of the hosts could always catch the ball and throw it to a good catcher. How often since, when I have discovered who my dinner partners were to be, I have wished that the rules governing House of Truth dinners could be enforced by some Emily Post. When we adjourned to the parlor some one guest, perhaps a well-known Senator, perhaps a Supreme Court Justice, more often a journalist newly returned from Europe, would be made the center and we would all have a try at drawing him out. There was one dinner, I remember, when unfortunately two guests of prominence had been invited and each considered himself the one entitled to the central role. The result was unfortunate.

In April 1917 we entered the war and at once the scene changed. For me the most important change was not so much the increased tempo and the vastly increased production as the new interest taken by my own profession in the protection of munition workers. While in England physicians connected with the Ministry of Munitions had been studying all forms of TNT poisoning and publishing their results, our doctors had been for the most part ignorant and indifferent, or secretive at the behest of their employers, who thought that frankness might frighten the men away. But when we were actually at war, the English example began to have its effect and this field to appear as a proper one for medical research. It was Dr. Richard Pearce who first offered me the help I so sorely needed and through his efforts the National Research Council was induced to appoint a committee of experts to act as a consultative body. Presently the committee made it possible for me to send into TNT plants medical students well trained in laboratory technique to study on the spot some of the unsolved problems, such as the influence of sex, of race and of youth, and of summer heat; the earliest symptoms of TNT poisoning; how long exposure lasts before such symptoms appear; how long it takes to get rid of the TNT that has been absorbed.

Our students unearthed some very shocking conditions, under criminally negligent doctors, all of which they reported to us, but even the committee backing me was not influential enough to bring about reforms. It is hard to believe that this rich and safe country should refuse to give its munition workers the sort of protection which France and England, fighting for their lives, provided as a matter of course. But it was impossible to overcome the arrogance of the manufacturers, the indifference of the military, and the contempt of the trade-unions for non-union labor. Grace Abbott and Felix Frankfurter on the War Labor Board tried to help but could only put the matter up to Gompers and there it rested. We physicians strove hard to get a mandatory code for the protection of TNT workers, then, when we saw that was impossible, to formulate one which the manufacturers would agree to follow, but the largest company refused and naturally that settled it. Only in April 1919 did Gompers finally publish a code, not as strict as the English, not mandatory, and issued five months after the Armistice.

The war did have a beneficial influence on industrial hygiene. If it increased the dangers in American industry, it also aroused the interest of physicians in industrial poisons. And that interest has never died down, on the contrary it has increased with the increasing complexity of methods of manufacture. A change took place also in the attitude of employers, for a large labor turnover was found to be not only wasteful but an unsatisfactory method of dealing with dangerous processes in industry. The Public Health Service had entered this field during the war and the medical journals had published articles discussing the action of the new poisons and various methods of preventing danger from the old ones. Industrial medicine had at last become respectable.

As I write we are deep in the second World War and our plants for the production of high explosives and of airplanes are working at a scale far beyond that of 1917–1918, they are employing many more men in this sort of work. But the picture has altered beyond recognition. It is true that the same products are needed — TNT, tetryl, military guncotton, smokeless powder, mixed powders, fulminate of mercury. Few new ones have been added, and all the important ones, new and old, are made with the use of nitric acid. The dangers we faced in the first World War are still there, but now they are largely theoretical. In no field of industry is there a more striking contrast between the two periods than in this one, both as to knowledge concerning the dangers and as to determination to control them. Our engineers have learned how to produce and use dangerous poisons without exposing the workers, we no longer have the bursting pipes and unexpected outpouring of gases that used to go with nitration processes, and the removal of poisonous solvent fumes is far more efficient. As for medical care, where earlier there was a great dearth of experts now there are hundreds of physicians who know what to do and are doing it. One branch of the Public Health Service is devoted entirely to industrial diseases, the Division of Labor Standards of the Department of Labor gives advice and help in the engineering problems, and the Army and the Navy have their own experts both medical and engineering. It is good to have one cheerful feature in this dark picture of a return to barbarism.

XII

"Dead Fingers"

My WORK in munition plants was interrupted toward
the end of 1917 by a summons to Washington from the Department of Labor, just at the time of our entry into the war.
As usual, I stayed with Julia Lathrop in her apartment in the
Ontario. The atmosphere in Washington was very tense with
excitement over the impending war vote in Congress. I have no
doubt the "little group of willful men" were besieged by both
sides; certainly the one war resister I knew in Congress, Jeannette Rankin, was. She was an ardent pacifist but she was
also an ardent suffragist, and she told Julia and me that her
worst ordeal came from her comrades in the suffrage movement who told her that if she voted against war it would be
taken as a proof of female emotionality and sentimentalism
and would set back the whole movement, nobody could say
how long. We did what we could to hold up her hands and so
did Mary McDowell and other women, and in the end the
first woman to be elected to Congress did register her vote
against our entry into the war.

To my surprise, my summons proved to be for a problem
quite remote from the war, and even from industrial poisons,
and it led me for a brief interval into an unfamiliar field, stonecutting. Formerly this work was done with mallet and chisel,
but during the last decade of the nineteenth century and the
first decade of the twentieth, the air hammer had gradually
found its way, first into the granite cutting branch, then the

marble cutting, and then limestone. The air hammer is driven by compressed air and delivers 3000 to 3400 strokes a minute while with hammer and mallet the cutter would hardly go beyond 150 strokes. Of course there was a great speeding up of the work and also a great increase in the dust produced. The men resisted the innovation as strongly as they could, insisting that the work was actually more tiring than before and that the hammer produced a killing cloud of dust. It was again the drearily familiar story that has followed the introduction of every labor-saving device, the men knowing that the disadvantages that came would be theirs and that of the advantages they would have little if any share; the employers insisting that the men cared only to hold their jobs and were incapable of understanding what progress in industry means. It is, of course, shortsighted of workmen to see only the unemployment and misery that threaten themselves and their mates, instead of rejoicing in the wonderful technological advances of the day, but that is the way working people are made. Incidentally, the prophecy of the granite stonecutters as to the increase of lung diseases which would follow the air hammer has been amply vindicated. It took twenty to thirty years to prove them right — but that is another story.

The complaint which led to my being sent on this new job came from the limestone cutters of Bedford, Indiana, who demanded, with the backing of the American Association for Labor Legislation, a Federal investigation of the injuries caused by the use of the air hammer, saying that physicians had told them its use would be followed by tuberculosis, paralysis, neurasthenia, insanity. A disorder known to the men as "dead fingers" was dwelt on especially. My chief handed over to me written statements from 68 stonecutters who said they had suffered injury from the air hammer and

from 29 who said they had not; from 20 employers who either
denied that their men had suffered any harmful effects at all
or said that the injury was negligible and the men's motive
in resisting the use of the hammer had nothing to do with its
physical effects. I had also the statement of a physician who
had examined a group of men at the request of the union
and found them "irreparably damaged," threatened with
neurasthenia and even insanity; also that of a neurologist who
had examined some men at the request of the employers and
found that few of them made any complaint at all and those
who did were not suffering from any pathological condition.
That is the sort of evidence that one must expect to find in
this curious branch of medicine, where the clear waters of
truth are so often muddied by mutual antagonisms, quarrels
over wages and hours, and over unionization, and also, I am
afraid, by the intense class consciousness of not a few
physicians.

In Bedford I met Mr. Sam Griggs, President of the Jour-
neymen Stonecutters' Association, a black-haired, blue-eyed
Irishman, one of the most likable men I have met in the
labor world and certainly one of the shrewdest. The weather
in January was perfect for my purpose, 14° F. to 34° F., and
early in the morning, the best time to see the men, the mills
were freezing cold. Limestone cutting is done almost entirely
with the air hammer, for roughing as well as for fine work.
This hammer resembles the jackhammer used in mining and
riveting and in cutting through city pavements, but it is much
lighter and is used differently. The stonecutter grasps the cutting tool, which fits into the hammer, in his left hand and
guides it, while his right hand holds the hammer, which is
delivering some 3000 strokes a minute. I tested several of these
hammers and at first the vibration in both hands was so severe

that I could not distinguish between them, but after a while I found that it was possible to hold the hammer rather lightly, which lessened the vibrations, but the tool in the left hand must be clung to with all one's might or the hammer would drive it from the hand, and it is the left hand that does the difficult work of guiding the cutting tool. This explains why the left hand is the one that suffers most, unless the man is left-handed.

The condition of which the men complained — and doubtless still do — is a spastic anemia of certain fingers, the ones most tightly cramped around the tool. It is caused by three factors — cramped muscles driving the blood from the fingers, cold which contracts the vessels, and the rapid vibration which sets up vasomotor disturbances. The men call the condition "dead fingers" and it is a good name, for the fingers do look like those of a corpse, a yellowish-grayish white and shrunken. There is a clear line of demarcation between the dead part and the normal part. I had provided myself with outlines on paper of right and left hands and when I examined a man I would make his record with a blue pencil on one of the sheets. The first man I saw came in from the bitter-cold morning air with the four fingers of his left hand a dead greenish white, quite without sensation and distressingly numb and cold. As he rubbed his hand and swung his arm about to restore the circulation the contrast between fingers and hand became startling, for the purplish and somewhat swollen hand met the white shrunken fingers abruptly, without any intermediate zone. The right hand was much less affected. After vigorous massage and beating his arms over his breast the blood gradually filled the fingers and they looked fairly natural, only rather purplish. This condition I saw again and again, differing only in intensity and distribution.

Dead fingers are not really painful as long as the anemia lasts, but cause enough discomfort to make the cutter stop work and get the blood back into his fingers, for the stroke of the hammer on the tool he holds is peculiarly intolerable when the fingers are white. Sharp pain comes when the blood flows back into the fingers but it does not last. However, the hand never feels quite natural and it is always "going to sleep," especially when holding a book or newspaper. Many men complained of loss of sensation in one or both hands, which made them clumsy in buttoning a coat or lacing a shoe, and some said they could not tell a dime from a nickel without looking at it. It seems that once the condition starts it persists even if the man quits stonecutting, for I found men who had not used the air hammer for eight or even ten years, yet in cold weather they would have typical dead fingers.

This condition was so unknown to the medical world that I had no authorities to fall back on and I did not feel competent to decide the question put to me, How much harm is there in this spastic anemia of the fingers? Obviously it did not prevent the men doing highly skilled work. I saw them carving the more-than-life-size figures which now adorn the façade of the Catholic Theological School on the North Side in Chicago and I was fascinated to watch their skill. Nor did I see any indubitable signs of a general effect on the nervous system, even though many of them had been frightened by rumors of cases of insanity and paralysis among stonecutters. I felt that more light was needed and asked the Bureau of Labor Statistics to let me send eight men who had striking cases of dead fingers to the Presbyterian Hospital in Chicago where Dr. Thor Rothstein could examine them. Dr. Rothstein found marked vasomotor changes and decrease of sensation, but no symptoms of a dangerous character and no serious effect on the general health of the men, though he would not say that after many years of work there might not be some unfavorable result.

Spastic anemia of the fingers has been observed of late years in Germany, not only in stonecutters but in shoemakers who press the soles of shoes tightly against a buffing machine.

The limestone belt having been covered, the Department of Labor sent me to Quincy, Massachusetts, and Barre, Vermont, to look into granite cutting there. In Quincy I met old James Duncan, head of the Granite Cutters' Union, who had been sent as the labor representative on that curious mission of good will, or, perhaps more truly, of encouragement to keep on with the war, which President Wilson dispatched to Russia in 1917. He was full of pride and joy as he told me about how he had explained the basic principles of the A.F. of L. to the revolutionary crowds in Moscow. "I got great applause," he said; "in fact I got a lot more applause than my interpreter did." And I was quite ready to believe him. In Barre, and Quincy also, the mills were largely engaged in making gravestones. I had little real knowledge about the danger of granite dust — the study of silicosis came after the war — but I knew that as far back as the days of Pliny the Elder, the consumption of stonecutters was classed as one of the diseases of slaves. In Bedford, talk of consumption was infrequent and vague, in Barre it was inescapable. A cutter would say, "Sure I know it will get me. It got my father, it's got my older brother, it's only a question of time when it will get me." Barre was a hotbed of pulmonary tuberculosis, yet the men had a high standard of living and were, as is true of all stonecutters, decidedly above average manual workers in education and intelligence.

There was something dreadful in the sight of a mill full of

men carving tombstones and, as they did it, preparing themselves for their own graves. If it had been something of undying beauty, a gift to the whole world, their sacrifice might have been justified, or if it had meant some invention to save others' lives, but granite tombstones! There is no excuse for them, they are ugly to begin with and will always remain ugly, for no moss or lichen can grow on that icy, polished surface. A tombstone should be perishable, so that after the people who knew and loved the dead are gone the stone would fall gently to oblivion, as do the marble and slate and Portland stone in our old graveyards. They are things of beauty and they fall into ruin beautifully. But granite, no, nothing can destroy or even soften it.

I was so obsessed by this vision of lives offered on the altar of uselessness and ugliness that when I was asked to speak to the Consumers' League in Baltimore I poured it out and begged my hearers never to fulfill their duty to their beloved dead by means of a granite tombstone. Nothing exciting was happening just then in Baltimore so the *Sunpaper* carried next morning a headline, "Wants to abolish granite tombstones," and this aroused the American Granite Association, who wrote, thanking me for my tribute to the lasting qualities of granite, but protesting against my "particularly unkind references," and denying that granite cutting was bad for the men's health. However it was only a few months after I had completed my study of stonecutters' dead fingers that the much more important problem of dust disease of the lungs was taken up seriously and I was asked to serve on a Committee for the Scientific Investigation of the Mortality from Tuberculosis in Dusty Trades, the work to begin in the stonecutting mills of Barre.

At our first meeting, at Lake Placid, we were told that thirty years had passed since the air hammer was introduced in the mills of Barre and during that time the death rate from pulmonary tuberculosis in Barre had risen steadily and was still rising, while the rate for the remainder of the state was falling, as it was all over the country. At that time rural Vermont had a tuberculosis death rate of 1.5 per 1000 males over 40 years of age, Barre stonecutters had a rate of 60.6 per 1000. There were more deaths from tuberculosis alone among stonecutters in a period of three years than in the general male population from all causes. This was, of course, infinitely more important an effect of the air hammer than the dead fingers I had studied, and the Public Health Service soon after inaugurated a three-year study of the Barre stonecutting industry and, with the help of the Saranac laboratory, provided a report which has been the basis of widespread reforms, not only in Barre but wherever the danger of silicosis exists.

XIII

Arizona Copper

THE REPORT concerning the effect of the air hammer on the hands of stonecutters was published by the Bureau of Labor Statistics in July 1918. Meantime, and up to the Armistice, I had gone back to explosives and aniline dyes and their intermediates, but with the end of the war came a summons to the copper camps of Arizona. The miners had seen the government bulletin about stonecutters' dead fingers and determined to have a similar investigation made in the Clifton-Morenci-Metcalf camps, for, they said, the air-driven jackhammer was destroying their health through its rapid vibrations. The stonecutters had had a Federal inquiry into their complaints of the vibrating tool, the miners had a right to the same treatment. So I was ordered out to Arizona in January 1919, and Clara Landsberg, who was living at Hull-House, decided to go with me on what promised to be an interesting journey.

This was a totally different situation from the one I had found in Indiana, Massachusetts, and Vermont. There the war had played no part in the labor situation. Nor was there much tension between the men and the employers, even in the limestone field, where a new wage agreement was being negotiated. But the copper-mining camps of Arizona had been the scene of bitter conflicts, accompanied by even more violence and lawlessness than is usual in American labor warfare. In the early summer of 1917 strikes had practically closed most of the mines for over three months, and this at a time when the demand for copper for munitions was most urgent. The feeling throughout the country was one of impatience and strong disapproval of the unpatriotic action of the miners in hampering our munition production simply because they wanted higher wages. The refusal of the copper companies to pay higher wages was not considered unpatriotic. Then suddenly the country, or at least the part east of the Rockies, was shocked by the tale of a mass deportation of striking miners, no less than 1186 of them, from Bisbee, Arizona, to the desert, where they were left for two days. That the soldiers from Douglas rescued them and escorted them to Columbus, New Mexico, where they were cared for by the government, did not make the conduct of the deporting authorities seem any less black. The strike, which had been on for some time, was not caused by any ordinary grievance the men had but apparently more because they knew the mining companies were making enormous war profits and believed they had a right to their share.

The deportation was carried out by the county sheriff under the direction of officials of the Phelps-Dodge Corporation and the Calumet and Arizona Mining Company. The sheriff had demanded Federal troops to control the situation but the governor refused, since an investigating officer of the U. S. Army had reported to him that troops were not needed or warranted under the existing conditions. So the sheriff took matters into his own hands, and early in the morning of July 12 he swore in some 2000 deputies, armed, of course, and rounded up the 1186 miners, put them aboard a train, and took them to a station in the desert — Hermanas, New Mexico. There they were dumped, and the deputies departed in the train, leaving them shelterless — in July! — and without "adequate food and water" for two days. The leaders of this enterprise even exercised censorship over telephone and telegraph lines, to prevent news of the deportation from reaching the outside world. How the story leaked out and who sent the soldiers to the rescue I do not know.

Lawlessness in labor disputes, even on the part of officers of the law, is an old American tradition and usually an outbreak does not attract much attention, but this was too highhanded and dramatically ruthless to be passed over. Moreover, Arizona copper represented 28 per cent of the nation's supply, and unless order could be brought back in that field there would be a serious shortage of this essential metal. So urgent was the situation that the Federal government was obliged to step in and a Mediation Commission which President Wilson had sent to the Pacific Coast to inquire into the notorious Mooney case was instructed to stop over in Arizona and report on the Bisbee deportation. The commission could only condemn the procedure as illegal, as a denial of rights safeguarded by the Constitution, a violation of the laws of Arizona, interference with interstate lines of communication, and so on, but no legal action was ever taken against the two mining companies or against the sheriff.

When I reached Arizona, more than a year had passed since the Mediation Commission had issued its report, but the shadow of the deportation still lay heavy on the copper country. There was a state of armed truce in the camps, everyone lined up on one side or the other, eyeing his adversaries with suspicion and hatred, peaceful for the moment, but ready to fight again at the drop of a hat. There were no neutrals anywhere. I asked the hotel clerk in Globe about physicians in the camp, or lawyers, or clergymen, whom I could interview, only to be told: "All the doctors here are copper, but they say there is one labor doctor in Miami. The lawyers are copper too, all but the one the union hires. They say Dean Scarlett of the Cathedral in Phoenix is labor, but most of the ministers are copper." Only one labor doctor could I find in all that region; the rest were deeply dyed copper, some of them more royalist than the king.

My first stop was in Phoenix where my cousin, Dr. Allen Hamilton Williams, was living, and he took me to see Dean Scarlett of the Cathedral (now Bishop of Missouri), who gave me a very sympathetic and understanding description of the labor war in that state. Allen also introduced me to a friend of his who was working in the New Cornelia mine in Ajo, and I decided to make my first inspection there. This miner was an Austrian nobleman, Count Coudenhove, who, in the summer of 1914, had been shooting in the wilds of western Canada with an English friend. They emerged from the wilderness to learn that their countries were at war. The Englishman helped Count Coudenhove to escape over the border into Montana, but the latter soon found himself quite without funds and the British Navy saw to it that none could reach him from Austria. I forget how he had worked his way down to Arizona, but there he was, with a job in the Ajo mine. He had come to Phoenix to consult Allen because, after working in the tank house at Ajo, he lost thirty pounds. He laid off a while and recovered weight, then went back and was losing it again. Allen suspected tuberculosis but it was not evident. When the Count described his job to me, I suspected slow poisoning from arseniureted hydrogen fumes, which would bring on a severe anemia and encourage a tubercular process. So, though there had been no complaint from Ajo about the jackhammer, I thought I had better go down and see if my theory as to arsenic was possibly right.

Ajo is very near the Mexican border, and to reach it my friend and I had to spend the night at Maricopa. There was no inn, only a long shed, with two rows of rooms and a passage in between. The rooms were really more like horse stalls; the walls were only about eight feet high, having a free space above, and there was no door, only a heavy canvas curtain. However, the very casualness was reassuring, and after all the room was as much shut in as is a Pullman berth. Anyway our night was quite undisturbed and we woke to see sunrise over the desert. The country was much more beautiful than that around Phoenix, and Ajo, when we reached it, was a surprise and delight — a little Spanish village which fitted so beautifully into the background of desert and barren mountains. The men in charge of the New Cornelia mine and leaching works told us it was the work of Colonel Jack Greenway, who had copied a village in Spain called Cornelia. It was he who had determined to exploit by a new method, used only in one mine in South America, the ore from a surface outcropping, and to do this he was obliged not only to build the plant and the village but to bring water from forty miles away. It was a great achievement and one would hardly have thought that a man who was faced with these enormous difficulties would have had time to think about beauty as well.

That same evening I was taken over the leaching plant, for Count Coudenhove had told me that the fumes in the tank house were worse at night. I am not a very courageous person and that visit was something of an ordeal. It began with a climb in the dark up to the third story of the crushing mill on a sort of glorified ladder running up the outside wall, with open treads and a high hand rail on one side only. Coming down was much worse than going up. The crushed ore was leached with dilute sulphuric acid and then by electrolysis the pure metal was recovered. The acid was in enormous tanks and I was escorted around them on a narrow path which ran along the edges, and here again there was only a hand rail between me and that evil-looking, dark, bubbling acid, and I had the feeling all the time that if I stumbled I could so easily slip under the rail and plunge into the acid.

It was here that, according to my theory, Count Coudenhove might have breathed fumes of arseniureted hydrogen, for in the electrolytic process nascent hydrogen is formed, and if any arsenic is present it will combine with the latter to form this very poisonous gas. Practically all copper ore has some arsenic in combination, but I could not get from the engineers in charge any admission that Ajo ore contained arsenic. There would have been little use in having a specimen analyzed; ore is not uniform, and a negative result might mean that I had hit on a lump which was arsenic-free. Only repeated analyses of the air of the tank house would settle the question and that, obviously, was not part of my job. I was sent to the copper camps to study the effect of the jackhammer, and so to this day I do not know if there is arsenic in the fumes from this electrolytic copper production. Count Coudenhove returned to his home soon after and is still living.

The next day we visited the open shafts on the mountainside and I watched the working of the jackhammer, which I found quite different from the stonecutters' air hammer. The jackhammer is big and very heavy, which in itself lessens vibration; the tool is not held in the hand but is inserted in the hammer, which is held in both hands and delivers less than half the number of strokes per minute that the cutters' hammer does. The work is also much less steady than that of the stonecutter; the miner is continually moving to another spot to drill. I tested the jackhammer and found the vibrations nothing like so great as in stonecutting, and I had to hold it lightly for if I pressed down hard on it, the tool stuck. When I asked the men about dead fingers, they looked at me in astonishment. Clearly they knew no such condition. In the stone mills every man knew. If I said to an Italian, "*Dita morte?*" he would hold up two, three, four fingers, according to the extent of the affection. This meant that my inquiry in the copper mines would probably not be very fruitful, but it must be completed.

As we walked back to the village along the railway tracks I asked my guides, three engineers and officials, if the miners were organized, and was not surprised to be told that the union was a thing of the past. We discussed it a bit and one of them said, "You say the men want more self-government; of course that means they want us to recognize the union. That is impossible — we can't deal with their leaders, they don't know anything about the management of a business, what demands are possible and what are impossible. Often they don't want to settle the trouble, but to make it worse, because they are dreaming of taking over the mines themselves. Why, when Colonel Greenway had pushed through this enormous enterprise, built this camp — and you have seen what it is like — right in the desert, run the works for years with no money coming in, what did the men do but come and say they wanted to be in on the profits, fifty-fifty, when they hadn't done a thing but mine ore? Well, we settled that in short order and we've kept it settled."

I did not ask how it was settled and after a short silence he began, to my great surprise, to talk about the Bisbee deportations. I said, mildly, that the story had rather shocked the East, and I wondered if there was another side to it. He replied with some warmth that Easterners could not be expected to understand. "I wasn't in Bisbee at the time," he went on, "and I didn't belong to either of the two companies, but all the same I stand by them. All I ask is, 'Who were the men that did it?' I know those men. They aren't just capitalists; lots of them are engineers, chemists, doctors, college-bred men, who couldn't act any way but white and square. There simply wasn't anything else for them to do. They knew the strikers had it fixed to tie up the mines, the government wanted copper for the war, and if they were to keep the mines running, they must get in the first blow. So they just rounded up the trouble makers and hustled them out on a train. Of course nobody died of thirst in the desert, the soldiers came and got them. No, the company men didn't know the soldiers were coming. I suppose they didn't stop to think what would happen — all they thought about was getting them out."

I made no comment and we walked on in silence for a while, then one of the engineers said: "Well, of course, it didn't do any permanent good, I suppose we must admit it did harm. But then, the Phelps-Dodge people never meant to deport so many — the thing got away from them. If they had got rid of fifteen or twenty of the agitators, it would have settled the trouble and there would have been no scandal. But they had brought in outsiders, deputy sheriffs, and those men went into houses and routed strikers out of their beds, raided poolrooms and took every man in them. Then when the mine officials saw what they had on their hands, the hundreds of strikers herded into the ball park, and mad as hornets, of course, they were up against it. For the moment they themselves were armed and the strikers were not, but once let the strikers out and they would be armed and it would be war. For two hours they kept them there and consulted, then they backed up a train and hustled them out. They gave them their chance, asked each man was he for the company, or for the strike, but not one, not even the really conservative men, would say he was for the company, so they all had to go."

"Well, what would you have done," I asked, "when it was put up to you in the presence of your comrades to choose between sticking to them and going over to the other side, with a war on?" "Oh well," he said, "I suppose I'd have stuck too. But it was a stupid affair. They lost a lot of first-rate men."

The Globe-Miami region came next. Allen Williams motored us up, a wonderfully beautiful drive over rather precarious roads. Nowadays one can reach Roosevelt Dam for lunch, go on to Globe and back to Phoenix for dinner, but we were lucky to make the dam by evening. We stayed seven days in Globe, for it is the center of a big mining district. Here I had my first experience of exploring a mine. Dressed in miner's overalls and helmet, the latter with a safety lamp fastened in front, we stepped into a "cage," which is a flimsy, shaky elevator, devoid of walls or anything else one can cling to, and dropped down into darkness. None of these mines is deep, as mines go, but in the first one, the Old Dominion, we dropped eight hundred feet, and that seemed a long way to me. Down in the mine I was expected to follow my leader, and I did — indeed I was pleased and flattered by the way he assumed that I was as good as a man, and could be trusted to look after myself. This attitude is found in its perfection out in the West, but it begins to appear in the Middle West, and only in the East and South does one meet with the tiresome tradition that a woman is something different and must be treated differently.

So I trudged along, stooping to avoid overhangs, and thankful for the protection my helmet provided against bumps, scrambling on hands and knees up into a stope to see the hammer at work, climbing down an eighty-foot ladder into a black pit, and, worst of all, crossing deep pits on rails which were so far apart I felt sure I could fall between them if I slipped. Some of the jackhammers had water attachments to keep down the dust and some of the mines were damp; in others dust was thick and often there was no effort to control it. The vibrating jackhammer, which was the object of my inquiry, seemed to me of far less importance than the dust which it produced. The Inspiration Mine in Miami impressed me then as the best as far as ventilation went, and the construction of drifts and tunnels, which were large and clean, also the signal system for train cars and the excellent modern change house for the miners. But several mines were devoid of either dust control or precautions against accidents which, even I could see, were needed.

My interviews with the doctors were not very enlightening. That they had never heard of spastic anemia of the fingers did not surprise me, for I was already convinced it did not exist in the copper camps, but I was irritated to find few of them taking the dust problem seriously. Most of them denied that there was any unusual incidence of tuberculosis among the miners. One man who admitted that he did see a good many cases said that these were consumptives who had come out to Arizona to get well. Several had the label of the "Loyal Legion," the anti-labor organization of the day, prominently displayed in their offices, which seemed a bit tactless. But tact has no place in war, and some of these doctors were passionate partisans, only too eager to discuss the strikes and to give me their side of the conflict. However, I did meet three well-trained men who were in a quite different class.

I was glad to find that in both Globe and Miami the union still survived and headquarters were still open, so for the first time I could get at the men in surroundings where they were free to talk and I spent a good deal of time interviewing the leaders and the English-speaking miners. Always I have found miners above the average of workmen in independence, resourcefulness, initiative, and pluck, and this is only to be expected when one thinks of what their work is like. A miner has no foreman to direct him, it is up to him to place his drills in the way he thinks will result in bringing down the most ore. The safety expert may instruct him in the principles of accident prevention, but their application depends on his judgment and decision. He works on his own and prefers it that way.

The men I met were Scotch, English, American, Spanish and Mexican. Few of them had been long in this camp, almost all had come in after the strike of a year and a half ago. There were at the time a couple of thousand men in the district, in underground work. I examined some thirty of them for spastic anemia of the fingers, but there was no sign of it nor had any man ever heard of it. Then we settled down to a discussion of the jackhammer and what was wrong with it. First, dust; there they were certainly right, it had increased enormously the dust from drilling. "But the employers tell me," I said, "that you refuse to use a wet drill which would keep down the dust." That brought prompt denials. If the company would make allowance for the extra time it took to work the wet drill the men would be only too glad to use it. But although the mining was done on a time, not a piece basis, a certain number of holes must be drilled or the man would be canned. Two drilling-machine jackhammers were in use, the stoper and the plugger, the latter much the more dust-producing. Both could be operated with water, and if an adjustment in wages were made to cover lost time, the men would be willing to take the responsibility of enforcing the use of the water attachment. This was agreed to by all the "white" miners. But it was admitted that the Mexicans did object to getting wet.

Then what about the complaint Washington had received, that the vibrations of the jackhammer were injuring the miners' health? From a host of statements I gathered that it was the vibration of the jackhammer when it was held firmly against the body that gave the men a strange sensation, and convinced them that lungs or heart or intestines or kidneys were receiving some sort of injury. The miner has to work in all sorts of positions and sometimes he has to press against the jackhammer with the upper chest, sometimes the lower chest, and sometimes the hammer comes against his abdomen. The discomfort is greatest in the last position. I tested this on myself, resting the heavy, jerking handle of the hammer against the three parts of my body. When it pressed against the breast bone and upper ribs it was not so bad, but the lower ribs furnished much less protection, and when it came to the soft abdomen I found the vibration quite intolerable. Lower down, against the thighs, it is again bearable. But I had no idea whether any real harm would be caused by it, and I told the miners that while I was sure the dust raised by the jackhammer was dangerous and the use of the water attachments must be worked out, I could not say anything definite about the harm done by pressing the tool against the body, for nobody knew. Later on, when I returned to Chicago, I consulted Dr. Thor Rothstein, who had examined the stonecutters. He said it was a totally new problem and he did not know the answer. Possibly the same form of spastic anemia seen in the stonecutters' fingers might be brought about in the abdominal vessels by the vibration of the jackhammer, but to answer that question either way would mean a long and complicated study.

Our next destination was a cluster of camps (mining towns out there are still "camps") at Clifton, Morenci, and Metcalf, which we reached at night, having made an early start by train from Globe to Solomon, a Mormon town, then by stage over the desert, with one breakdown, to Gila where we took train to Clifton. The next morning, after a miserable breakfast — wretched coffee and condensed milk served in its original can, all sticky with trickles down the sides — I went to call on the head of the Arizona Copper Company, a Scotch concern, one of the largest in Arizona. The general manager, Norman Carmichael, was Scotch. I sent in my government card and when he entered the room he said, very surprisingly, "How do you do, Miss Addams?"

I said, "My name is Hamilton, Mr. Carmichael." "Oh yes, of course, I know. You see, I associate you with Miss Addams and so when I saw you, the name slipped off my tongue." "But," I said in complete bewilderment, "why did you associate me with Miss Addams, how did you know I live at Hull-House? How do you know anything about me? I've just come." "Oh, my dear lady," he laughed, "I know all about you, your past history, when you reached Arizona, where you have been and whom you have talked to — everything. We think it wise," he concluded more gravely, "to know as much as we can about people who come to this state on errands like yours."

The experience of being followed by spies was not entirely new to me, for I had had it in German-occupied Belgium in 1915. But then I was an intruding alien, and it was war. Here I was in my own country on a mission from my own government. It made me curiously angry at first, then it began to seem amusing. Never before had I been treated as a dangerous plotter whom even great commercial bodies feared and felt they must protect themselves against. Years afterwards, in Boston, I met an elderly retired mining engineer and, to amuse him, I told him this story. He took it in entire seriousness. "Yes," he said, "I remember that, I was in Arizona at the time. We thought you might be a trouble maker, but in the end we found you were perfectly impartial and fair." He had no feeling that there was anything strange in setting spies to dog the steps of a Federal agent.

The Clifton-Morenci-Metcalf camps are more remote and isolated than the Globe-Miami region and the mine villages were almost completely Mexican. Morenci is on a mountainside and then had only enough level space to provide a little plaza and school playground. To reach it we had been driven in Mr. Carmichael's car through a narrow canyon, where the mine railway ran. Here, Mr. Scotland, the manager of the Humboldt mine, told us, the miners took possession during the strike of 1917, tore up the rails, cut the wires, and had the camp at their mercy, for this was the only road out. We lunched that day at the house of the company doctor, and his wife told us that she and the children had been driven by night up the mountain to a solitary ranch, but the doctor had returned to take his luck with the other mine officials. Eventually, they too were obliged to make their escape over the mountains and leave the camp to the strikers. "Deportations," Mr. Scotland said, "are not uncommon in Arizona, nor confined to one side. In this strike the white miners were deported by the Mexicans, cleared out of the camp because they had no use for the Mexicans who were running the union and would not join it. There was plenty of violence in that affair. This has been a Mexican camp ever since."

The Arizona Copper Company's mines and the Phelps-Dodge Corporations were excellent places to study the working of the various machines: the water-lines; the different varieties of jackhammer, weighing from 40 to 70 pounds, mounted so that the man need not hold them against his body, or unmounted, so that he must, some with water attachment of one kind or another, some without; the stoper, wet or dry; the Sullivan rotator, and so on. My notes are full of the discussions I held with managers, engineers, and doctors over the dust problem, for all the practical men recognized it, especially in the mines where the ore matrix has a high proportion of quartz. I saw a great variety of devices for wet drilling, but there was general agreement that only white miners would use water, the Mexicans said it gave them rheumatism; they were much less afraid of the dust.

As to the vibrating jackhammer, the men's complaint was held to be justified. It did no harm to brace the hammer against the thighs, but some men were actually nauseated when they pressed it against the body. In one mine they provided short boards which the men could use as a shield, but all the officials admitted that only mounting or suspending the hammer would prevent the trouble, and that was a difficult problem in practice. I watched one man drilling a hole, with the jackhammer braced first against his thighs, then his lower abdomen, and by slow stages mounting up to the level of his shoulders. He stood with his feet braced back, his body strained forward and shaking. It certainly looked like strenuous work.

Our visit to Clifton-Morenci closed with a dinner at Mr. Carmichael's with two Phelps-Dodge officials. By that time I had quite forgiven him for having set spies on my trail and we parted good friends.

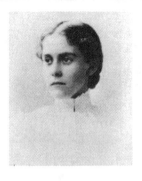

Alice Hamilton at twenty-four, the year she graduated from medical school (1893). Courtesy of The Schlesinger Library, Radcliffe College.

Medical Clinic at Michigan. Alice Hamilton is third from left in front row. Courtesy of University of Michigan Medical School Collection, Michigan Historical Collections, Bentley Historical Library, University of Michigan.

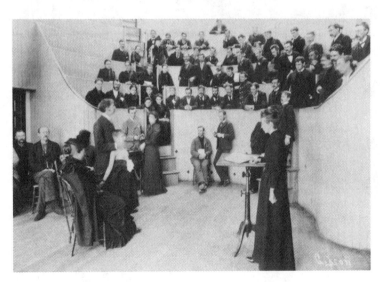

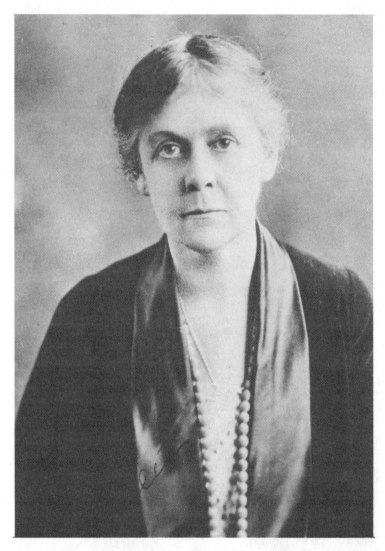

Alice Hamilton c. 1925. Courtesy of The Schlesinger Library, Radcliffe College.

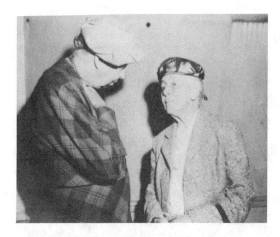

Alice Hamilton and Eleanor Roosevelt at a meeting of The International Relations Club, Connecticut College, October 1958. Courtesy of The Schlesinger Library, Radcliffe College.

Alice and Margaret Hamilton in Hadlyme, Connecticut, in 1959. Photograph by Paul J. Maguire. Courtesy of the *Boston Globe*.

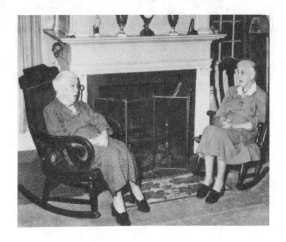

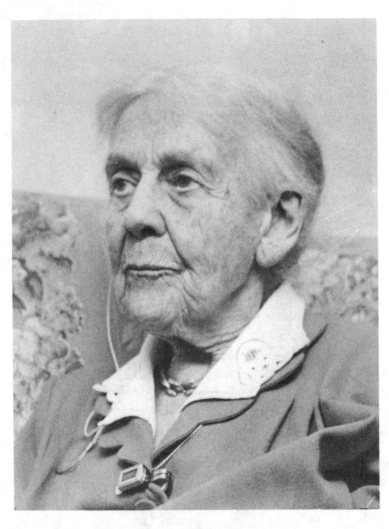

Alice Hamilton in 1959. Photograph by Paul J. Maguire. Courtesy of the *Boston Globe.*

XIV

Europe in 1919

CLARA LANDSBERG and I returned to Chicago from
Arizona the last of January and two very busy months followed, with preparing my report on Arizona copper mining
for Washington and taking part in the preparation of a
report on the question of health insurance for Illinois. The
state legislature had appointed a committee to inquire into
the necessity for such legislation, for at that time, 1915 to
1917, there was a good deal of public interest in the lack of
adequate medical care, especially for the near-poor, and a
number of states took up the question. Then we entered
the war and feeling against Germany was so bitter that it
was easy for some of the large insurance companies to put
a stop to the whole movement simply by denouncing it
as "made in Germany." Only lately has public interest in
the subject been revived. Our committee consisted of the
usual assortment, an employer, two A.F. of L. representatives,
the head of the Visiting Nurse Association, a delegate from
the State Medical Society, a social worker, and myself. Professor H. A. Millis of the University of Chicago was our secretary and supervised the work. We made a fairly thorough study
of typical regions in the city, and certainly to me the evidence
was conclusive that some form of health insurance was needed.
Indeed, my life at Hull-House had convinced me of that
already. But Gompers's A.F. of L. had declared against it,
which meant negative votes from Matthew Woll and Mary

McEnerney; the State Medical Society was equally opposed and so was the Illinois Manufacturers' Association. So the social worker, John Ransome, and I had to content ourselves with a minority report.

Early in April I met Miss Addams in New York and on April 9 sailed with her on our old friend the *Noordam*, which had carried us to Holland in 1915. We went to attend the first meeting of the Women's International League for Permanent Peace since the one in The Hague in 1915. Miss Addams had kept in close touch with the groups of pacifist women in all the different countries, even after our entrance into the war, for the Dutch, Swiss, and Scandinavian women acted as go-betweens. It had been settled at the 1915 meeting that the next one should be held at the same time and in the same place as the conference to settle the terms of peace, for we all assumed that this would be in a neutral country and that it would be really a peace conference, with both sides represented. But when Paris was chosen and it was clear that only the victors were to participate, the plan was given up. The German and Austrian women could not possibly go to France, so Zurich was chosen instead.

There was quite a little group of Peace Congress women on the *Noordam* — Mrs. Florence Kelley, Emily Balch, Rose Nicholls, Mrs. Lucia Ames Mead, Mrs. Louis Post, Mrs. John J. White, Jeannette Rankin. Our passage was smooth and there was opportunity for much eager talk about the war and the coming peace and reconstruction, and about the plan for a League of Nations. Of course there were many different opinions, especially with regard to the way the defeated Germans should be treated, and Miss Addams implored me to be discreet, which I was for most of the time. Indeed, the only indiscreet statement I remember making was to a clergyman who had upset me by saying that Germany was a country which had lost its soul. I told him that Lenin was the greatest man who had emerged from the war, and we separated in mutual disesteem.

In Paris we met young Lewis Gannett, then a foreign correspondent, who promised to go to Zurich and give the Congress as much publicity as he could. We stayed in Paris some seventeen days, including a five-day trip through the devastated regions. The Versailles Conference was on, and one met everywhere Americans who had come because of it, to bring protests and petitions, or simply to watch and report what was happening. My diary is full of records of lunches, teas, dinners, even breakfasts, with those we knew or came to know — with Lincoln Steffens, William Allen White, Henry Nevinson, Frank Simonds, Manley Hudson, Charles R. Crane, Felix Frankfurter, Judge Julian Mack, Henry Morgenthau, Senior, Oscar Straus, Lillian Wald, Ida Tarbell. We met also Ethel Sidgwick, Fridtjof Nansen, and Romain Rolland and his sister, Madeleine. Rolland had come back to Paris for the first time since the war, to see his dying mother. He made a very striking impression, tall, blue-eyed, more like a Scandinavian than a Frenchman. Indeed, there was something of a resemblance between him and Fridtjof Nansen, the same burning blue eyes, the same impression of strength both physical and spiritual, and the same intense absorption in a cause. But Nansen had his feet on the earth. One was not sure Rolland had. Nansen's cause was entirely objective — the relief of the starving; Rolland's cause, aversion to war, was closely bound up with his own personality.

Our talks with most of these people confirmed the misgivings we had felt as to the coming treaty of peace, for we found a general distrust of the three men who held the destiny of the world in their hands: Clemenceau, strong-willed, vengeful, taking short views; Lloyd George, far more astute and alive to realities, but too ready to compromise on crucial matters; Wilson, arrogant but bewildered, ignorant, yet unwilling to consult his own experts, and never realizing the power he could have wielded. There were many in Paris then who were watching with dismay the way things were shaping themselves, but who could not even get a hearing. Some of the most disillusioned men we met were newspaper correspondents who seemed able to get access to all the undertones of the conference and to grow more cynical the deeper they went. They kept saying that if Wilson would only threaten in real earnest to leave Versailles and go home, he could bring Clemenceau to terms. Charles R. Crane told me that the war had started in a Balkan mess and bade fair to end in a worse one if national rights were ignored in favor of the victors. We could not feel pride in the part Americans were playing in the formulation of the peace terms, but at least we were asking nothing for ourselves. The way the former German colonies were being allocated to the victors was shocking, the worst instance perhaps being the transfer of part of German Africa from Germany, which was "unfit to rule over blacks," to Portugal. And this after Nevinson's revelation of the atrocious treatment of the Negroes in Portugal's cocoa plantations. Nor were these transactions bettered by Philip Kerr's covering note to the Germans in which he assured them that colonies brought no advantage to the ruling country, only a heavy burden of responsibility. I have always resented the phrase "Anglo-Saxon hypocrisy," but I had to accept it then and admit that Orlando's blunt admission of "sacred egoism" was more to be respected.

The newly invented "mandates" were also a stumbling block,

for the promise to respect the will of the people in the choice of the mandatory power was not being followed. We saw a good deal of Alexander Rhibany, who had come on behalf of the Syrians, and who told us that they would not object to becoming a "mandated country" if the United States were the mandatory power — they would even accept England, but France, never. And, of course, France was what they got.

I remember a luncheon Juliet Rublee gave, where we met Nansen, the Frank Simondses, William Allen White, and Dr. E. J. Dillon and his young wife. The talk turned on Bolshevist Russia and on the Allied blockade, the *cordon sanitaire* which was shutting out not only foodstuffs but essential medical supplies, antiseptics, anesthetics, quinine. Frank Simonds defended it; starvation was the only way to bring Russia to her senses (and we were eating such abundant and delicious food!). Dr. Dillon, who had just published his *Eclipse of Russia*, was not so sure but quite willing to play with the idea. William Allen White, who sat next me, was so disturbed and wretched that he could not eat, but it was Nansen who burst out in a tirade of indignation against the cold-blooded cruelty of such a policy. I wished then, as I did so often during that journey, that I belonged to one of the small neutral countries which had kept their sanity and their human capacity for pity and kindness during those savage years. They seemed to me like wise and experienced old women looking on while a crowd of hotheaded youths cracked each others' heads, knowing that they had no strength to stop the senseless fight, but ready to step in and bind up wounds when it was over.

Something had happened that winter before we left home which etched in sharp lines on my mind the contrast between my own country and the neutrals in Europe. We Americans had not been told that the Armistice was not followed by a lifting of the blockade, although that was the promise made to Germany. On the contrary, the cessation of the war and the surrender of the German fleet made a complete blockade of the North Sea possible for the first time, and all supplies of sea-borne food could thus be kept out of Germany. The Allies understood very clearly that Germany would never accept the peace terms they were planning to offer unless she were forced to do so by her starving people. But most of us did not know this and it was a complete surprise when a group of prominent German women, in December 1918, cabled two American women, Mrs. Woodrow Wilson and Miss Addams, begging them to protest against the seizure of 3000 milch cows in Germany destined for France and Belgium, and reminding them of the plight of the starving German children. Miss Addams was never allowed to receive the cable but the newspapers did and when they printed it the reaction of the public was such as to shake one's faith in one's fellow countrymen. Not indignation over the broken promise to Germany, not pity for the starving. No; instead, a wave of rage seemed to roll over the country. Miss Addams's mail has often brought her angry and even scurrilous letters, but except for the time of the "bayonet charge" episode, I never saw anything so full of hate and bitterness as the letters she then received, all of them from people of the educated, well-to-do class.

Nothing could have shown more clearly the searing effect of war than this attitude on the part of Americans whose kindliness and generosity have been proverbial. The neutrals were caring for the sick, the children, the aged, regardless of which side they were on. They were behaving as children of our Father in Heaven, who "maketh His sun to rise on the evil and on the good, and sendeth rain on the just and on the unjust." And there were Americans who, living in a neutral country, caught this spirit. In Berne we met Dr. Alfred Worcester, who was with the American Red Cross. He told us that the state of the Austrian children who were sent to Switzerland was so shocking that the Red Cross workers believed thousands of them left in Austria must die unless the peace treaty were signed quickly so that food could be sent in. "A trainload of food was waiting on the border," he said, "and when word came that peace was here, we cabled to the State Department asking that it be ordered at once to Vienna. Then we had word that not a pound of food was to go to Austria. We simply could not understand it."

My brother Quint turned up while we were in Paris, waiting to be demobilized and sent home. He was with the Red Cross, acting as a liaison officer, for his specialty is Romance languages, and he had left his chair in the University of Wisconsin when we entered the war and had sailed for France soon after. Throughout his stay in France he had written us in full about the economic and political situation there, but the only letters that reached us were those which told of his influenza, his plans, his personal experiences. It was plain, as we talked it over, that the French censorship had been thorough.

We had some pleasant excursions together while Miss Addams was occupied with the French W.I.L. women and interviewing important people. One was a Sunday excursion with M. and Mme. Flateau to their château in Bellevue, one of those typical French châteaux with pepper-box turrets, built for the Abbé Boileau in the seventeenth century. The Flateaus had adopted Quint, after the kindly custom of the French during the war, and had been very good to him. Mme. Flateau asked me if it were really true that during the war we Americans had voluntarily restricted our food, gone without meat, wheat flour, sugar. I assured her we had. "But,

not when you had guests?" she asked. I said that then above
all times we would not have dared serve meat on a meatless
day, or more than a spoonful of sugar, or we would be dis-
graced. "Oh well," she sighed, "we French are not that way."
Yet she had lost her only son in the war and made no open
lament.

That evening Quint took me to dine in a restaurant which
he knew from his student days and had come back to with
pleasure, for it was frequented by professors from the Sor-
bonne, and he had made the acquaintance of a number of
them. As we sat down a young woman, very attractive, and
gentle-looking, was making her way out, and was exchanging
friendly *bonsoirs* with everyone. I asked Quint who she was,
and he said she was a young war widow who was left with a
little son and a very inadequate pension. "She has been obliged
to become the mistress of a rich old man whom she cannot
possibly like and everyone admires her, for it is only devotion
to her little son that makes her do it." The French are different — there is no denying it.

We were told repeatedly while we were in Paris that we must
visit the devastated regions, that until we had seen the destruction we had no right to criticize the French for their bitterness
and vengefulness. Then the Red Cross, I think through the
prompting of Miss Wald, offered a car and a chauffeur to
take us on a five-day trip, Miss Addams, Miss Wald, Jeannette
Rankin, and myself. It was the last week in April, but bleak
and cold, gray skies all the time, rain often. It was weather
appropriate for such a trip; it made us realize the misery borne
by the soldiers in the trenches much more sharply than we
could have done if we had gone in late spring, with sunshine and sprouting green and soft air. Many tragic pictures
rise before me as I think back over that journey. One is the

picture of Vimy Ridge where the Canadian Army suffered such heavy losses. Our car broke down there and Miss Addams and I walked along the ridge with its ghastly, shell-shocked skeletons of trees, to where Chinese laborers were digging graves for the bodies of English soldiers. Just after a battle the bodies were buried hastily, without coffins sometimes, and it was the work of the Chinese indentured laborers to dig them up and give them lasting burial. It was work only the Chinese would do. The skies were gray above us, the earth barren and scarred, the wind was piercingly cold; the whole made a scene of unrelieved tragedy.

We spent that night in Lille, where my friend Mabel Kittredge was feeding children under Hoover's Committee for Belgian Relief. She took us to see a school clinic and there I saw for the first time what I was destined to see so often in Germany, the child victims of long starvation, for these children of Lille had suffered from the scarcity of food, as had the German children, up to the Armistice. But then relief had come and though I was shocked at their emaciation, their condition was not nearly so bad as what I saw later in Germany. The doctor who was examining them could speak only in a whisper, for he had lost his voice through nervous shock when Lille was taken by the Germans. It was a strange scene, carried on in whispers, for the children, not understanding why it was a secret, accepted the fact and whispered back. Later on we saw them sitting at table, eating thick soup and bread, a very comforting sight. I had been much interested to watch the making of that soup. The Lille women used meat and vegetables as we would, but instead of adding water they put a quantity of green leaves of all kinds, the outside leaves of cabbage and lettuce, and a lot of what we should call weeds, through a grinding machine which reduced them to a fluid green paste, and that provided almost all the liquid needed, and of course doubled the value of the soup.

We passed Ste. Menehould and the Argonne the following day and reached the headquarters of the Quakers at Grange le Conte, where we found Margaret Curtis of Boston and Mr. and Mrs. Charles Rhoads, and William Scattergood of Philadelphia. That evening a group of some sixty young Quakers assembled in the big room. They were English and American, working under a former Warden of Toynbee Hall, rebuilding ruined houses in the villages and farms, putting up temporary refuges for those who had already come back, and supplying the essentials which would make life possible.

Miss Addams had lost a nephew in the war, John Linn, an Episcopal clergyman who had gone as chaplain to the front and was shot down as he was passing from one "fox hole" to another. Somewhere in that region he was buried and she wanted to find his grave, so the next day Mr. Scattergood drove us in search of it. Here the battlefields were hardly cleared at all; one saw tin hats, canteens, knitted socks, lying in the mud as they had fallen. It was mud everywhere, deep, slimy mud, and it rained again and the cold seemed more piercing than ever. We found the grave, at the far end of a ruined farmyard. There were three rows of iron crosses, each cross with an identification tag hanging on it. John Linn's cross stood between that of a Greek-American soldier and that of a Polish-American.

Before we left Paris for Switzerland we went to see Robert Cecil, who was Minister of Blockade during most of the war. It was the threatened confiscation of milch cows from Germany that induced Miss Addams to call on him and beg him to use his influence against a move so disastrous for a country that had been suffering hunger for three years or more. Robert Cecil, now Viscount Cecil, is a striking-looking man, very tall and stoop-shouldered, with deep-set melancholy eyes, ugly in a strong, attractive way. We did not succeed in our errand. Lord Robert's feeling was that the devastation wrought in invaded France and Belgium by the Germans must be, so far as possible, repaired by the Germans, that this was simple justice, and Miss Addams's protest that the punishment was falling not on those responsible for the destruction but on guiltless babies did not change his attitude.

Zurich was a great relief after France. We stayed in a simple, pleasant "hostel," the Glockenhof, where most of the delegates were housed. Food restrictions were more evident there than in Paris — no white rolls for breakfast, no cream for coffee, little butter. But there was a delightful atmosphere, which came partly from the lovely hospitality of the Zurich women, and partly from the relief of finding oneself at last in a circle of like-minded people who took it for granted that war was an unmixed evil and that to treat the conquered with vengeance was only to prepare for another war. The English had sent a delegation of very unusual force and ability. No other country was so brilliantly represented. Mrs. Pethick Lawrence was there, Hilda Swanwick, Mary Sheepshanks, Chrystal Mac-Millan, Mrs. Despard, Margaret Ashton, Katharine Marshall, Kathleen Courtney, Dr. Ethel Williams. From Ireland came the Irish Quaker, Louie Bennett, who told me, when I said I had never heard of Irish Quakers, that there were several colonies of them, founded at a time when intolerance drove them out of Protestant England but Catholic Ireland welcomed them. She told me also of the tragic Easter uprising and the repression that followed. She and some other women pacifists had urged the Irish to offer passive resistance to the English authorities, to refuse to run trains carrying soldiers, or military supplies, to bring all services to a standstill so long as a region was occupied, but never to resort to violence. It was not a program that appealed to Irishmen, no matter how sensible it sounded.

Our French colleagues had been refused passports by their government, but the German women came, Gertrud Baer, Anita Augsburg, Lida Heymann, also the Austrians, Yella Hertzka and Leopoldina Kulke from Vienna, Paula Pogany and Wilma Glucklich from Budapest. It was pleasant to meet again our traveling companion of 1915, Dr. Aletta Jacobs of Holland. There was, of course, not the least hostile feeling on the part of the women from the victor countries toward those of the vanquished, only an eagerness to renew our ties with them and even a sense of apology, of embarrassment, because we were the fortunate and the safe, they the helpless who did not yet even know what fate awaited them. They showed the effect of the war privations as none of us did, and though they said little about their sufferings, what they did let fall was all the more poignant. I was getting on a street car with a Viennese woman and as we took our seats she said, "It is so wonderful here, nobody pushes and shoves and swears at you, everyone gets on quietly." "Well, it is not crowded," I said, "there is room for all." "Oh, but that did not keep us in Vienna from pushing and swearing," she said. "I suppose it was because our nerves were so on edge all the time, we lost our habits of courtesy. You see, we could not think of anything but food, all the time, scheming and contriving and failing almost always. That makes one a primitive creature again; one's civilization is lost."

In Miss Addams's *Peace and Bread in Time of War* she has given a full account of the Zurich conference, and I will not attempt to do more than give a few of my impressions. I remember a speech of hers in which she likened the fanatical nationalism of the day to the fanatical devotion to the medieval Church, which demanded worship for its own sake, demanded that the individual submit to its authority in every walk of life and do all possible to increase its power and wealth. The crime of heresy was now called disloyalty, treason, but it was the same thing, a holding of opinions not permitted by those in authority. And the State held, as the Church had, that all things were permissible which worked for its advantage. I remember, too, the warm discussions that were held with regard to the League of Nations. I was one of those who would have none of it, thinking it would be only a League of the Victors, a second Holy Alliance. Miss Addams, as always, was for accepting even a quarter-loaf, and doing as much with it as could be done. But she did lament the sheer unwisdom of the course followed at the founding of the League. She thought that if only it had taken as its first problem the feeding of the hundred million people in Europe who needed food; if the coal, the iron, the oil, as well as the food, had been distributed under international control to the nations most in need, the League would have restored normal human relationships between the divided peoples and laid the foundations for its future task of bringing peace and security to a war-torn Europe. Instead, at that very time a starvation blockade was being enforced against Russia, in spite of poor Nansen, and against Bolshevist Hungary, in an attempt, as Miss Addams said, "to settle the question of the form of government in a country through the starvation of its people."

The Treaty of Versailles was made public while we were in Zurich and was greeted with dismay by the women of the victor countries, with despair by those of the vanquished. I

think I shall give only the brief preamble to the resolutions
we passed, though a reading of the full text is worth while
if only to see how accurately this obscure group of women
foresaw what results would follow the decision of the famous
statesmen who sat in Versailles: —

This International Congress of Women expresses its deep regret
that the Terms of Peace proposed at Versailles should so seriously
violate the principles upon which alone a just and lasting peace
can be secured, and which the democracies of the world had come
to accept.

By guaranteeing the fruits of the secret treaties to the con-
querors, the Terms of Peace tacitly sanction secret diplomacy,
deny the principles of self-determination, recognize the rights
of the victors to the spoils of war, and create all over Europe dis-
cords and animosities, which can only lead to future wars.

By the demand for the disarmament of one set of belligerents
only, the principle of justice is violated and the rule of force continued. . . .

With a deep sense of responsibility this Congress strongly urges
the Allied and Associated Governments to accept such amend-
ments of the Terms, as shall bring the peace into harmony with
those principles first enumerated by President Wilson upon the
faithful carrying out of which the honor of the Allied peoples
depends.

Soon after our return we received a call from the Quakers
to go to Germany and look into the condition of the children,
especially the effect on them of the long years of underfeeding,
and to report back to the Quakers in America how the need
could be met practically. Carolena Wood brought us this
request, saying that the English Quakers were sending a small
group for this purpose and that Herbert Hoover had suggested
to her that Miss Addams be asked to go on behalf of the

American Society of Friends. Mr. Hoover was in Paris and we went to see him. He told Miss Addams that he hoped she would undertake this mission. "Germany needs not only food," he said, "she needs people of good will to bring her back to normal relations with the rest of the world. It is bad for a man to feel that he is a social outcast, it is bad for a nation to feel itself a pariah among the nations." Of course Miss Addams could not refuse. We had planned to sail for home at the end of the week, but she offered to stay on for another fortnight, thinking that we could, in three weeks' time, make a fairly useful survey in the larger German cities. But it was dismaying to find that Mr. Hoover would not consider sending us in before the Peace Treaty had been signed by the Germans. It would be too dangerous. One could not tell what would happen over there from day to day. The German Government was struggling to hold out against the terms of peace, but whenever it seemed that a refusal was impending, the mobs would form in the Alexander Platz in Berlin and march on the Wilhelmstrasse, demanding peace and an end to starvation. It was clear that the victors had calculated well when they maintained the food blockade all those months.

We promised Mr. Hoover to consider it, although an indefinite stay in Europe was dismaying to our minds and to our pocketbooks. But that same afternoon we had a long tea conference with one of our French colleagues, Mme. Duchêne, and with William Bullitt, Felix Frankfurter, and Dr. Alonzo Taylor, Mr. Hoover's food expert, at the end of which we were both convinced that the need was too great, the chance to help, even a little, too tempting to be refused. We would wait on in Paris and, if our permits did not come soon, go over to England where Miss Addams had many friends and where I could visit chemical and dye factories. Dr. Taylor's account of his experience in Germany was very interesting, for the picture it gave us not only of conditions there, but of what may happen to a thorough conservative when he comes up against a human situation quite new to him. For though he was what one might call a Hoover Republican, he was all for revolution in Germany, revolution of the Left-Wing Socialists against Ebert's Right Wing. He told us that food was beginning to go into Germany but the people could not buy it and the government ought to distribute food free, using the property which rich Germans held in the United States to pay for it. Ebert's group had not the courage to do this and was really not a revolutionary government at all, just the old bureaucracy relying on the old military system under Noske. The rich Germans he denounced as selfish and blind. They had never tolerated any interference and they refused to make reasonable concessions to labor in order to get industry started. The Americans had tried to act as mediators but the industrialists would not yield an inch and Dr. Taylor could see no hope without a revolution led by the extreme radicals.

There was a long wait for our permits and often we were on the point of giving up and taking passage home, but that seemed cowardly. Finally, as the days went on I grew restive and decided to go over to England, Miss Addams promising to meet me there in a fortnight, if the way to Germany did not open up before then.

The morning after my arrival in London I went to the Home Office to talk over my plans with Dr. Thomas Legge and Dr. John Bridge of the Factory Inspection Service. I always enjoy my visits to that part of the Home Office, it is such a contrast to anything we have over here. The rooms are pleasantly old-fashioned and informal, with open fires often, and somebody is always making tea. I am strong for the English worship of tea and I believe that if our workers in office and factory took five minutes off morning and afternoon for a cup of tea with milk and sugar, and a sweet biscuit, it would make work easier and less tiring, which means more efficient.

Dr. Legge advised me to see Professor Stanley Kent of Manchester University, who could tell me more about the chemical works in the Midlands than anyone else. He was staying in Salisbury at the time and I was only too glad to embrace the opportunity to spend the week end in that lovely little city, so I went down Friday afternoon and had three nights at the Old George Inn. It was perfect weather and Salisbury was a haven of rest and beauty. I went to the Cathedral service Sunday morning, and was struck by the absence of mourning in that great congregation of women. In Notre-Dame and in St. Sulpice almost every woman was in deepest black; here no one was. Dr. Kent, when I spoke of it to him at tea that afternoon, said that he supposed hardly a woman in the church had escaped the loss of someone dear to her in the war. But it was looked on as cowardly to proclaim one's loss, one bore it in secret.

The service made a curious impression on me. In Salisbury Cathedral, more than in most, the choir is shut off from nave and transepts by great screens. The procession of clergy and choirboys marched in, ascended to the choir, where they were hidden from our view, and then the service was carried on by men, without any part in it for the women, who sat outside the sacred precincts, meekly listening. No woman's voice took part in the choir singing, yet had it not been for the women the service would have been without an audience, the men and boys would have intoned and sung for themselves alone. It made me think of the Jewish synagogue in our Hull-House neighborhood and of the Orthodox Greek Church there, where

I had sat in the gallery with the women, spectators of the men's worship. Then followed nine days in Manchester, Liverpool, Huddersfield, days of factory visiting under the guidance of factory inspectors who were scholars and gentlemen, such as we did not then find in similar positions in the United States. Miss Margaret Ashton's is the figure that rises to my mind when I think back over those days. I had returned to Manchester from Huddersfield to find that no hotel would take me in, and when Miss Ashton discovered that I had gone to most dubious-looking lodgings, she took me out to her pleasant house in Kinnaird Road for the week end.

Like most of the English Miss Ashton was very casual about her own achievements and still more so about her sufferings in the various causes she had espoused. She was a suffragist and though she did not belong to the militant group, had never smashed windows or poured treacle in letter boxes, she had suffered much rougher handling than had ever been the lot of our most violent militants. Repeatedly she had been dragged out of halls and thrown down the stairs, simply for calling out "Votes for Women." "Was it the police who treated you so roughly?" I asked. "Oh no," she said, "the police do not keep order in our meetings. That is done by wardens selected by the group which holds the meeting. Sometimes it would be Conservative gentlemen, members of County families. But the police would be brutal too, when we would try to march to Parliament to present a petition. Most of us gave up wearing hats, for one does look so drunk and disorderly when one is dragged through the streets with one's hat all awry. The worst thing was the pelting. Once a big, hard gooseberry struck my right eye. It does not seem a dangerous weapon but really I almost lost that eye." I looked at her in wonder, a tiny woman, delicate and gentle, with a weak heart. What could explain such an attitude on the part of Englishmen, such a fierce sex antagonism? Three years before I had been given the vote in Illinois and though I knew that many women in that state had worked hard for it, none had ever been roughly treated, none had ever been jailed.

Miss Ashton was also an avowed pacifist throughout the war and as such she was expelled from the School Board of Manchester, lest she corrupt the minds of the young, but she was allowed to head the group appointed by the city to feed babies and expectant mothers and she was very proud of the record made, a lower infant death rate than ever before.

She took me on Sunday morning to her Unitarian Church on the outskirts of the city. "Do you see the steeple?" she said. "Isn't it lovely?" I said it was a nice steeple. "Ah, you don't know what that steeple means to us. We Unitarians were not allowed to have a steeple when the church was built, nor to build the church within four miles of a parish church. My father might not attend a public school or a university; my brothers did go to the university, but had to go to Europe for their school years. And of course we Unitarians had to pay tithes to support the Church of England. Not till 1890 were all our disabilities removed."

When I returned to London Miss Addams was there, staying with Mrs. Ayrton Gould, who gave a lunch for us, inviting Bertrand Russell, Lowes Dickinson, Norman Angell, H. Brailsford, and Hilda Swanwick. These had all been opposed to the war and were then opposed to the Versailles peace and fearful lest the outcome of it all would mean America's withdrawal from Europe in disgust, leaving the terrible aftermath to be settled without her help — exactly what did happen. All the people we met there belonged to that school of thought. Another interesting lunch was at the "1917 Club" to which J. A. Hobson invited us, to meet Henry Nevinson. We asked why the club had that curious name, and were told that it was founded at the time of the Kerensky Revolution in Russia; everyone who was in favor of the revolution was eligible to membership. "Was there any difference of opinion?" we asked. "At home everybody was enthusiastic over the downfall of the Czarist government." "Indeed there was," answered Mr. Hobson. "Many people here said that the Czar had been a good friend to England and that the revolution would be disastrous to the war effort of Russia, as indeed it proved to be."

Some of the pacifist women were, of course, extremists. Sylvia Pankhurst for one, Emily Hobhouse another. The latter introduced us to Olive Schreiner, who told us quite dispassionately about the Boer War, the devastation of farms and orchards, the gathering of women and children in concentration camps where those who had menfolk at the front were given less food than the others, and her own experience as a hostage. She would be made to sit in the engine cab with the engineer to protect him against Boer bullets.

One cannot be in England or meet English people without making comparisons between them and ourselves, perhaps because they are so like and so unlike — while Europeans are just frankly unlike. What struck me most forcibly on this particular visit was the fairness, the moderation, of these people who had suffered so much more deeply from the war than we had. There had recently been a meeting of 20,000 women in Trafalgar Square to protest against the prolongation of the blockade. That was simply unimaginable in our country. Lord Parmoor was heading the "Fight the Famine" fund, Mrs. Charles Roden Buxton the "Feed the Children" fund, both for Germany.

While we were in London I spent a day going down to Oxford to see Sir William Osler, whom I had known when I was a student in Baltimore, and loved and admired as all his students did. He had lost his only son, Revere, in the war, but I found not a trace of hatred for the Germans. On the contrary, he approved heartily of our plan to help get food into that country. "And for heaven's sake," he said, "don't let them take cows away from Germany. That would be terrible. I have just been writing to Robert Cecil begging him to stop it." That was only about three months before he died. I never saw him again.

We had practically given up hope of getting permits to make our German survey and we crossed to Holland and went to The Hague — for if the German trip must be given up, we could sail home on a Dutch steamer. Finally, on July 6 our passports came. We were told that they were the first civilian passports issued since the signing of the peace treaty. Mr. Hoover's word was law in Europe then, much more authoritative than that of any government executive — at least, that is what everyone believed. It was said that no freight car moved without his permission, that embargoes and blockades broke down before him, and if he did not personally put through our passports, everyone believed he did.

Carolena Wood, Dr. Aletta Jacobs of The Hague, Miss Addams, and I were in Germany from July 6 to the twenty-third. We saw Berlin, Halle, Leipzig, Chemnitz, and Frankfurt am Main, with visits to near-by villages and one trip up into the Erzgebirge near Chemnitz to the village of Bärenstein. These cities were chosen by our advisers as typical — Berlin, Frankfurt — or as places which had suffered the most extreme hardships — the Saxon cities and villages. Our advisers were Elizabeth Rotten and Sigmund-Schultze and the physicians to whom they introduced us. The English Quakers were Joan and Ruth Fry, Marian Fox, and Thompson Elliott. We met them in Berlin but after that our ways parted.

In Berlin we made our first acquaintance with wartime food — heavy, soggy, black bread which was said to contain sawdust and bark, dried cabbage and turnips, potatoes, sauerkraut (very small helpings of those last two), and various loathsome-looking ersatz meats and sweets, soft, sticky, and dyed a deep red, which we could not bear to touch. Our breakfast would consist of a bitter "coffee" made of roasted beans and cereals, no milk, saccharine tablets for sugar, black bread, and a marmalade made of beets and turnips with some flavoring extract and saccharine. By noon I would begin to feel that I had had no breakfast at all and I shall never forget the day Joan Fry, the English Quaker, noticing my "peaked" look, gave me a dozen raisins. There is an emergency food which rivals sweet chocolate.

Our midday and evening meals would be practically alike, a big plate of watery soup with some pieces of potato or perhaps a big spoonful of sauerkraut, or of dried cabbage, black bread, and the offer, always declined, of ersatz meat or fish. Dr. Jacobs, a very practical person, had brought in with her a big hunk of Edam cheese, another of cold boiled bacon, and some hard biscuit and sweet chocolate, so we usually made one good meal in the evening in our rooms. One afternoon two Chicago men, Richard Henry Little of the *Tribune* "Line o-Type" and Ben Hecht, came to call on us and Miss Addams was so moved by their description of the meals they had had ever since they came to Germany that she sent me for the cheese and crackers and fed them thin slices of cheese as long as it lasted, to her joy and theirs too.

I had not taken all the cheese down that time, which was lucky, for an even hungrier guest came the next night, Frau

Minna Cauer, one of the leading women Socialists in prewar Germany. She was on the editorial staff of a Socialist paper and was the one chosen to "sit" — that is, go to jail when somebody had to go because the paper had offended the Kaiser's government. She was a tiny little thing, shy and gentle, anyone more harmless-looking I never saw. Dr. Jacobs had known her through the Woman Suffrage movement and when she saw her she exclaimed with horror over her emaciation and promptly produced cheese and cold bacon, which she cut in tiny pieces and fed to Frau Cauer, as a mother bird might feed her young. Cold fat bacon would be hard for me to swallow but the poor lady ate it with an avidity that was revealing.

We asked her if she had had trouble during the war because of her pacifism. Not much, she said; only once was she arrested. That was in the first year of the war. She had translated into German the Christmas 1914 prayer of the Archbishop of Canterbury, in which he prayed for the Germans as well as the English, and had printed it and distributed copies. For this she was arrested, and when she was brought before the judge he asked her if she had not known she was breaking the law. "I thought for a moment, and then I said, '*Ich kenne höhere Gesetze als die geschriebene.*'" (I recognize laws higher than those that are written.) "Of course he knew his Sophocles and he was ashamed not to let me go." Miss Addams and I exchanged glances, which meant, "Lucky for her she was not in the United States. How many of our judges would 'of course know their Sophocles'?" It was Antigone's speech before Kreon she was quoting, when Antigone has broken the law to do her sisterly duty by providing burial for her brother's body.

My German diary is a succession of pictures of starvation, as seen in crèches and kindergartens and schools, in hospitals and sanatoria for the tuberculous, and in outdoor day camps for boys and girls. I saw then face to face what I had never seen before except in the illustrations in medical books — extreme cases of marasmus. We visited two "Air Cure" parks, on the outskirts of Frankfurt, where children of primary-school age spent the day, the girls in one, the boys in the other. All were naked, for they must get the sunshine on their bodies, to make up in part for the lack of fats, so we could see plainly the little sticklike legs, the swollen bellies, the ribs one could count, the shoulder blades sticking out like wings. And we saw them eat their midday meal, a bowl of "soup" — hot water with coarsely ground grains, chopped green leaves, and a few drops of margarine.

Although all had the same food, it was easy to see that the boys were more emaciated than the girls, a fact which I noticed again and again. The doctors to whom I mentioned it said it was quite true and could not be accounted for by the boys' activity, for they were all listless and quiet. Evidently women have more viability; more girl babies survive the accidents of birth than boy babies, and the girl child can stand starvation better than the boy. Nature sees to it that she is preserved.

It was Frau Professor Edinger, the widow of my old teacher, who had induced the city to open these parks and herself bore the expense of running them. Later, under the Republic, the grateful city placed a marble bust of Frau Edinger (she was a beautiful woman) in the Rathhaus and named a street Edingerstrasse, but when I was there in the summer of 1933 the Hitler *Gauleiter* had sent word to her daughter to come and get the bust if she did not wish it to be thrown out on the dust heap, but luckily Frau Edinger died before that.

The blockade affected not only the poor. It is true that a certain amount of smuggled food could be bought for a price, but not much, and there were conscientious Germans who would not eat smuggled food. Frau Edinger laid her husband's death to his scruples on this score. He knew she bought it for the three children and he did not interfere, but he would have none of it himself. Then, when he was much depleted, he underwent a fairly simple operation and died of heart failure.

Old people are to me only a little less appealing than children and one of my most vivid memories is of the almshouse in Neukölln, a working-class suburb of Berlin. It was such a pitiful place because it was at once so poverty-poor and so kind. I knew our poorhouse in Chicago, big expensive buildings with good furniture, good bedding and central heating, and abundant food, but so bleak and cold-hearted. All the bedside tables must be tidy and bare, everything put away in drawers. Here in Neukölln there was a cluttered, untidy, homelike air in the ward, the poor old women could have about them the messy things they loved, they could go around in shabby faded wrappers instead of our chilly seersucker dresses. One bed had a great baby doll lying in it and the superintendent said the feeble-minded woman really believed it was her baby. He was such a kindly person. He said, "No, we have not had nearly enough food even for our children, that is true, but we could not think only of the young. What sort of people would we be if we let our helpless old ones die?" I think of him now when it seems as if all Germans were following Hitler's program of "ruthless brutality," so passionately advocated in *Mein Kampf*.

The Germans we met were very kind and courteous and only a few of them wanted to parade their miseries; the majority left us to gather our own impressions and some even tried to cover up the grim truth — to give us better food though it meant a great effort. In Leipzig the Oberbürgermeister gave us a lunch in the Rathhaus, with meat, potatoes, fresh cabbage, and two kinds of wine. I sat next a city official, a pleasant person who startled me by saying quite calmly that he remembered Lille very well — he had been asking me where we had gone — because he was one of the officers in charge of the notorious Lille deportation, when in the last year of the war the Germans seized men and women in that French city and took them off to labor camps, for hard manual work. "It was not a pleasant job," he said. "We were ordered to round them up at night and that meant arousing the household, picking out the able-bodied, forcing them to come with us to some unknown destination. You can imagine the distress of the family left behind." I certainly could and I must have shown it in my face for he shrugged and said, "Well, that is a soldier's life. One obeys orders." We had all heard of that utterly unjustified act on Germany's part and I knew it was not only the able-bodied who were seized. The wife of the great French bacteriologist, Calmette, was one. She was seventy years old and was put with a group of women who were working on the railroad tracks.

We went to Halle chiefly because a famous Swiss chemist, Abderhalden, was professor in the university there and had been for some time at the head of the organization which sent sickly children to Switzerland. He had been able, as a Swiss citizen, to receive packages of food from Switzerland throughout the war and his children were quite normal. He told me that under the stress of the blockade German botanists and chemists had tested every kind of tree foliage and every weed, and even the inner bark of trees, in the effort to discover some new food, but they had found none. Mankind, he thought, had for centuries gone through famines and had chewed whatever could possibly be chewed, so that long ago man had discovered everything that would sustain life, no new discoveries could be made in that field.

The scarcity of soap was a feature of the blockade we heard about from the women especially. German women do so respect cleanliness. In the hospitals it amounted to a calamity. Antiseptics cannot take the place of soap, and the allowance of the latter represented from one twenty-fourth to one-thirtieth of the normal. I meditated on those Englishmen who had kept up this situation for almost eight months after the war was ended. They were high-minded, religious men, doubtless they went to church regularly and prayed for "all women in the perils of childbirth, all sick persons and young children," yet it was just those people who were suffering most from the blockade.

The Quaker relief began before we left Germany, indeed the English Friends had already, in May, succeeded in sending cod-liver oil to Berlin. The American organization allowed Carolena Wood and Miss Addams to buy $30,000 worth of condensed and dried milk from Holland, as a small beginning of what soon developed into the famous Quaker feeding in Germany and Austria. The Germans invented a new verb, quäkern, which meant to be fed by the Quakers. When I was in Königsberg in 1933 a handsome young Nazi told me he would have been a weakling if he had not gequäkert in his boyhood.

When we left Germany, it was to return to The Hague and to sail for home, but another delay came, a strike on the Netherlands-American Line which held us up for eleven days. When I expressed my feelings pretty warmly to the company on the ninth day, I was told severely that it was all the fault of the United States, the La Follette Act for the protection of seamen had put foolish ideas into the heads of the Dutch sailors and made them discontented.

We were not idle that week, for our report had to be written and we had a number of acquaintances in The Hague. Mme. Pelenyi and her son John were there, exiles from Hungary so long as the Karolyi regime lasted. John Pelenyi introduced us to a Count Banffy, also an exile, living in poverty in an attic but happy because he could for the first time do as he pleased and paint pictures instead of leading the life of a Hungarian noble. We invited him with the Pelenyis to dine at our very modest vegetarian hotel restaurant where the food was excellent but unexciting. Two years after, in 1921, when Miss Addams and I were in Budapest, we received an invitation to dine with the Minister of Foreign Affairs and it was our friend Count Banffy, no longer cold and hungry, but also no longer a painter.

Much more moving and troubling was our meeting with Baron Frantz of the Austrian Legation. He came to us, I think, just to pour out his distress over the fate of his beloved country to sympathetic ears, for he could not hope that we could really help. But Austria, that great country, and Vienna, the city beloved of all the world, were being mutilated almost to the point of death. The Czechs, under the fanatically nationalistic Krammarcz, had just succeeded in swallowing up the last remaining beet-sugar factory, on the pretense of straightening the boundary line. Of course the men in Paris knew nothing about Austria's beet-sugar industry, and if the experts did, nobody listened to them.

Baron Frantz spoke with warm gratitude of Archibald Coolidge and his efforts to stem the Czech aggressions, but they were in vain. He spoke of the concessions the Austrians had made to the Czechs in recent years: they had their own language — even the German names of streets in Prague had been removed — their schools, university, churches, and practically self-government, yet they seemed to cherish an undying hatred of all things Austrian. It made me think of Ireland as I saw it in 1912, for there too all sorts of concessions had been made by the victor to the conquered; indeed the Irish peasant had his rights more strongly secured than had the English tenant farmer, but the feeling of the Irish was not thereby softened. In both countries, Bohemia and Ireland, I think the grievance of the subject nation was based not so much on actual tyranny as on the sense of being held in contempt by their lords. For while he who hates his brother is in danger of judgment, he who calls his brother a fool is in danger of hell-fire. Hatred may go with respect, so may fear, but contempt sears the very soul.

One imperative duty in The Hague was a visit to a skin specialist, for I came out of Germany with a strong suspicion that I had picked up the unpleasant little creatures which had several times infested my hair in the early Hull-House days, before I had learned not to be too affectionate toward Italian babies. Miss Addams's experienced eye failed to find them but I decided to consult a famous dermatologist before we sailed. He was a rather unresponsive gentleman, perhaps because his English was not fluent, but he knew his job. After a careful examination of my head he pronounced his verdict: "I do not see ze beast but I see ze egg and wizout a beast zere is no egg." So he gave me spirits of camphor and told me to rub it on the scalp each night and tie my head up in a silk handkerchief, which was just as efficient and much pleasanter than the fishberries or larkspur or kerosene that I had used at Hull-House.

XV

Boston

DURING the fall of 1918, on one of my trips to Washington, Dr. David Edsall, Dean of Harvard Medical School and one of my advisers on the National Research Council's Committee, had asked me if I would come to Boston in April and give three Cutter lectures to the Medical School. My astonishment can be imagined, for Harvard was then — and still is — the stronghold of masculinity against the inroads of women, who elsewhere were encroaching so alarmingly. Of course I was both pleased and proud to accept and I worked very hard on those three lectures, but before I left for Boston the Cutter lectures had come to seem almost unexciting compared to the much greater event of my appointment to Harvard as assistant professor of industrial medicine.

Harvard had not changed her attitude toward women students in any way, yet here she was putting a woman on the faculty. It seemed incredible at the time, but later on I came to understand it. The Medical School faculty, which was more liberal in this respect than the Corporation, planned to develop the teaching of preventive medicine and public health more extensively than ever before. Industrial medicine had become a much more important branch during the war years, but it still had not attracted men, and I was really about the only candidate available. I was told that the Corporation was far from enthusiastic over this breaking away from tradition, and that one member had sworn roundly over it. "But then," said my informant, "you know, he always swears." Another member had asked anxiously if I would insist on my right to use the Harvard Club, which at that time had no ladies' entrance, and did not admit even members' wives. One of my backers had promised them I never would nor would I demand my quota of football tickets, and of course I assured him that I should never think of doing either. Nor did I embarrass the faculty by marching in the Commencement procession and sitting on the platform, though each year I received a printed invitation to do so. At the bottom of the page would be the warning that "under no circumstances may a woman sit on the platform," which seemed a bit tactless, but I was sure it was not intentional.

Dr. and Mrs. Milton Rosenau were my hosts in Boston when I went to give the lectures, and were very good to me, as were the Edsalls and Shattucks and Drinkers and Hunts, who made me feel that coming to live in Boston was not nearly so formidable a prospect as I had been thinking. The men took me to laboratories and hospitals and their wives asked me to luncheon parties. One of these, I was told, was at a "Brahmin" house, an expression new to my Midwestern ears. Here I did meet some rather formidable ladies, and had the impression that a reputation for radicalism had preceded me. An elderly lady sitting opposite me brought up the subject of Bolshevism. "My niece said to me the other day, 'Auntie, I am a Bolshevist.' I said, 'My dear, you deserve a good spanking.' I don't know what the young are coming to. She told me Bolshevism means the dictatorship of the prot-e-larians." The word did not sound quite right and she hesitated a moment, but then plunged on resolutely, glaring at me, "The dictatorship of the protelarians — well, I said, if I must live under a dictator, at least let it be one of my own class." I was rather overwhelmed till I heard my neighbor murmur comfortingly, " 'Never mind, they're only a pack of cards.' " She was the charming and humorous Mrs. Harvey Cushing, herself from the Middle West, but at home anywhere, and I felt very grateful to her.

My appointment to Harvard Medical School began in the fall of 1919, but I did not at once sever my connection with the Department of Labor — not till the beginning of the Harding Administration — so that I was able to complete a study of aniline-dye manufacture and one on carbon-monoxide poisoning. This last was in response to a resolution which was passed at the first meeting of the International Labor Office, requesting all the industrial countries to investigate the occurrence and the proper control of this dangerous industrial gas. That meeting was held in Washington, in a pitifully futile attempt to enlist American interest in at least one activity of the League of Nations. Of course it failed. Henry Cabot Lodge and his following were at the height of their power, our State Department did not even dare to answer official letters from the League Secretariat, and, as far as the I.L.O. was concerned, neither trade-unions' nor employers' organizations were in favor of any kind of internationalism. The trade-unions held that if international standards were formulated, American standards would be dragged down to the level of the "pauper labor of Europe"; the employers denounced the I.L.O. as under Bolshevistic influence, though Russia was not a member of the League.

That meeting, as I remember it, was distinctly uncomfortable for us Americans. The hostility toward our foreign guests was not even thinly disguised, and no amount of cordiality in private could make up for the rudeness of many of the public speeches.

The resolution as to a carbon-monoxide study was not incumbent on Americans, since we refused to join the I.L.O., but I had always been given a free hand in the choice of fields to investigate. Explosives being no longer important, I decided to take up this industrial poison, which is really the most widespread of all, except lead. It is not, strictly speaking, a poison; it is an asphyxiant. Its action produces an effect like that of strangulation, because the supply of oxygen on which life depends has been shut off. This it does by displacing oxygen from the red blood corpuscles, which have a far greater affinity for carbon monoxide than for oxygen and readily become saturated with monoxide. Then the body undergoes oxygen starvation. A mild form of this is mountain sickness, from which the scale runs up through mounting stages to the rapidly fatal form which may be caused by blast-furnace gas in steel mills, by gas in flues and pipes of illuminating gas works, or that produced by the burning of celluloid films as in the famous Cleveland Clinic disaster, or by wood burning with too little air, as in the Iroquois theater fire.

The most prolific source of carbon-monoxide gassing in industry is mining, especially coal mining. When blasting takes place carbon monoxide forms; a blast of dynamite produces a gas which contains as much as 34 per cent CO. This is why the miners' unions always insist that the shots must be fired all at once, at the end of the shift, and an interval be provided for the ventilators to work before the next shift comes on. In coal mines there are added sources of CO. The slow combustion of veins of coal without enough air may send the gas seeping into working galleries, while a sudden explosion of coal dust may result in the formation of enough gas to kill the miners if they cannot escape at once.

Carbon monoxide gives no warning of its presence, for it

is not irritating and it has no odor. When one smells escaping gas, it is not CO but the other constituents in the mixture that cause the familiar odor. It has a slow, insidious action, which affects the highest centers first, the seat of judgment, resolution, initiative, so that the very qualities needed to effect escape from the deadly air are the ones to fail first. We have several careful descriptions of the onset and course of severe CO poisoning, written by educated men who were caught in an accident or deliberately experimented on themselves. One of them noted that, while he could reason logically and realize what was happening to him, he had not resolution enough to climb the ladder which was quite near him. Glaister, the great English authority on colliery gassing, says that coal miners have told him they had had a feeling of weakness in the legs which they knew was a warning sign of danger, but the gas had so dulled their minds that they kept on working mechanically till they lost consciousness.

If rescue comes in time and the men are given the treatment which has been carefully worked out and which not only rescue crews but policemen and firemen are now familiar with, then as a usual thing recovery is complete and the victim can go back to work in a day or two, apparently none the worse for his near brush with death. But sometimes the cells of the body do not recover from the oxygen starvation, especially if it has lasted for some time. This is most likely to be true of the cells of the gray matter of the brain and of the ganglia at the base of the brain, and once those are killed there is no new formation of cells to take their place. The cells which form the walls of the smaller blood vessels may also be destroyed, so that a sudden rise in the blood pressure may cause a rupture with hemorrhage. This means that severe gassing which does not kill may be followed by mental symptoms, by palsy, by an apoplectic stroke or an injury to the heart, to mention only the more striking possibilities.

There are a number of industries in which milder forms of CO gassing occur; in fact, any kind of work which uses illuminating or producer gas as a source of heat or energy is likely to poison the air of workrooms more or less, unless ventilation is well planned. Printing, pressing clothes, type founding, lead molding, cooking and baking, laundry work, all these may come under the head of gas-using industries. The French, who use charcoal so much in cooking, write of the *"folie des cuisiniers,"* which is undoubtedly caused by carbon monoxide. But garage workers are probably the most seriously affected, for exhaust gas may run as high as 12 per cent CO.[1]

This was a very big field to cover and I was spending half the year teaching at Harvard. I doubt that it would have been possible for me to complete it before my connection with the Department of Labor ended if Dr. Henry S. Forbes of Harvard, who was interested in the pathology of carbon-monoxide poisoning, had not volunteered to cover the mining industry, especially west of the Mississippi. That left for me the steel mills in the region around Chicago, in the Pittsburgh region, in South Bethlehem, and in the soft-coal fields of Illinois. What we were chiefly interested in was the question of permanent damage following acute gassing.

It was a curious and depressing experience. The great steel strike of 1919 had just ended in complete defeat for the men, who had gone back, sullen and embittered, to the twelve-hour

[1] The standard established as a result of many studies is the following: For an exposure of several hours one part of CO to 10,000 parts of air is safe; for one hour only, four to five parts. Unpleasant but not dangerous symptoms are caused by one hour's exposure to 10 parts and death follows less than an hour's exposure to 40 parts per 10,000 of air.

day and the seven-day week, to a system of blacklist and espionage probably more complete than anywhere else in American industry. For the first time I found resentment against the government so high that I could expect no help from the steelworkers. They believed that the Department of Justice had worked for the steel companies, even to the extent of sending *agents provocateurs* into the field to incite the strikers to violence so that martial law could be invoked. This belief appeared credible to me, for we were told at the time by some of Hull-House's Russian neighbors that certain White Russian spies well known to them were working for the government in South Chicago and Gary.

Whether it was true or not, the men believed the Federal government had thrown all its weight against them. They would have nothing to do with me. Nor could I find any of them assembled together, in union or lodge headquarters, where I could talk to them. An inquiry about any such meeting met with silence or denial. The atmosphere resembled what I found in Germany, among non-Nazis, in 1933 — suspicion, mistrust, bitter humiliation. I had to turn to doctors, apothecaries, priests, ministers, social workers. In South Bethlehem I remember meeting a spirited Alsatian priest and a sympathetic Slovenian Lutheran minister who had championed the cause of the strikers at a decided risk to themselves, for this was during Mitchell Palmer's time and accusations of radicalism led easily to deportation.

American steel towns are not attractive places. Gary looks fairly well from the railway station, but the steelworkers' houses are not visible from there. When it was built by United States Steel, we thought that it was to be a model town, like those abroad, but apparently it is un-American to build model towns for working people. Gary is like any other industrial

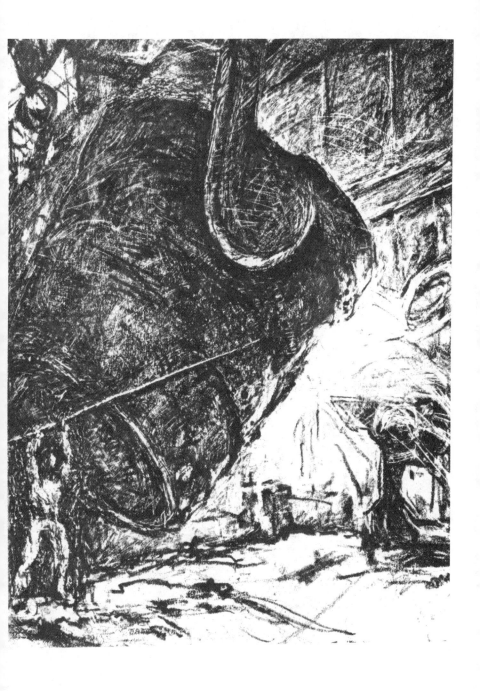

town, although it is not so blackened as those that huddle round Pittsburgh, because it is not so old. South Bethlehem is etched most deeply on my memory, perhaps because of the contrast between the upper town, with Lehigh University and the pleasant houses and smooth lawns of the upper class, and the lower town where the mill workers live. Here down by the river are the great mills, as formidable as a fortress, stretched out for miles along the bank; here are the rows of sooty, unpainted houses facing the mills, no trees, no grass, not even decent cleanliness. In 1919 (has it changed since?) the sewage system served only the upper town. At that time one was not supposed to think of Germany except with contempt; but as I looked down on those wretched streets I thought of the Essen of Krupps, with its charming houses and its admirable sanitation, and I wondered at the American fear of "paternalism," which can make a steel company refuse to surround its workers with health, comfort, and beauty, and can permit it to crush out all trace of independent unionism among them and reduce them to the helplessness of single individuals face to face with a great corporation. The German workman under the Kaiser had freedom to combine with his fellows but not to live in sewerless streets; the American had just the reverse.

It is twenty-three years since then, and in those years changes have come in the steel industry. The twelve-hour day and seven-day week were given up in the early twenties, which was a great boon to the workers but marked no real change in their condition of feudal dependence on the voluntary beneficence of their all-powerful employers. Unionism had been crushed under Carnegie and Frick in 1904, again under Gary and Schwab in 1919, but the passion for freedom was never really quenched and as the years have gone on it has grown much stronger. At long last, with the help of the Wagner Act, the steelworkers have won their freedom from industrial feudalism, but it has been at the cost of much privation and much violence. No one who knows the inside history of American steel can ever wonder at the bitterness and hatred of the revolting workers. It is a black chapter in the history of American labor.

My search for cases of permanent injury following severe gassing was almost fruitless, yet I am sure that had they existed I should have found them, for the people I interviewed were close to the workers and most of them were sympathetic in attitude. When I had gone into a lead-smelting town and inquired about lead colic or palsy, or "lead fits," everyone knew what I meant and many could tell me of individual cases. But in these steel towns, and in the soft-coal towns of Illinois, my inquiry as to mental symptoms or palsy in men who had been gassed aroused only puzzled surprise. Dr. Forbes had the same experience and Cecil K. Drinker's study of the victims of gassing, accidental or suicidal, treated in New York hospitals is another confirmation of the fact that such cases are very rare in this country.

It was not possible to extend the investigation into those industries where exposure to carbon monoxide is continuous, though too slight to cause severe symptoms, but this was soon done with great thoroughness by State Labor Departments, which have investigated garages, traffic tunnels, and even the air of congested street corners. The Holland Tunnel afforded a wonderful laboratory for Yandell Henderson and H. W. Haggard of Yale; the Bureau of Mines and the Public Health Service have devised methods for the accurate determination of the amount of CO in the air, and have tested various concentrations on animals and human beings. Through the combined studies of several scientists an efficient method of re-suscitation has been devised. Carbon monoxide presents practically no unsolved problems any more, and if miners still are killed by this gas, it is not because of ignorance on the part of owners or inspectors.

That spring and summer I had spent in Europe with Miss Addams and I went to take up my new life in Boston in late September. The autumn of 1919 was one of unrest and even rebellion all over the country. William Z. Foster had led the great steel strike, which had been crushed with the help of Mitchell Palmer's Department of Justice but had left the men sore and hostile. The strikers had called for "one big union," as had the I.W.W., and that was held to be Bolshevism. I had myself seen the armed truce in the copper country. The Plum plan for the nationalization of the railroads and the rise of the Non-Partizan League in the Dakotas seemed to many people a plain threat of state Socialism. The American Legion added fuel to the flames everywhere, for the soldiers who came home were not only used to violent methods of carrying out what they thought right, but filled with un-reasoning rage against any suggestion that what they called "the American system" could be in need of change. Curiously enough I had heard in England a warning against this very thing. In London I met an English labor organizer, Stella Franklin, whom I had known in trade-union circles in Chicago, and who had gone back to England when the war broke out. "I've seen a lot of your doughboys," she said, "and I warn you there is going to be a conservative reaction when they get home. They simply hate everything in Europe and they hate any thought of changes at home. They want to cut loose from Europe and let her settle her ugly messes in her

own ugly way and they are ready to fight anybody who says
there is anything wrong about the United States." I often
thought of that shrewd forecast as I watched the career of
the American Legion.

Boston, like all the rest of the country, was in the throes of
this antiradical agitation, panic about the subtle, underground
infiltration of Bolshevism in the working class, and a passionate longing to get back to "normalcy," to the old ways, the
old security. The Federal government was in apparent sympathy with this widespread apprehension and certainly did
nothing to quiet it. The Lawrence strike of textile workers
typified the postwar attitude of the country. New England's
textile industry had had strikes before, but the one of 1919
was different; it was profoundly alarming, because it was not
only over the old complaints about wages and hours, but for
something more. It was led by well-known radicals, Ettore
and Giovannitti and Elizabeth Gurley Flynn, who, Boston
was sure, were planning a Bolshevistic control of the industry.
This strike would be the opening wedge. The strikers proclaimed their belief in "one big union," and that was abhorrent
to the A.F. of L. as well as to the public. I remember an
elderly woman telling me of a speech which William Burns,
the famous head of a detective bureau, made before her club.
He told them that the country was riddled with Bolshevists,
that they were living over a volcano which might break out at
any moment. He tapped his vest pocket and said, "Ladies, if
you could see the evidence I carry about with me in this pocket
you would not have another peaceful night." Two of the
women fainted and the meeting broke up in terrified disorder.

That strike in Lawrence was broken, and with violence.
The governor sent in the state troops and their officer charged
the crowded sidewalks with his men on horseback. The stories

I heard reminded me of those we used to hear about the Pennsylvania Mounted Constabulary in strikes of coal and iron workers. In the Hammonds' book on the rise of the industrial age in England there is a quotation from an official of the government in the early years of the nineteenth century concerning the handling of strikers. "Put your men on horseback. If a man is on a level with the crowd he may hesitate to attack; he may even feel one with the men near him, but let him tower over them on a horse and he will ride them down without mercy."

Even more frightening to Bostonians was the police strike which came in September of that year. The men, most of them Irishmen, had perfectly legitimate grievances but nobody paid any attention to their protests so they formed a union affiliated with the A.F. of L. But the Police Commissioner was uncompromising and in a fit of anger the men struck, led probably by a minority and those younger men. There were some days of great confusion, there was some looting, there was a hurried call for state troops and volunteers; the strike was broken, but not till it had shaken Boston to its foundations. This had happened just before I reached Boston. I was staying at the Women's City Club, that attractive place on Beacon Hill, till I could find a permanent home. Feeling lonely one evening, I went to a meeting I had seen announced on the bulletin board, of the newly formed League for Democratic Control. It seemed very homelike; I could imagine myself back in Chicago at one of the meetings of liberals to protest against something. John Codman was presiding and they were discussing the recent strike, its causes, the parts played by Governor Coolidge, by Police Commissioner Curtis, and by Mayor Andrew Peters, how great the danger had actually been, and how the whole thing might have been averted. That evening was my introduction to a circle of people who became my most intimate friends, for Mrs. Glendower Evans was there and Gertrude Winslow, Margaret Shurcliff, and Katherine Bowditch Codman, in whose home I lived for all the fifteen years of my Boston sojourn.

I had gone to live in Boston with some little apprehension. That I should enjoy my work at Harvard I felt sure, for the men on the faculty had shown themselves most friendly at the time of the Cutter lectures. But I had, as most ignorant Midwesterners have, a picture of a city aloof, indifferent to outsiders, self-contained, quite devoid of the warm, easy cordiality of Chicago. My experience was just the opposite, perhaps because I was so completely a foreigner — at least that is what one Bostonian suggested. "You see," he said, "you come from the Middle West. Now if it were Haverhill or Lawrence, it would be quite different." Whatever the reason, I met only warm kindness from Bostonians, with very few exceptions. After the emergence of the Sacco-Vanzetti case I began to be classed with the radicals and the attitude of a few people toward me changed, but that was true of all the champions of that cause, far more so for most of them than for me.

I found in Boston more of the old American respect for individuals' rights, more willingness to go against the stream, than I had found in Chicago. Always there was a group of eminent men and women who could be trusted to stand up publicly for civil rights, even in behalf of people for whose views they had little or no sympathy. When an attempt was made to pass an antisyndicalism law, such as had long since been adopted in many states, a little committee of courageous opponents took Alice Stone Blackwell to the hearing in the Statehouse. That stately woman, who looked like incarnate

Victorianism, spoke solely for the traditional liberties, for
the traditional principles and ideals of Massachusetts. She
called on pride in a glorious past, she denounced any action
which would sully that past, and she carried the day without
having said a word that could be called radical. And her hearers
responded to-an appeal to their deep-seated traditions. At the
time of the policemen's strike young Harold Laski, who was
then teaching at Harvard, made a speech at one of the strikers' meetings, to Boston's deep indignation. A demand for
his dismissal, signed by members of the faculty and of the
Board of Overseers, was sent to President Lowell, but his answer was to invite Mr. and Mrs. Laski to dinner. Nobody could
call Lowell a liberal, but he had his tradition of respect for
free speech. There were state universities in the Middle West
which were not held back by any such feeling.

Attorney General Mitchell Palmer's "raids on the Reds"
began early that winter and culminated in mass arrests made
during the first three days of 1920, when over six thousand
"radicals" were arrested. The situation was very bad out in
Chicago, as I heard from Miss Addams and from Grace Abbott. As head of the Immigrants' Protective League, Miss
Abbott knew in shocking detail what suffering police ruthlessness and stupidity were causing to helpless immigrants. The
possession of Herbert Spencer's books was proof enough of
dangerous radicalism; so was Omar Khayyám's *Rubáiyát*, which
the police recognized at once as Russian. People were herded
into crowded police stations and held incommunicado. It
was impossible to make a public protest. Miss Addams and
Miss Abbott tried to have a mass meeting, to protest against
police methods — not against the Federal department's policy, only against the way it was being carried out — but they
found it impossible to get a hall. In Boston, there were raids,

but police violence is not traditional in Boston. The Federal Judge was George Anderson, a really great judge, and under him most of the arrested were released. The ones who were held were decently treated on Deer Island. And a big mass meeting of protest convened, with highly respected citizens on the platform. Yes, Boston showed a courage and independence which I had not found in Chicago.

My appointment to the faculty of Harvard Medical School had caused a great sensation, not only among my own friends but among the general public, yet when I took up my work there it was perfectly simple and pleasant. There was one episode at the outset that might have been painful but was not. A very patriotic lady who habitually contributed to the budget of the Medical School wrote to a member of the Corporation saying she would never again give a penny to Harvard so long as a pro-German who went about rousing people's sympathies for Germany was on the faculty. The gentleman came at once to see me and to get a denial which he could show her. When I was obliged to tell him that much of the letter was true, that I was speaking as often as I could on the subject of starving German children and raising money to help them, he went to Dean Edsall about it. But the only result was an emphatic refusal on Dr. Edsall's part to interfere with me in any way. More than one faculty member took occasion to assure me that academic freedom was one of Harvard's cherished traditions and even more of them told their wives to ask me to dinner at once.

The pro-German activity of which I was accused kept on all that year, for Miss Addams and I had come back resolved to do what we could to soften the postwar feeling toward conquered Germany and to raise funds for the Quaker feeding centers which were being opened that fall. Often my audience was German, but sometimes I was asked to speak to Americans. A Congregational minister once presented me to his colleagues as follows: "You know that when a saint is to be canonized by the Holy See, there is always present an 'Advocatus Diaboli.' Well, we have today an *Advocata Diaboli* in the person of Dr. Hamilton, for if Germany is not an incarnation of the Devil, who is?" All the same, the clergymen were the easiest to convert to a merciful attitude. I remember one tremendous individual, with a booming voice and a manner of unquestioned authority. "The Germans are still our enemies," he said. "Then," I answered, "as Christians we are obliged to feed them if they hunger." He stared at me for a moment. Then he drew a paper toward him, wrote on it, and handed it to me. "That will start your subscription list," he said.

The one thing about Boston which is really hard for a Midwesterner to accept is the attitude toward women, partly because it is so unexpected. We all think of Boston as the home of progressive movements. We know also that she has been the home of more famous women than any Western city, and that the proportion of women in Boston is much higher than in the West. So it seems incomprehensible that this enlightened city should have opposed woman suffrage long after Chicagoans had won it (I voted for Wilson in 1912), and that women doctors should be less recognized in Boston than they are in New Orleans. No woman can be on the staff of any important hospital in Boston, but in New Orleans she can. I think it is the influence of Harvard, really a deeply pervading influence on the mind of Boston. I was at a medical dinner in Boston where the guests of honor were two public-health men from Yugoslavia. Someone spoke of the exclusion of women from Harvard. The two foreigners could not believe their ears. "Harvard not admit women! If we should tell that at home nobody would believe us. Why, even Turkey admits women to her universities."

When Edith and I were students in Germany, we were told that even if other German universities opened their doors to women, Bonn never would, for it was the stronghold of the *Junker* aristocracy. Then under the Weimar Republic Bonn did, and so did all other institutions in Germany. A very attractive German woman doctor came to Boston when she and her half-Jewish husband had had to leave Germany, and after much difficulty she secured some work in the Outpatient Department of the Children's Hospital, for she is a child specialist. She was astonished at the contrast between Boston and Berlin. There she was on the staff of a big children's hospital where the majority of the doctors were women because work with children is a specialty appropriate for women. In Boston she found women could hold only the most inferior positions in such hospitals with no hope of going higher.

Most people think that women in medicine have now attained equality with men — but that is true in one country only, Russia. In the United States a woman finds it harder to gain entrance to the medical schools than does a man, much harder to get her internship in a first-class hospital, and difficult if not impossible to get on the staff of an important hospital. Yet without such hospital connections she can never hope to reach the highest ranks in her profession. As for private practice, I sometimes wonder whether it was not easier to make a start in the old days, when a woman doctor could count on the loyalty of a group of devoted feminists who would choose a woman because she was a woman. We do not find their like now.

Yet I must admit that though I have seen the difficulties

women doctors have to overcome, I have never suffered from them myself. During the period of my laboratory work I could join any scientific society and speak and publish as freely as if I were a man. And when I went into industrial medicine I often felt that my sex was a help, not a handicap. Employers and doctors both appeared more willing to listen to me as I told them their duty toward their employees and patients than they would have if I had been a man. It seemed natural and right that a woman should put the care of the producing workman ahead of the value of the thing he was producing; in a man it would have been sentimentality or radicalism.

Once in the days before the suffrage amendment I stood beside the manager of a big celluloid factory at his office window, watching the workmen pouring out of the plant. He turned to me and asked: "Are you in favor of woman suffrage?" "Yes," I said, "I have always been." "So am I," he said. "I want women not only in politics but in industry, because we need the woman's point of view. Now take this crowd. As you look down on them you see so many fathers and husbands and brothers and sons, real men, individuals. Don't you? All I see is a lot of my hands, a part, and a bothersome part, of my machinery, and that is the way most men feel. Until we get into industry the woman's way of looking at people we shall never run it as it ought to be run."

The woman's way. He was right. It is different from the man's and it should be. In Zurich in 1919, Hilda Swanwick, that delightful Englishwoman, told me of a visit she had made to an English school for boys and girls modeled on our George Junior Republic, with the police, the courts, and the jail all under the management of the youngsters themselves. She asked if there was any difference between the girl and the boy judges. "Yes, there is," her guide answered. "A boy judge will ask, 'What did he do and what is the penalty attached to that offense?' The girl is likely to say, 'Why did he do it? Did it do anybody any harm? If it did not, why punish him? If it did, let him make it good.' "

Boston is a lovely city and one that is content to remain very much as it is, without the violent upheavals that keep New York constantly in a condition of untidy transition. My home with Dr. and Mrs. E. A. Codman at 227 Beacon Street is still my home whenever I return to Boston, one of those stately houses with two great rooms on each floor and endless stairs to reach them. Amory Codman, who died in November 1940, was a very unusual man, to me both stimulating and lovable. He was a rebel, a nonconformist by nature; his life was largely a battle for reforms in hospital management, especially in the surgical department, for he was a surgeon.

I have known a great many crusaders but I never met one who was so wholeheartedly indifferent to the condemnation of others, even of the men in his own circle, nor one who was more completely unconventional in his outlook. His wife told me a characteristic anecdote of him. Just after our entrance into the first World War, one of his colleagues said tauntingly, "Well, Amory, are you as pro-German as ever?" His answer was, "Yes, I haven't changed." Naturally his wife demanded to know why he had said that and he answered that he never had been pro-German, he had only protested against silly things people said about Germany, but if that meant being pro-German, all right, then he was.

Amory Codman was one of the early explorers in the use of the X-ray; he became a unique specialist in the pathology of the shoulder, but his chief interest was in standardizing hospital efficiency by what we have come to call "the end-result system." He insisted that hospital trustees were responsible for the sort of service they offered the public and that they must rate the success of their surgical staff by the "end result," that is, by following up their discharged patients to discover the final outcome of the operation. This "end result," not just the condition on discharge, must be the basis of the published report. Hospitals should also encourage a surgeon to specialize in a fairly narrow field, making himself master of it instead of claiming to be competent in all fields. All this is familiar and accepted now, but it was revolutionary in those days.

In spite of his crusading zeal, Amory Codman did not take himself too seriously, as so many crusaders do. He could often laugh at himself even when the clouds of controversy were heavy over his head. And he could get completely away from the battlefield by plunging into the woods with his gun and his dog, for his second passion was hunting. The first time I saw him was in a characteristic pose. He had just come back from a shooting trip and he stood in his shabby hunting suit and high boots in front of the fire with his bird dog at his feet, a tall, wiry figure with sunburned skin, smoking a cigarette and exhaling with every breath a sense of deep comfort and enjoyment. It was on days like that, he told me, stalking through the woods with his dog at his heels, that he felt most completely alive and himself.

As for his wife, Katy Codman, it is quite impossible for me to tell how much she did for the happiness of my life in Boston, making 227 Beacon Street a warm and welcoming home and giving me a precious comradeship. She and I agreed on almost all subjects and I could always count on her ready sympathy and understanding when I felt driven to espouse some unpopular cause, as she could on mine when she took the unpopular side. We went together to meetings of all kinds, Old South Forums, Ford Hall Forums, Foreign Policy lunches, and Statehouse hearings on everything from Birth Control (my specialty) to the Abolition of the Death Penalty, which was one of hers. Amory would listen to our fervent discussions, sometimes tolerantly, sometimes challenging us to give facts and figures, a wholesome check on our enthusiasm. Katy was always ready to laugh with me over Boston's singularities, though she might not have noticed them unaided, being a Bostonian from way back. Even when I find them amusing I like those characteristic Boston ways, and I have a great respect for the George Apleys. There is something very fine in their indifference to outward show, though I admit it may be founded on a deep, subconscious assurance that their way is best because it is their way. Still it helps to create manners that are serene without arrogance and independent without combativeness.

Both the Codmans loved outdoor life and I soon began to go with them to spend Sundays at their place in Ponkapoag, where we would light a fire in a small cabin near the big house, cook our lunch over the coals, and spend the day tramping or chopping down dead scrub-oak trees or smearing creosote on gypsy-moth eggs. Sometimes, if the autumn leaves or the new-fallen snow were tempting, I would sketch till I was too stiff with cold to keep on. Those Sundays were a deep refreshment to body and spirit.

Cambridge is a separate city, but to me it seems as much a part of Boston as the South Side of Chicago with the University is a part of that city. All my friends there were Harvard people, of course, and the atmosphere took me back to Ann Arbor days, for university life is much the same all over the country. Always, whether in Cambridge, or Ann Arbor, or

Urbana, or any other college town, one meets men and women from all over our own country and from abroad, so that even a small town has none of the provincialism which can be found in many a large city. Always there is a conspicuous lack of money worship — people are not graded according to their incomes, their cars, their houses. Indeed there is little evidence of any "keeping up with the Joneses," since everyone knows what salary a man has; if his wife indulges in extravagant display, that is no cause for envy, only for pity for her husband. It may be that in the Old South there are still places where money counts for as little in people's standing in the community as it does in a college town, but it is not true of any other part of the country.

When I went back to Boston in the fall of 1921, I first heard of the Sacco-Vanzetti case, which was to overshadow our days for seven long years, the clouds seeming to lift sometimes, only to grow darker. Mrs. Glendower Evans drew Mrs. Codman and me into the circle of those who from the first believed that the men did not have a fair trial, and who soon came to believe passionately in their innocence. Later on she literally forced in Felix Frankfurter, who was reluctant at first but then so firmly convinced that he became the Zola of the American Dreyfus case. This comparison between the French and American cases was often made, especially at the end of the seven years when all efforts to secure a new trial were failing, and it was a comparison which made Americans ashamed, for Dreyfus had been condemned by both the military and the civil courts. To grant him a new trial meant discrediting the military caste, uncovering scandals in army circles, yet France faced it and came out with honor.

The case is far too well known to need discussion here.

During those years the whole world was following it with indignant interest. I was in Europe in 1926 and again and again I had the mortification of reading in French, Italian, and English papers new protests against what Europeans held to be persecution for anarchistic beliefs, not a trial for murder. The list of protesters was long, and it included the Pope, Mussolini, Masaryk, and a whole host of eminent men and women. To us it seemed incredible that these names should have no influence — but perhaps they had, only it was just the opposite of that which was intended. When Miss Addams wrote Senator Borah, hoping to enlist his aid, he answered her in a public letter in which he declared that it would be shameful if Massachusetts paid any attention to criticism from foreigners. That was curious when one remembered the many times Americans had sent protests to foreign countries against actions Americans disapproved of: the Dreyfus case, the imprisonment of Gandhi and of Francisco Ferrer, the Black and Tan campaign, the hunger strike of Mayor MacSwiney, and all the pogroms in Russia.

As the years went on our hopes would revive when new evidence was brought to light, when new proof of the judge's prejudice came out, and when the case passed into the hands of able and devoted lawyers. But Massachusetts law is amazing; it was the judge himself who passed on every motion for a new trial; it was he and he only who could decide whether the trial had been fair, whether the new evidence counted, and even whether he himself had been impartial and just. It seems unbelievable but it is true. There was an appeal to the State Supreme Court, but it could pass only on technical questions of legality.

Then came Governor Fuller's appointment of an advisory committee, known always as the Lowell Committee, to review the record and to determine whether the men had had a fair trial. We all breathed more freely for a while after that, though not all of us were really hopeful. And then that too failed and the men were sentenced to die on August 22, 1927. There were frantic last-minute efforts to bring about at least a commutation of the sentence; there was the hurried trip of Arthur Hill to the summer homes of the Justices of the Federal Supreme Court; the securing of 505 signatures of men and women all over the country, a list which reads like a *Who's Who* of American intellectuals, beginning with Jane Addams and Felix Adler.[2]

Finally Paul Kellogg of the *Survey* and John Lovejoy Elliott of Hudson Guild resolved on an eleventh-hour personal appeal to the Governor, and they wired me to meet them in Boston on the morning of the twenty-second. Margaret and I went up the night before, and early the next morning we went to the committee's headquarters in the Bellevue Hotel, to meet Kellogg and Elliott. There we found Waldo Cook of the *Springfield Republican*, who had carried on a seven-year crusade against the court of Judge Thayer, Reverend Edward Drown of the Episcopal Seminary in Cambridge, and John F. Moors of the Harvard Corporation, who had persuaded the Governor to appoint the Lowell Committee. Mr. Moors had secured the Governor's consent to see us and he led us to the Statehouse. It was a painful experience, quite hopeless from

[2] These are some of the other names: Charles Beard, Bruce Bliven, C. C. Burlingham, Ruth Standish Baldwin, J. McKeen Cattell, Henry Sloane Coffin, John Dewey, Haven Emerson, Glenn Frank, Mrs. Malcolm Forbes, Ernst Freund, Zona Gale, Lewis Gannett, William Green, Norman Hapgood, John Haynes Holmes, W. E. Hocking, David Starr Jordan, Florence Kelley, George Kirchwey, Julia Lathrop, John Howland Lathrop, Agnes Leach, Hendrik van Loon, Robert Morss Lovett, Mrs. Lawrence Lewis, Alexander Meiklejohn, Bishop McConnell, Mary McDowell, Fremont Older, Father John Ryan, Mary Simkhovitch, Margaret Shurcliff, Henry R. Seager, Graham Taylor.

the first, but worse than hopeless to me, for I realized for the first time what a terrible thing it is to have the lives of men depend on the will of one man, a fallible human being, swayed by feelings of pride and anger and self-love and deep-rooted prejudices. The Governor was deeply angered, his face was flushed, he was hostile and clearly had no patience to listen to us. We were tools of Felix Frankfurter, he insisted, who was at the bottom of this whole mess. The atmosphere was not helped by his secretary, who accused Waldo Cook of having taken a bribe of $20,000 from the Defense Committee for his editorials. We got nowhere, the Governor took refuge behind the Lowell report, and our words did not reach him.

As we walked from the Statehouse to the Bellevue we saw Beacon Hill crowded with police and with demonstrators carrying banners. Margaret had waited for me there and when I joined her she told me that she had seen men and women arrested right and left. I believe some hundred and fifty were arrested and taken to police headquarters but there were propertied people there waiting to bail them out. We went to the Women's City Club where we met Mrs. Glendower Evans. Her friends had begged us to see her through this last day's ordeal and so we sat with her through the afternoon while people came and reported what was happening or simply came to share their grief with us. William G. Thompson's aide, Herbert Ehrmann, was there, and Felix Frankfurter, Jeannette Marks, Powers Hapgood, and Mary Donovan, before they too joined the army of the arrested — which included Edna St. Vincent Millay, John Dos Passos, Dorothy Parker, Ruth Hale, Lola Ridge, and gentle, white-haired Professor Ellen Hayes of Wellesley College. Mrs. Borden Harriman was one of those who came to plead with Fuller, but she was not arrested.

Our last hope, a faint one, lay in the visit of Sacco's wife and Vanzetti's sister who had just come from Italy. By evening we knew that too had failed. Mrs. Evans could not sleep till it was all over, so we went with her up to the roof of the Club, looking over the Basin to Charlestown Jail and up the Hill to the Statehouse, and there we waited in the still August night, saying very little — everything had been said long ago; counting the quarters of the hour as they rang out from the Church of the Advent below the Hill. Midnight came and we knew it was Madeiros to go first, the young Italian gangster who had confessed to being part of the Morelli gang when they committed the payroll murder, a confession ignored by Judge Thayer and by the Lowell Committee. At a quarter past twelve, Mrs. Evans murmured, "Good-bye, Sacco." At half past twelve she rose to go. Vanzetti had died, it was all over, and she went quietly with us down to her room. Our fear that she would "go to pieces" had ignored her New England upbringing.

This case had made a cleavage in Boston and I think all over the country, dividing friends, even members of families, into two hostile groups, and it was bewildering to watch the make-up of these groups; people one had not credited with much interest in impersonal affairs became warm partisans of the accused, while others who had a long history of aggressive liberalism went over to the side of those who believed that the death of two innocent men would not be so terrible as the admission that Massachusetts justice might err. Mrs. Codman told me of her effort to persuade an old lawyer who for years had championed the cause of the underdog to read the record of the case, only to meet with a fierce refusal. "If the men were Negroes or Filipinos or even Bravas," she said, "he would have taken up their cause at once. It would be following the tradition of his whole life. But Italian anarchists, no." My sister Margaret told a college friend of hers, a Boston woman, of our visit to Boston to plead for clemency and her friend said she was glad Margaret had not tried to see her. "If I had known what brought you to the city, I would never have opened my door to you."

Some time after, I talked it over with Alfred North Whitehead, the English philosopher at Harvard. On his return to Boston from a visit home he had been deeply shocked at the appalling gulf between the classes in the United States which the Sacco-Vanzetti case revealed. His American friends belonged to the upper classes and among them he found a fear and hatred of lower-class radicals which he had never known in England, even at the time of the General Strike. John Dewey also, in an article in the *New Republic,* said that to him the most momentous thing was the revelation of the psychology of the dominant, cultivated class of the country, as revealed by the Lowell report. But I think Whitehead and Dewey were wrong. The District Attorney, Katzmann, was no aristocrat; the lawyers for the defense, William Thompson and Arthur Hill, were. The men and women who signed the petition for clemency and those who marched on Beacon Hill were among the most eminent in our country. And I came back to Hadlyme to find little sympathy from any of my neighbors, rich or poor, for the strange errand I had just been on. No, it was not a class cleavage — it was individual. But it lasted a long time. I used to be invited to "Sacco-Vanzetti dinners," where the congenial could discuss past history freely. Even out in St. Louis I remember my cousin, Tyrrell Williams of the Washington University Law School, whom I was visiting, telling me we were to dine at Dr. and Mrs. Gellhorn's. When I asked whom we should meet there, he said, "I don't know, but they will all be on the right side on the Sacco-Vanzetti case."

My last formal connection with the case was two years after the execution, when I was asked to speak at a memorial service to be held in Boston. But it could not be held there, no public or private hall could be found which would permit so dangerous a meeting, and the indomitable Gardner Jackson moved it to New York. There Gertrude Winslow, Morris Cohen, and I spoke to a fairly large audience of the public and an appalling number of uniformed policemen. As Gertrude and I went to the platform we passed through a side room, packed with them. I think I have never felt so small and feminine as I did when I squeezed through the crowd of huge, formidable creatures, assembled, so they said, to protect me against communist violence.

My exploration of dangerous trades did not stop with the appointment to Harvard. The study of carbon monoxide has been described already; then came the completion of a study of aniline oil and aniline dyes which I had covered in part while I was studying explosives. That was by far the most complicated industry I ever undertook to master and I was thankful for the foundation Ann Arbor had given me in organic chemistry, but a great deal had to be added to that foundation. Then in 1923 I had an opportunity to enter a very interesting field, that of the mercury-producing and mercury-using industries. This is one of the oldest of the industrial poisons, for quicksilver was mined in Almadén, Spain, in Roman times, and even then mercurial poisoning was rife among the slaves who worked those mines. Later on convict labor was used and then free labor, but always there was much sickness among the miners. Since nobody knew how to get rid of the danger, they did the next best thing: they shortened the hours of work. A tradition grew up in these Spanish mines which was still in force when the last published description appeared (in 1921) that eight days of four hours each should constitute a month's work. The same method of protection was introduced as long ago as 1665 in the Austrian mercury mines of Idria in the Upper Isonzo, now Italian. This is said to be the very earliest instance of legislation to deal with the poisonous trades.

One reason why work in the Spanish mines is so dangerous is the presence in the ore of droplets of pure quicksilver. Mercury ore is chiefly red cinnabar — mercury sulphide — which is quite harmless. That is the form in which it is found in most of our mines, in California, Nevada, Texas, Oregon, but there are some in which "the silver runs free," as the miners say. During the first World War, when there was a tremendous demand for mercury fulminate to make detonators for high explosives, these mines were opened for a while, but work in them was so dangerous that they had to be closed down again. I talked with a man who had worked in such a mine in Sonoma County where the silver runs free and the temperature is over 90 degrees. He became severely poisoned after two weeks' exposure. One of the doctors told me of miners who not only became poisoned themselves but carried home so much quicksilver in their overalls that their wives contracted poisoning through washing the clothes. Drilling for the charge and blasting the rock produces a fine dust which is full of tiny droplets of mercury; these flow together and collect in pools on the floor to be scooped up. The heat volatilizes the mercury so that the air is full of it. They tried working the men in two-hour shifts with two hours off, then another short shift; they provided hot sulphur baths; they posted signs urging the men not to exert themselves too much, but it was all of no avail. Mercury poisoning has always been notorious and conspicuous because it is easily recognized. Not only miners, but felt hatters, makers of thermometers, of dry batteries, of amalgam, all know the symptoms. They call it "salivation," though most of the victims of chronic poisoning do not suffer from an excess of saliva; dry mouth is more common, but the old name survives. In mercury poisoning there are swelling and pain in the gums and lips, jerking of the limbs, a fine tremor which grows worse the more one tries to control it, and a characteristic psychosis which has been called "erythrism" from the Greek word for red, because of the blushing embarrassment so often seen in the victims. If you try to examine such a man, you find that instead of dwelling on his distressing symptoms, as most nervous persons do, he will make every effort to hold his arms steady, to speak distinctly, and then perhaps he will suddenly fling away, declaring that he won't stand being looked at. I have seen hatters, who could do their work satisfactorily at the accustomed bench when nobody was noticing them, go to pieces and shake like a leaf if I asked them to stop and show me something. In one of the Oranges I heard of a hatter whose muscles jerked so violently that he could walk to work only if he pushed a baby carriage in front of him, but once his mates had guided him to his sizing bench, he could carry on.

The mental symptoms caused by chronic mercury poisoning have been known for centuries as a feature in the hatters' trade, as witness the old phrase "mad as a hatter." Nowadays a mercurial psychosis rarely progresses to actual insanity, but it is bad enough to rob the victim of his zest in life, his contentment, his initiative. His disposition changes — he is depressed and full of fears, of a sense of unworthiness, or he is irritable and easily angered; he will not take orders, he cannot work in peace with others, or he is dull, apathetic, even somnolent. But unless the case is very serious, withdrawal from the poisonous fumes usually brings recovery. Nowadays one rarely sees a serious case of mercurialism even among metallurgists.

This country is the third most important source of mercury in the world, Spain coming first and Italy second. But although there was plenty of opportunity to discover all about our mercury production, especially during the war, I could find in the literature only one reference to mercurialism in California miners and that was from the Eleventh Census Report. Of course I was keen to explore this unknown area and in 1923 I got the chance. Dr. Henry S. Forbes of Boston had become interested in this form of industrial disease and, being struck by the scarcity of information about its occurrence in this country, he offered to finance a study of mining and metallurgy, and the making of felt hats, trades in which we might expect to find cases. So I went out that summer to California, knowing only that I wanted to visit the New Almaden mines in Santa Clara County and those of New Idria in San Benito. The first was easy to find, but nobody seemed to know where New Idria was, not the railway people, not the hotel clerks, nor the automobile association. They all assured me that California's mercury mines were the biggest in the country, which was of course what one would expect of everything in that state, but the nearest to directions I could secure was the advice to get to Fresno and inquire there. I reached Fresno at seven in the morning and hopefully asked the stationmaster where to find the mines. "Well now," he said, "I ought to know. They use this station all the time but I never thought to ask them how they get here. The best thing you can do is to take a taxi. I'll find you a good man, and see if he can't find the way." The taxi man was willing but hazy and we traveled till nightfall before we found New Idria, which was really only seventy miles from the station by the right road. It was a wonderful drive over mountain and desert — only it was not really desert. My driver resented my calling it that. "Why, this is pretty good land," he said. "Forty acres will feed one head of cattle." I was just as stupid about recognizing highways. Our directions at the last ranch — they were miles apart — would be "when the road forks keep to the highway." Then when we came to the fork, one road would have the tracks of two cars, the other of only one. We decided that the two-car road must be the highway and followed it. We were almost twelve hours finding New Idria.

I had assumed that there would be at least a small commercial hotel where I could spend the night, but the young engineer-manager who came to meet me was overwhelmed at the suggestion. "I'm so sorry," he said. "There are only three American houses here — mine, the storekeeper's, and the doctor's. I'd love to invite you to my house, but my wife has gone to the rodeo in Stockton" — and he paused uncertainly. I told him that I was old enough to be his mother, needed no chaperon, and would be glad to accept his hospitality. He brightened at that and said we would have supper with the storekeeper's wife and breakfast too, so all was settled. They were an intimate group at supper that night, like a little colony of aliens in a strange land, for the miners were Mexicans or California Spaniards and there was no settlement near by. They were very likable and glad to talk and I learned a great deal about mining and ore reducing and mercurialism. I learned that it takes only a moderate heat (less than 400° Centigrade) to reduce the ore and get quicksilver. Therefore it is risky for a man to handle his tobacco, to roll his cigarettes, for if ore dust is on his hands and gets into the tobacco, the heat will free the quicksilver and then volatilize it. Spanish miners insist on doing this and Americans always advise them to take to chewing tobacco instead. I learned also that the metallurgical works are always close to the mines because it is much cheaper to get the quicksilver out and ship it in flasks than to transport the ore. Many curious stories were told me about this fascinating metal. It can penetrate anything, iron, vitreous tiles, firebrick, and, of course, wood. It has been found thirty feet down under an old furnace; and all the wooden floors and the condensers have to be torn up and put through the furnace sooner or later. Mercury begins to volatilize at about 40° Fahrenheit, so that it is impossible to keep the air clean unless all the work is done in an airtight apparatus — and this is simply impossible.

I saw plenty of opportunity for poisoning when I went over the premises the next day and my talks with the men brought out many stories of cases, most of them in men who had had to quit because they did not know how to protect themselves or were oversusceptible. The experienced men were very careful to have their working clothes washed often and never to wear them home, not even the cap. When they felt an attack coming on — usually soreness of the mouth was the warning symptom — they would ask to be transferred to the mine for a spell to "sweat it out." Fortunately the buildings of these California recovery works are very open, some of them mere sheds, so that the dangerous fumes are diluted. But furnace doors must be opened to feed in the charge, condensers are rarely completely fume-tight and they must be cleaned out once in so often because the fumes from the furnace carry soot as well as quicksilver and it must be treated to get the metal out. Since quicksilver vaporizes at ordinary temperature, even filling the flasks for transport is not free from danger. The making of electrical apparatus and of mercury lamps requires the use of mercury and of course much is used in laboratories; in fact, laboratory technicians are often exposed to dangerous fumes because of careless spilling of quicksilver on benches and floors. I had a curious experience, which showed the penetrating power of this metal, in a large factory for electrical supplies. On the second floor I had seen a process that required fairly large quantities of quicksilver and I had warned the manager of the danger of having a wooden floor in that room. Then I went downstairs to see, right under this room, the shower baths for the women employees. At the door I met the matron carrying a piece of stiff paper with a big globule of quicksilver on it. I asked her where it came from. "Off the floor," she said. "Don't ask me how it gets here from that room upstairs. All I know is I find some every morning and I scoop it up and carry it back to them." In one such plant, the Cooper-Hewitt, which makes mercury lamps in New Jersey, I saw what appeared to be complete protection for the workers against poisonous fumes. The apparatus is closed and every precaution is taken against the escape of mercury — but all the same a man sweeps the smooth linoleum floor all day long with a soft brush, and every day the workers are looked over by the company nurse, to detect the first sign of a sore mouth.

None of the other mercury-using trades is so interesting as mining and recovery. The most important one, if we consider the quantity used, is making mercury fulminate, which I had already studied among the explosives. Next to that I believe comes the making of felt hats. Real felt, as distinguished from wool felt, is made from the soft fine hairs of animal skins, chiefly rabbit skins, those soft hairs you see when you brush back the surface coarse hairs. The legend is that Saint Clement the Roman, who is the patron saint of felt hatters, once on a pilgrimage lined his sandals with fine hairs to ease his feet and that the heat and sweat and pressure produced a sole of firm felt. Those are the factors still used in making felt. How early the acid nitrate of mercury was introduced to help the felting process I have not been able to discover, but we do know that in the seventeenth century this method of preparing skins for felting was a secret of French Huguenot hatters. When they were driven out of France by the revocation of the Edict of Nantes, they carried the secret to England and for almost a century thereafter the French were dependent on England for their felt. In France the mercurial fluid is still called *le secret*, the process is *sécrétage*, the workers are *sécréteurs*. But in English-speaking countries the term "carrot" is used, because the pelts take on a carroty yellow color, and we speak of "carroters" and "carroting."

The function of the carrot is to make the hairs of fur limp and twisted and rough, which renders felting easier. As soon as the long hairs have been removed (by hand plucking in Europe, by machine shaving in this country) the carroters brush the pelt with the mercury solution and from then on, through all the complicated process, mercury is slowly given off, until the finished hat is practically free from it. Making felt means matting fine hairs together and shrinking and pressing them till the mat is firm and hard. I saw in Russia the primitive method of felting, still used in the Orient. A pile of loose fur, cut from the skin by hand, lies beside a cone-shaped form. The hatter fills his mouth with water, strikes a bowstring, the vibrations of which blow fur into the air, and as it settles on the cone he squirts water over it from the corner of his mouth, presses it gently with a moist cloth, and carries on till the cone is covered with a thick layer. This is what we now do through a series of complicated machines. Nevertheless, hand work does persist somewhat. The hand-plucked pelts are still considered the best, and, although one finds sizing machines widely used, the most expensive hats are hand-sized. Sizing means shrinking the soft, floppy cone down to the proper size and thickness, which is done by repeated plunging in hot water and kneading and pressing.

In 1921–1922 a group from Harvard, including the late Dr. Wade Wright, undertook a study of a hat-manufacturing community, choosing Danbury, Connecticut, which is pretty much a single-industry town. My share was the inspection of factories, while Dr. Wright and his associates examined something over a hundred hatters. We found that this old hatting center had a long tradition of mercury poisoning, many tales of hatters' shakes and of eccentricity, but those stories belonged to the past. In late years the trade had improved so much that serious cases no longer occurred. Dr. Wright did find forty-three of the hundred men with some evidence of mercurialism, inflammation of the gums or tremors or psychic irritability, but no case was serious.

My study carried me into other centers — the Oranges, Philadelphia, New York — and as usual I found all sorts of conditions, ranging from almost intolerable dust and steam to cleanliness, air conditioning, dust-tight apparatus. I had already visited European plants, seen the little primitive French factories, the uniformly well-managed ones in England, and two beautiful plants, the famous Borsalino factory in Alessandria and Hückels Söhne in Neutitschein, Moravia. Only the French were as bad as our worst, but in Philadelphia, Orange, and Danbury I found some of ours which measured up to the Borsalino standard, though none surpassed it.

After the first World War a change for the worse came in

the hatters' trade and serious cases of mercury poisoning re-appeared — not only here but in Germany, and probably else-where. This was because in every country very cheap felt hats were made and that means using all sorts of shoddy mixed with a little real fur: to make felt of it the carroting fluid must be much stronger. Not long ago I saw a New Jersey hatter who had worked for years in an excellent factory and had never been ill, but then a branch was opened for making cheap felt and after only eighteen months there he was poisoned. When I saw him he was helpless; the least disturbance or effort would start arms and legs jerking violently, and he was so ashamed of his want of control that the tears ran down his cheeks as he talked to me. It is certainly one of the most distressing of the industrial diseases.

There have been many efforts made to get rid of mercury in the making of felt hats, especially in France, and a number of chemicals have been found which act on fur much as mercury nitrate does. But the use of the latter is strongly entrenched in the industry — all the processes, all the timing, the different temperatures, the periods of ripening, everything, are based on the use of mercury carrot. I was always told that to give it up would be to revolutionize the methods. Only in Russia did I see felt made without mercury. There, before the Revolution, this was a home industry and there was a shocking amount of poisoning, family poisoning really, in those peasant homes. Now they use caustic potash. The felt they showed me was pretty stiff and ugly, but when I said so I was told severely that in Soviet Russia human lives were more precious than pretty hats. I felt justly rebuked.

That was in 1924. Now, some seventeen years later, what we thought was impossible is taking place here in this country. American manufacturers of felt hats are about to give up the use of nitrate of mercury and substitute some nonpoisonous carroting fluid. This great reform must be put to the credit of the industrialists themselves and of the Division of Industrial Hygiene in the Public Health Service and the Connecticut Bureau of Occupational Diseases. In 1937 a study made by the two Services showed that among 534 hatters there were 59 cases of chronic mercurialism and 49 "borderline" cases. The number of men affected was roughly proportional to the amount of mercury in the air of the workroom. The physicians and the ventilation engineers decided that the only method of preventing mercurialism in this industry would be the universal use of a nontoxic carroting agent. Now, we are told, the leaders of the industry have entered into a gentlemen's agreement to do this very thing, troublesome and expensive as the necessary changes will be. So one more poisonous trade promises soon to pass over the border into the safe trades.

XVI

Social Trends

IN 1923 Gerard Swope asked me to become medical consultant to the General Electric Company, of which he was then president, to visit all their plants and report on conditions as I found them. This I did for the next ten years, and it was a new experience in many ways, for I was not dealing with a dangerous trade — the real dangers were only in certain spots in certain plants — and I was dealing directly with the men in authority so that I was always sure my advice would be heeded. For the first time I found myself obliged to go into the less obvious and less direct hazards in industry, such as the underlying causes of fatigue, improper seating, dazzling lights, noise and vibration, lack of a nourishing midday meal and such, factors I had never paid much attention to when my mind was riveted on lead and mercury and nitrous fumes and benzol. It was also the first time that I had dealt with large groups of women workers. I had time too to look into systems of employee management, personnel work, medical examination for employment, so although the General Electric Company afforded me no opportunity to gain new knowledge about dangerous gases and fumes, it did give me a chance to learn a good deal that was new to me about the industrial world.

The General Electric plants were not unionized then, though many of the employees belonged to craft unions. I found employee organizations in most of them, sometimes paternalistic, sometimes fairly independent. One I remember especially was run by a man who had once led a strike in the plant. When I talked with Gerard Swope about trade-unions he told me he would gladly let all the plants organize in one all-inclusive union, like Sidney Hillman's Amalgamated. What he objected to was twenty or more separate craft unions with no place for the hundreds of unskilled and semi-skilled. I thought of that years later when, the C.I.O. having made his program a reality, he had a vote taken in each plant on the question of joining the C.I.O. I think that now all are affiliated with it.

The spirit I found in the General Electric is best shown by two statements that remain in my memory because they pleased me so much. At a meeting of heads of departments in one of the larger plants the discussion turned on the underlying cause of accidents in industry and one of the younger men said, "I think what causes most accidents is the determination of the man to do a good job. He is so absorbed in his work that he forgets to look after his own safety." The other statement came from Gerard Swope at a conference in the Harvard School of Public Health. One of the doctors present said that an industrial physician must always be alert to detect malingerers. Mr. Swope said he thought that of little importance. "Most men are pretty honest," he said. "In business you have to assume that you are dealing with decent people mostly and in your relations with your men you have to do the same. I don't believe malingering amounts to much." He turned to me for confirmation and I gave it gladly, for in my experience workers are more often likely to conceal illness, out of fear of losing their job, than to exaggerate it, to say nothing of deliberately cheating about it.

I had another job at this time which lasted two years, from the spring of 1930 through 1932. In 1929 President Hoover

asked a small group of men to examine and report on recent
social trends in the United States. This group, which came
to be known as the "President's Research Committee on Social
Trends," consisted of Wesley C. Mitchell of Columbia University, Charles E. Merriam and William F. Ogburn of the
University of Chicago, Shelby Harrison of the Russell Sage
Foundation, and Howard W. Odum of the University of
North Carolina, with Edward Eyre Hunt as executive secretary.
The following year the President decided that there had better
be a woman on the committee and the members selected me.
It was one of the pleasantest things that have happened to me
as a reward for having been born a woman. I knew already the
two Chicago men, Mr. Merriam was an old friend of Hull-
House, and I knew Mr. Mitchell, whose wife was at Farmington with my sister Norah, and Mr. Hunt, whom I had seen
in connection with Hoover's Belgian Relief Work. We met
every few months, in New York or Chicago or Washington,
discussed the subjects that were to be covered and to whom
they should be assigned, and then, as the chapters began to
come in, they were divided among us for review and criticism.

My contribution was chiefly that of an enthusiastically interested listener, for most of the subjects were way outside
my field. Only the chapters on medical practice, national
vitality, labor, and women were entrusted to me, but the discussions which covered the whole range of national life were
absorbingly interesting, and, since we were a small and intimate group, quite informal. No man I ever met has a more
delightful personality than Wesley Mitchell and as chairman
he dominated the atmosphere of our meetings.

The reports covered the widest range of subjects, really
everything pertaining to our national life, from natural resources to the influence of the automobile on family life, from

distribution of population to the rise of trade-unionism and the entrance of women into industry. I became fascinated by a continually recurring contrast, the contrast between advances and lags. Surprisingly enough it is in the field of man-made governmental institutions that progress seems to be incredibly difficult, while the basic factors of human life can undergo great changes quickly. The automobile can loosen family ties and church ties, it can practically wipe out neighborliness, it can revolutionize the structure of cities, but it cannot make a dent in the system of county administration, that expensive burden on the state which provides a county seat and a staff of county officials based on the distance that can be traveled in a day by a horse and buggy. Think of the radical changes that have taken place in the relations between the sexes, in the relation of parents to children, of servants to masters, in the last hundred years, and then think of states such as Illinois and New Jersey which have never been able to change their constitutions although these are based on England's constitution in the days of James the Second.

When our work was finished we were invited to dine with Mr. and Mrs. Hoover at the White House, my first inside view of the Executive Mansion.

All through my years at Harvard I kept in close touch with the dangerous trades, especially those in which poisons are used or produced. More and more this came to mean the solvents, for as the years have gone on and the well-known poisons — lead, mercury, wood alcohol, benzol, carbon monoxide — have come under a large measure of intelligent control, our attention has turned to a group of industrial poisons which increase in number and complexity every year. These are the volatile solvents which are used in the widest variety of industries, for coatings of all kinds, lacquers, Ducos, plastics, as well as shellac, paint, and varnish; and nowadays practically everything we use, from a pencil to an automobile, must be coated. Then there are the dry-cleaning industry, which depends entirely on volatile solvents, the rubber industry, the production of machinery which must be degreased, the production of artificial leather and fabrikoid, of celluloid and nonshatterable glass, and a host of other processes which require one or more of these solvents.

A good solvent acts quickly and strongly on fats, oils, grease, gums, lacquers, and other coatings, and then it dries quickly, but both these properties spell danger to the worker, for such a solvent has an affinity for the fats in the human body, and when it is breathed in and reaches the blood stream it makes for the fatty substances in the brain. This is the basis of the anesthetic action of ether and chloroform, and all the industrial solvents have a narcotic action, some strong, some very weak. The quicker the solvent evaporates, the greater the contamination of the air of the workroom, which means that a coating or a degreaser which is advertised as a powerful, quick-drying fluid is one that must be regarded by a physician with suspicion.

Before the first World War the solvents used in American industry were few and simple — petroleum distillates, turpentine, wood alcohol. We did not produce the coal-tar solvents in this country; we bought what benzol we needed from Germany and it was expensive. But a great demand for benzol, phenol, toluol, aniline, came with the war and it was met by the construction of chemical plants which, when the war was over, had to find new markets for their products. The petroleum solvents, naphtha, benzine, petroleum ether, and the like, are relatively harmless in comparison with the coal-tar solvents, especially benzol, and most unfortunately benzol is an ideal substance for many manufacturing processes. During the ten years following the Armistice benzol came into wide use in industry and often it was used by girls, especially in the form of rubber cement, in shoe factories, rubber factories, and in those producing tin cans for food containers.

Benzol is a narcotic, as are all fat solvents, but in industry it is easy to guard against an exposure great enough to make a worker lose consciousness. Much more serious is the chronic form of poisoning, which is slow and insidious and sometimes, by the time it is discovered, has gone so far that it cannot be checked but progresses even after the victim has been removed from his dangerous job. Benzol attacks the marrow of the long bones and thus, because the marrow is the tissue which produces the red blood cells and most of the white cells, it brings about anemia; no new red cells are formed, and no new phagocytes, those white cells on which the body depends to defend it against invading germs such as streptococcus, staphylococcus, pneumococcus. It also causes hemorrhage, for the substances which bring about clotting of the blood are also formed in the marrow. This is often the first thing that sends the victim of benzol poisoning to a doctor — uncontrollable bleeding from the gums, or the nose, or under the skin, or from the uterus, but by that time the damage done to the marrow is already serious.

As long ago as 1897, at an international medical congress in Moscow, a Swedish physician, Santesson, described this form of poisoning in young girls who had been making rubber tires for velocipedes, but it was not till 1910 that American attention was called to this new industrial disease. In that year Lawrence Selling of Johns Hopkins reported three cases, two of them fatal, in girls between fourteen and sixteen years of age who had worked in a can factory through a hot Maryland summer, sealing the bottoms of the cans with rubber dissolved in benzol. Selling worked on benzol poisoning for the next six years and a number of research students followed in his steps, so that when the war was over we had enough data on this dangerous solvent to make us do all we could to limit its use. In this we were helped by the National Safety Council, which made a very thorough study of the benzol-using industries in 1924. Many manufacturers voluntarily gave it up, at a decided financial loss, but others did not and it continued to be a serious danger for some years.

Then a safe substitute was found which could be used in both the rubber industry and the sealing of cans. This was nothing else than the untreated, liquid latex from the rubber tree. Instead of first coagulating this latex, then shipping it to the United States and turning it back to liquid form by means of benzol, rubber importers found they could keep it a liquid, transport it in tankers, and deliver it in liquid form for use. Cans now are sealed with this harmless latex, rubber goods are cemented with it, and it is used to make all sorts of dipped and spread rubber products which formerly needed some one of the volatile solvents. That is one of the great reforms in industry. Yet latex cannot displace benzol in many processes, and that the latter still is a danger in American industry is shown by a joint report published in 1939 by the Departments of Labor of Massachusetts and New York, on benzol poisoning in rotogravure printing and in making artificial leather.

The newer solvents belong to the petroleum series, chiefly, and they are far too numerous and complicated for discussion here. Our industrial chemists are introducing new ones continually about whose effect on human beings we know very little. The Public Health Service in Washington does its best to keep up with these rapid changes and when a new solvent is introduced it is tested as soon as possible, on animals in the laboratory, but that gives us only the acute action of the solvent, it tells us nothing about the far more important aspect, the effect that may be slowly produced by exposure for months or years to quantities in the air too small to be noticed by the worker. The workers themselves must serve as laboratory material and it is only by constant vigilance on the part of the plant doctor that they can be protected from harm, for a solvent which is not a powerful narcotic may have a slowly destructive action on kidneys and liver and blood.

Even when there is enough of an acute poisonous action to give warning of danger, that may not be enough to save the workman from havoc. For instance, some years ago we all felt justified in assuring manufacturers that a solvent known as Dioxan (diethylene dioxide) could be used without danger because the Public Health Service had found that before the fumes in the air reached a dangerous point there would be enough irritation of eyes and throat to give ample warning. Then we had a report from England which showed that under actual working conditions such a warning cannot always be depended on. Five men were working on a rush order, working overtime for extra pay. It was just before Christmas, the money was especially welcome, and the job was especially precious since unemployment was rife. So when the exhaust apparatus got out of order, the men kept on working, in spite of burning eyes and throat and dizzy spells. Within a fortnight all five were very sick and all died after a few days, of hemorrhagic inflammation in liver and kidneys. This is an unusual accident, but it goes to prove what we should never forget, that even with all the help the laboratories can give us, it still remains true that for most of our knowledge concerning new compounds in industry we must depend on human experiments, the workman himself is the guinea pig. This is especially true of those volatile solvents which do not seem harmful when used a short time but about whose action over a prolonged period we know little.

XVII

The League of Nations

IN 1924 two very exciting things happened — the first, an invitation from the Public Health Service of Soviet Russia to visit that country and see what they were doing in the field of industrial hygiene, the other my appointment by the Council of the League of Nations to the Health Committee of the League. I accepted both eagerly and in the fall of that year I went to Geneva, for the first time since the war. The League of Nations was at that time severely ignored by our government, which, I was told, would not even permit a letter addressed by the League to the State Department to be answered, and this attitude was accepted without protest by the majority of Americans. It lasted for many years and when, after 1924, I took every chance to speak in public about the Health Committee, I always felt that the very words "League of Nations" made my hearers' minds close with a snap, so skillfully had they been conditioned against it. So I always began by saying that it was only the work of the Health Committee that I meant to discuss and always I would find that in a short time they were listening eagerly to a wonderful story, one which should have been familiar to all Americans but which was obscured by the black mantle of anti-Wilson hatred and of resolute isolationism and xenophobia which descended on us after the war. One of the most striking results of the second World War is the change in our attitude toward narrow nationalism and the general acceptance of the fact that after this war some kind of international organization must emerge. And surely among the first tasks that will face such an organization will be the control of epidemics and the restoration of public health service, and that is why I wish to describe the way this work was carried on between the two great wars.

The Covenant of the League had made provisions for an international commission of medical experts which the Council of the League was to appoint, for they knew well that of the pressing problems facing Europe in 1919 none was more urgent than that presented by the epidemics which had invaded Russia and were threatening that vague line separating Poland and the Baltic States from Russia, for the strict sanitary cordon which Germany had maintained during the war had broken down. Across the boundaries everywhere, returning soldiers and refugees were pouring, most of them diseased and half starved, and there was an appalling dearth of doctors and nurses, many having died of these diseases; there were no medical supplies, no disinfectants, no soap even.

In Russia, before the war, typhus claimed about 90,000 cases a year, but in 1920 the officially reported cases were about 3,000,000. To the credit of Soviet Russia it must be said that all measures were taken which were possible under the financial and social difficulties in that country, and in 1921 there was a decided improvement, only 600,000 cases of typhus being reported that year. But then came the famine of 1921 which started mass migrations to the northwest, and at the same time the repatriation of war refugees was continuing. Millions of the populations of Poland and the Baltic States had been forcibly evacuated by the Czarist armies into Central Russia and even to Siberia, and they began to return to their homes, destitute and often starving. All this overtaxed the newly created Public Health Service of Russia, and there was a sudden and violent recrudescence of typhus and relapsing fever and cholera.

Early in 1919 the Red Cross had tried to cope with the situation and had sent doctors and nurses (many of them American) into Poland, but the task was too great for a voluntary body to undertake and in 1920 the Council of the League hastily appointed an Emergency Epidemic Commission, also with American members, which did brilliant work for the two following years. I believe that their most remarkable accomplishment was the staging in Warsaw, in the early spring of 1922, of a Health Conference which was participated in by twenty-five European countries, by the city of Danzig, the Ukraine, Japan, and Turkey. Those two bitter enemies, Poland and Russia, were there; so were the new Baltic States, and the new "succession states," and while statesmen of these countries could not even agree upon boundaries, the health authorities did agree to send their exchanged prisoners and repatriated refugees through jointly controlled quarantine stations.

As I read the official report of the Warsaw Conference I was struck by the tone of courtesy and respect in all the dealings with that pariah among the nations, Soviet Russia, and this at a time when most of Europe was eager to force her to submission by war or by starvation. Only the medical profession recognized the fact that disease is no respecter of nationality, nor of victory or defeat.

The Epidemic Commission also went to Greece to help in the terrible situation which developed there in the fall of 1922, when more than a million refugees from Asia Minor, fleeing before the Turkish Army, poured into Greece, bringing with them cholera, typhoid fever, and smallpox. There were American physicians helping in this work also, and indeed Americans as individuals have co-operated eagerly in all the health work of the League, even when our government was holding itself very much aloof.

By 1924, when I received my appointment, these urgent emergencies had been brought under control, and when I went to Geneva for the autumn meeting it was to find a new set of problems waiting to be handled. The members of the Committee were then twenty in number (this varied from time to time), most of them from European countries, two, an Englishman and a Frenchman, from Africa, one each from Japan and South America, two from the United States. Surgeon General Cumming, then head of our Public Health Service, was one of the vice-presidents, and I was the second American on the Committee and the only woman. It seems that at the time of the organization of the Committee some good feminists persuaded the Council to provide for the appointment of at least one woman and, since they were then still hopeful of our joining the League, they turned to the United States and chose Dr. S. Josephine Baker, the child specialist. But Dr. Baker was unable to accept the appointment, and since they had no member from the field of industrial medicine they passed the invitation on to me for two three-year periods.

I went to Geneva full of eagerness to see the League and to meet the group of eminent experts from all over the world, but I did not look for anything exciting in the meetings, where I should probably have to hear reports, largely statistical, sent in by health inspectors, with all the vividness and human interest carefully deleted. But from the very first meeting I found myself in for an extremely interesting experience. We met in a long room in the old Palais des Nations, sitting around three tables which were arranged as three sides of a square. Our presiding officer was a Dane, Dr. Thor Madsen, gentle, aloof, judicious, liked by everyone.

There was absolutely no touch of narrow nationalism, perhaps because these men did not represent their governments (of course Dr. Cumming and I could not have, nor could the German member); they had been chosen by the Council because they were experts in some field of medicine, not because they were French or British.

The first meeting was given over to a Malaria Subcommittee which had just finished a journey through the most heavily infected areas of southern and southeastern Europe. I was astonished to learn that, the epidemic diseases having been brought under control, malaria had become the most serious postwar problem in Europe. Of course I had read of its prevalence in the Campagna and the Maremma, in Corsica and Sardinia, but this report covered Serbia, Croatia, Dalmatia, and Albania, Macedonia, Thrace and Greece, Bulgaria and Russia. It seems that malaria was always endemic in those countries but the war had caused an enormous increase, partly because anti-larval measures had stopped, doctors, nurses, and quinine were lacking, but also because the forced migration had brought people with no immunity into infested regions and people with infection into regions hitherto free from malaria. And of course undernourishment, wretched housing, and exhausting suspense and grief added their share. An American physician I met on the steamer going home told me that in Russia he had seen fulminating forms of malaria which at first he had diagnosed as encephalitis.

The system of malarial control advocated by the Malaria Commission at that first meeting was the one which is considered most practicable in poverty-stricken countries where large-scale, anti-larval measures cannot be undertaken — that is, the tracking down of cases and their thorough and prolonged treatment with quinine, also prophylactic doses of quinine for the prevention of infection, and the instruction of the people on the part played by the mosquito. The treatment of the malaria patient must always come first. Even for the prevention of malaria, this is the first step, to kill the parasite in the blood of the carrier. It was Robert Koch who introduced this method in Italy, because it is more immediately practicable than the enormously expensive drainage of swamps to get rid of mosquitoes, for if the plasmodium is not present in the blood of people of the region, the bite of the mosquito loses its danger. Even this simple system was costly and there was not nearly enough quinine to fill the need, so the Health Committee had inaugurated a study of the mixed alkaloids of cinchona bark, testing them in hospitals in Italy, Rumania, Spain, and Jugoslavia.

Although at my first meeting all the stress was laid on quinine treatment and little was said about measures to destroy mosquitoes, at my second visit the Malaria Commission reported on the anti-malarial work in Palestine, made possible largely by the contributions of American Jews, and announced that at last they had seen an ideal system actually carried out, malarial control by every possible method. Quinine prophylaxis, while helpful, proved often disappointing and it can never take the place of drainage, poisoning larvae, protecting the people by screens and nets, all of which were in use in Palestine. But no European country was then willing to assume the expense of such a program.

During their journey through the malarial countries the Commission was struck by the scarcity of doctors with skill in diagnosing and treating malaria and therefore urged the Health Committee to offer anti-malaria courses for the training of experts. Here as in many other instances the Rockefeller Foundation came to the rescue and by means of fellowships made it possible for physicians from the backward lands to attend such courses in Hamburg, Liverpool, Rome, and Paris. More than two hundred and fifty attended these schools.

I have gone into such detail concerning malaria because the work done in that field is typical, but I must mention also the second subject which chiefly engaged our attention in 1924. The Mandates Commission of the League had demanded from the three great African powers, Britain, France, and Belgium, an accounting of their administration of public health in the mandated areas (the former German colonies), especially with regard to tuberculosis and sleeping sickness. Those countries appealed to the Health Committee, which sent a commission of French, English, and Belgian physicians to Equatorial Africa to make a survey, and report. The results of this survey were read to us. It was a gloomy story to which we listened, a story of tuberculosis introduced into Africa and meeting a population which had no acquired immunity and spreading far and wide.

The English experts reported that the disease used to be absolutely unknown among the native populations, but it was then spreading rapidly and was prevalent in the mines of the Rand where there was every opportunity for its spread. The original infection was traced to the Hindu, Greek, and Syrian immigrants, but the course of tuberculosis is much more rapid in the African than in the European or the Asian. The infection proceeds inward from the coast in proportion to what the report called the "advance of civilization, that is, the use of strong alcoholic drink, the increase of poverty, the change from healthful ways of life to unhealthful, and the increase of moral and physical degeneration." The Belgian expert's report was similar. At the beginning of the present century human tuberculosis might be said to be nonexistent in the Belgian Congo, but of recent years the disease had been introduced from Europe, often by returning recruits, and was rapidly fatal, for the natives have as yet acquired little or no resistance to it.

The sleeping sickness of Equatorial Africa is quite distinct from the encephalitis lethargica of the temperate zone, which is sometimes called by the same name. It is caused by a protozoan organism, a trypanosome, which is carried by the tsetse fly and transmitted to man and to animals by the bite of this fly. The authorities tell us that it was brought over to America by African slaves, but fortunately the tsetse fly was not. Sleeping sickness is native to Africa but up to 1888 was confined to a small area on the west coast of Equatorial Africa; then Stanley's explorations transmitted it to Uganda and Central Africa, and all the later opening up of the country has caused it to spread far and wide. In 1903, Castellani, the great authority on tropical diseases, discovered the cause and the mode of transmission by the fly. The victim suffers from irregular fever, weakness, wasting, increasing apathy, somnolence, and usually succumbs after about a year or eighteen months.[1]

The report of the British experts revealed the effects of white civilization in increasing the disease, for they found that it follows trade routes, villages far distant from the main roads showing less infection, and there is even evidence that tsetse flies have been carried by train and motorcar. The effect of the war was seen in the report from the Sudan, where 800 natives,

[1] The scientists of the Rockefeller Institute made a great contribution to the control of sleeping sickness when they produced the compound tryparsamide. Dr. Louise Pearce and Dr. W. H. Brown took it to Africa and started its use there.

levies from local chiefs, were taken to an area very heavily infected, and on their return they scattered to their homes and had since produced a rich harvest of cases, and sleeping sickness after that was definitely established in the Sudan.

The French expert said that in order fully to appreciate the importance of the control of sleeping sickness it must be remembered that in the regions affected by it, the birth rate is less than the death rate because the malady results not only in a high death rate but in sterility and abortion. In one region, watered by two large rivers, the infection reached 64.5 per cent of the population, and in another 90 per cent.

The record of work done by the French during the two years preceding the report was very impressive, and in some regions the death rate from sleeping sickness had been reduced by 45 and by 65 per cent. It was evident, however, that the fly was gradually encroaching on new areas, continually attacking new and nonimmune populations, especially in the neighborhood of the main traffic routes. I remember that the report of the experts closed with this significant comment: "If we should put on opposite sides of a ledger the benefits and the evils which have come to Equatorial Africa as a result of the invasion of civilization, we should be obliged to say that the evil overbalances the good."

Four years later, at the meeting in 1928, we heard a very heartening report on the results of this international co-operation. Six nations had met at Entebbe and had agreed to co-operate. Observation posts and sanitary posts were to be established on either side of frontiers and no native allowed to cross without a medical passport. Difficulties that seemed insuperable had been overcome, such, for instance, as the moving of whole villages from infected to healthful areas. In Tanganyika, 14,500 people were moved from fly-infected forest to fly-free clearings, and yet so carefully was this done that the tribal organization was maintained and the people still live under their own chiefs. The breeding places of the tsetse fly are the shady banks of streams and lakes where the natives love to linger because of the coolness. They breed also in thickets and tall grass, and the pupae die when exposed to sunlight. Wide-open spaces were made around fords and watering pools, grass was burned, thickets destroyed with fire, chemicals, and tractors. The French had established voluntary segregation villages where families could go and have land to cultivate, supplies to carry them till the first harvest, and no head tax. The French also found that they could win the confidence of the natives by treating frambesia, or yaws, a loathsome skin disease which yields quickly in a few days to arsenobenzol. When the native sees that disappear under the white medicine, he is usually willing to take the treatment for sleeping sickness.

Through all the discussions, especially of plans for future activities, the Health Committee was faced with the difficulty of finding physicians and sanitary engineers adequately trained for public health work. Here again the Rockefeller Foundation stepped in and furnished traveling fellowships for men and women who were to be selected by their governments and sent to whatever country offered the best instruction in the particular field to be studied, the students pledging themselves to return home and enter the public health service. I had a number of these men and women in my classes at Harvard and it was a pleasure to teach them, for they were so eager to learn. I remember one class which had representatives of thirteen different nationalities, among them a Chinese, the ablest of them all. He told me of the appalling need of public health work in his country where, for over 400,000,000 people, there were only some 4000 doctors trained in Western medicine and almost all were in the coastal cities. He was not the only student who gave me a picture of primitive conditions. When I asked a Serbian what was the most pressing public health problem in his country, he replied, hydrophobia from the bites of dogs who had been bitten by rabid wolves.

In addition to the program for the training of public health experts, that 1924 meeting saw the inception of a great scheme to obtain and broadcast all information concerning the outbreak of epidemics. Never had it been possible to make governments exchange this sort of information; on the contrary, every effort had always been made to conceal an outbreak of cholera, plague, typhus, smallpox. People of my generation will remember the time when California refused to recognize an epidemic of bubonic plague, lest tourist and real-estate interests suffer, so that Washington had to send William Welch and Simon Flexner out to the Coast with authority to deal with the situation.

That had been the way all the countries had acted, but suddenly, perhaps because of the terrible experiences during the war, that form of isolationism broke down and the governments of the Asiatic countries as well as the European, and our own for the Philippines and the Canal Zone, agreed to exchange as promptly as possible all information concerning the five epidemic diseases, cholera, typhus, smallpox, bubonic plague, and yellow fever. In later years others were added — encephalitis, meningitis, infantile paralysis, influenza. Singapore was selected as the center for these reports, which came from Vladivostok on the north to the Southern Archipelago and from Suez on the east to the Canal Zone, and were transmitted from Singapore by wireless to public health stations everywhere. In this way, an outbreak of cholera or plague in a remote part of China or India could be broadcast all over the world. The monthly, printed reports used to come to me regularly. It is tragic to think that all that service is now at an end.

On my second and third visits, I found the Health Committee swamped with pleas for assistance. No longer did we have to approach governments tactfully and suggest that perhaps some expert advice might be helpful; the governments themselves were pleading for it. They asked us to look into their appallingly high infant mortality rate, and incidentally to tell them how to collect vital statistics; they told us confidentially that their budget for malaria control was small and that the big landholders wanted to spend it on large schemes of drainage which would benefit them and leave nothing for quinine for the poor, or that the government had decided to ignore malaria and spend the money on irrigation. We were asked to back up the health authorities with the prestige of the League and in both those instances this was done successfully. A request came from South America for the appointment of a Leprosy Commission, to determine the best method of control and to study the action of chaulmoogra oil, which so often proved disappointingly ineffective. Brazil, it seems, has a serious leprosy problem, an aftermath of the slave trade, it is said. In certain regions there is one case to a thousand inhabitants; in a single region it is one to five hundred. Argentina, Venezuela, and Colombia also have many cases. This request was backed by the Oriental countries.

Then there were pleas for the standardization of therapeutic sera and vaccines; for a commission to test and pronounce on the value of the various tests for syphilitic infection; for another to study the efficacy of vaccination against cholera by mouth instead of by injection; the use of dried smallpox vaccine lymph, so much more practical in the Orient; the value of bacteriophage in combating cholera and dysentery. The Pacific powers, France and Britain, asked advice on how to stop the depopulation of the Pacific Islands, where white invasion had been followed by a rapid decline in the native population. This request revealed a tragic picture of what O'Brien called "White Shadows in the Orient": the introduction of new diseases to a nonimmune people; the forced deportation of men to work far from home, leaving the farms and fishing grounds to the women, which meant that canned food bought from the traders took the place of fresh food; the inevitable change in living habits; in short all the blessings of civilization imposed suddenly on primitive people. Measles, influenza, bacillary dysentery, are deadly to these people. In former times leprosy existed on the islands, but it did not spread much because the different tribes were always warring with each other and this constituted a sort of quarantine. Now leprosy has increased greatly, especially in New Caledonia. Tuberculosis also is increasing, although the Commission reported that it is not so bad as it might be because the natives do not have time to become tuberculous, those with a poor physique and poor resistance die of bronchial pneumonia, which is the most frequent cause of death among them.

The measures which the Health Committee's Commission recommended did not strike me as very hopeful; physicians, health centers, quarantine stations, insane asylums, can hardly do much to save these people so long as the real cause, the sudden, enforced introduction of Western ways, still remains. The Commission urged the governments to send out European-trained nurses to travel about the colonies, since they found that the natives, especially the women, can be reached by nurses much better than by doctors. Much more fundamental were the recommendations for "a rational and humanitarian utilization of native labor, with a period of recruitment limited to two years, and the emigrant laborer allowed to take his family with him." An inspector of labor should be appointed and medical care for the emigrants should be provided.

It was at the 1928 conference that I noticed a significant change in the attitude of some of the members toward public health education for the masses. This was regarded as an American idea and at first it was opposed and sometimes ridiculed by the Europeans. Thus at the first meeting I heard Dr. Stampau, the chief health officer of Jugoslavia, say that he expected to spend his malarial budget on free quinine, rural dispensaries, and visiting nurses to instruct the people, whereupon a French professor exclaimed: "Educate the people! But you cannot make peasants understand such things. You must issue your orders and follow them up with police power." Dr. Stampau retorted that he could do it and had done it; that he had taken the Malaria Commission into peasant schools and shown them how boys and girls could draw on the blackboard pictures of culex and of anopheles and tell which was the one which always must be killed. Four years later this same Frenchman said to me, "This afternoon you will see what you Americans call a health propaganda film, on tuberculosis. It is the Americans of the Rockefeller Foundation who have taught us how to do such things." And we did see a very nice film of a country hospital for tuberculous mothers and of the placing and supervising of their babies in peasant homes.

An urgent request was sent to us in 1928 by Greece, which was in the grip of an epidemic of dengue, so severe that in

September of that year — we met in October — no less than 86 per cent of the population of Athens and the Piraeus were infected, the infection being transmitted by mosquitoes and biting sand fleas. When the Greek delegate came to Geneva in October he reported no less than 850,900 cases with 1378 deaths. Greece had no public health service, and no trained personnel to man such a service. The Health Committee promptly appointed a commission, with two Americans, Haven Emerson and Allan McLaughlin, an Australian, and a Croatian. These men organized a public health service for Greece and arranged for the training of personnel in schools abroad, the work being carried on temporarily by imported experts, who would also organize a School of Hygiene, this last as well as the other activities to be turned over to the Greek students when they returned from their training abroad.

The report of this inquiry was presented in October 1930, when a picture was given of the vicissitudes of public hygiene in Greece, beginning with the Balkan War of 1912, increased by the World War and even more by the Greco-Turkish War and the forced exchange of populations in 1922, when 1,300,-000 refugees, all but 200,000 of whom were Armenians, were dropped upon Greece, a country of only 5,000,000 inhabitants. All these refugees, the majority of whom were women, old people, and children, depleted by famine and grief and absolutely poverty-stricken, had to be accommodated somehow in the various Greek ports. They brought with them much disease to a country ill equipped to deal with it. Even the task of feeding them was enormous, and the water supply insufficient in Athens, in the Piraeus, in Salonika, and in the Macedonian plains. Then there was the problem of housing. In Athens and the Piraeus alone the population rose in one year from 300,000 to 1,000,000. Needless to say, hospitals, insane asylums, and all other institutions were hopelessly inadequate.

The 1930 report, however, was by no means all dark. In eight years the Greek government had built 180,000 dwellings to house a million refugees, and the last budget contained provision for the construction of more cheap dwellings. The health situation was improving gradually, as material conditions for the refugees improved. Thus in Macedonia, where 60 medical centers had been set up, the mortality rate, which in 1923–1924 had reached the terrible figures of 30 to 50 per cent in the refugee villages, had now fallen to 17 per cent. It was also discovered that though the refugees had at first constituted a formidable burden on the Greek state, little by little they had become a valuable productive element, introducing the carpet and silk industries, developing the preparation of raisins and figs, increasing the yield from fishing, trebling the production of tobacco, and adding 60 per cent to the production of cereals. This is a record that should be seriously studied by our Congressmen, especially those who wish to keep our doors barred against all refugees.

When my second term expired in 1930 I had heard reports from all these commissions, most of them very heartening, and I had seen the beginning of an interesting study of infant mortality — the first report of which reached me two years later.

The Health Committee had long wished to make such a study, to discover which country had the lowest mortality rate and then to adopt as standard the infant welfare measures used in that country. But at the outset it was found that one could not compare the death rates of countries because of the difference in their systems of vital statistics. Finally it was decided to adopt the method originated by our Children's Bureau which resulted in those very valuable infant mortality reports from cities and towns and urban regions in this country — namely, to chose typical regions and make in these a detailed study of the circumstances attending every baby's death during the preceding year. This means inquiry into the family's standard of living, the father's earnings, the mother's work, whether in or outside the home, breast or bottle feeding, whether the child was the first or the twelfth, and so on.

The countries selected were England, Norway, Holland, France, Germany, and Austria, city and country and small-town areas. The reports are extraordinarily interesting reading, bringing in all sorts of intimate details of the life of these people. The lowest death rates were found in England, Holland, and Norway, with the last standing at the head; the highest were in France, Germany, and Austria. Poor Austria came out at the foot in both city — Vienna — and country — the mountainous regions of Gründen, Schärding, and Engelhartszell, so movingly beautiful, but of great poverty, with a population of small farmers and landless agricultural laborers, where women's work is excessive during pregnancy and immediately after, breast feeding is rare and artificial feeding is inadequate, there is a high percentage of illegitimate births, and midwives are unusually poor.

Poverty emerged as the most important factor but a close second was bottle feeding. Breast feeding proved to have much more influence on the death rate than had so-called infant welfare work. At the discussion in committee M. Velghe, of Belgium, said that during the German occupation the baby death rate fell in Brussels, in spite of the hardships of the people, simply because the women could not get work and had to suckle their babies; and Dr. Chodzko, of Poland, remarked that the same thing was noted in Warsaw under the German occupation.

In France there is a far higher infant death rate in Normandy than in the wine-producing regions of the South, although the Norman peasants are wealthier than the Provençals. But they are hard-working and avaricious, the women will not suckle their babies because it interferes with their work in the fields. The Southerners are easy-going and breast feeding is universal there.

The League of Nations was in principle an international organization devoted to the welfare of all, but nationalism is deep-rooted and "sacred egoism" is to most "patriots" the first duty. I went to some meetings of the Opium Control Committee and I met members of the Committee on the White Slave Traffic, and in both it was only too clear that some, if not all, the delegates from certain countries had the interests of their country in mind far more than the welfare of the whole world. They could not forget that they represented their countries and must defend national interests. But when I entered the great room where the Health Committee met I could breathe at once a different air. For here nobody represented his government, all had been chosen on the basis of their scientific standing, and all were working for the control of disease no matter where. Countries were rated only according to their need for help or their ability to give help. Those nations which had received help understood its importance and when, in 1928, England, under Sir Austen Chamberlain, began to sabotage the League and attempted to cut the budget of the Health Committee, a storm of protest arose, especially from the countries of South America and the Far East. These delegates said that the only activity of the League their people knew anything about was the health work. The budget was saved.

The Health Committee still exists though it has not met since the autumn of 1939. There are still some four or five members of the Secretariat left in Geneva and epidemiological reports were still sent from Singapore to Geneva and from Geneva to the United States up to December 7, 1941. Then that last international service ceased.

But it will be restored some day. The task that will face us after this war will be far, far heavier and more widespread than in 1919. When the first war ended we discovered the ravages that starvation had caused in Germany and Austria. But what shall we find in Poland, Greece, and Spain? Indeed almost all of Europe has suffered as much from lack of food as did Germany and Austria under what we then called the greatest mass starvation the civilized world had ever known. If Serbia and Montenegro were typhus-ridden then, they must be so now, and to them are added the Baltic States and Poland, and probably Rumania. Doctors and nurses must have perished in as great numbers as then. We know much less now about life in the conquered countries than we knew in the first World War, but it is not hard to imagine the plight of refugees who have spread over all the face of Europe and much of Asia. We need only think back to Greece after the Turkish war when the hordes of Near Eastern Greeks and Armenians were driven into that little country and then we must multiply that number by hundreds of thousands in country after country. But we know that the task that will face us can be done; we can point to the work of the Health Committee of the League of Nations as a proof, and we can go forward on the path it blazed.

XVIII

Russia in 1924

IN THE summer of 1924, as I have said, I received an invitation to visit Russia. It came from Dr. Kalina of the Department of Health, writing on behalf of the chief of that department, Semaschko, who wished me to make a personal survey of what Soviet Russia was doing in industrial hygiene. This was a very tempting invitation. Russia was still a land of mystery and terror; few outsiders had come back with descriptions of it which one could accept without question, for if they were not uncritically enthusiastic, they were uncritically condemning. It seemed to me unfair to expect much from a country which had gone through what Russia had — seven years of war, foreign and civil, and the complete destruction of her social system and her commercial relations with the outside world. We did not think it strange that the South took years to recover from a like experience which was far less deep-reaching and prolonged.

So I was prepared to view tolerantly a great deal of inefficiency and did not expect to find industrial medicine on a high plane. But the chance to visit the factories and to see for myself what life there was really like attracted me enormously. I had not the courage, however, to go alone; I persuaded three friends to come with me, three whom I could describe to Semaschko as "experts in social administration": Mabel Kittredge, who started the housekeeping centers of the public schools in New York City and was connected for years with the public school lunches; Edith Hilles, who was working with a fruit raisers' co-operative in Pennsylvania; and Louise Lewis, who lived at the Lighthouse Settlement in Philadelphia and had specialized in work for the unemployed. We decided to go in the fall, when I was due to go to Geneva for the meeting of the League of Nations Health Committee, whose work I have just described.

Our country did not then — nor for years after — recognize Soviet Russia. Americans who wished to enter that country had to get visas from a Russian embassy in one of the European countries which did recognize it. We decided on Warsaw, and as soon as my work in Geneva was over, we journeyed to that city via Berlin. Dr. Rajchman, the Polish director of the Geneva office of the Health Committee, had been very much interested in our venture. He strongly advised us to join the Quaker groups in Russia. "You will find," he said, "that they are the only foreigners the Russians trust. There were several foreign groups who went in to help during the great famine of 1921, but though they did wonders in feeding the children, especially the American Relief Administration, the Russians never believed they were disinterested. They thought these people had come to spy out the land and report its weaknesses. But they trust the Quakers."

It was a long journey to Warsaw from Berlin, which we left in the evening. I woke early and watched from the window the sunrise over that great, sad Polish plain that the Tharauds describe in *L'Ombre de la Croix*. The shadow of the Cross was often to be seen, a great wooden cross, so poor it was not even painted, but very high, towering over the roadside. It was a poor land, sandy to the west, with scrubby pine trees, miserable little farms with too many people to a field,

working barefoot and in rags. It made me think of the West
Country in Ireland for poverty, but it must have been partly
the result of war, for we saw old trenches and ruined houses
only half rebuilt. It was perfectly flat, marshes here and there,
no forests, nothing. Then farther east the land grew better
and there were big estates, well farmed, even with machinery
and grand houses surrounded by trees. The big estates had
not been partitioned in Poland; partition had been promised
but the aristocracy fought it bitterly and successfully.

The night before I left Geneva I dined with Dr. Rajchman,
Professor Nocht, Dr. Cantacuzene, and Dr. Cumming. Mme.
Rajchman is a very intelligent and cultivated Polish lady
and she told me many things about the country. Dr. Cumming said I must be sure to see the great Russian church,
the most interesting thing in Warsaw. Mme. Rajchman's
face stiffened as she said, "We are tearing it down. You will
see only the skeleton." We all exclaimed in dismay. Why
could it not be kept as a national monument, for its historical
value? She said, "It is not national; it is Byzantine. It was
built to crush us, to impose on us an alien religion and an
alien art. We cannot breathe while it is there." And the first
striking thing we saw as we drove through the shabby, undis-
tinguished streets of the city was this half-dismantled hulk
of a church.

We went to the Hotel Bristol, an amusing mixture of attempted gorgeousness and actual shabbiness and primitiveness
— plenty of plush curtains but filthy rags on the floor, broken,
chipped tableware on the breakfast tray, pillowcases for towels
when the latter gave out, and a water supply which consisted
of a tap out in the gilded corridor.

We went at once to call on the Quakers and met there a
Russian-Polish refugee, a Pani Jagmin (*Pani* is "Madame"),

who took us completely under her wing for the whole week, which meant that we met many Polish people informally and saw everything we were interested in. The Poles were very friendly and all of them spoke some language besides Polish, sometimes skipping from French into German into English and back again.

The day after our arrival I had to present my letters to the Minister of Health and of Labor, and then go all over the building of the Hygienic Laboratory and meet every single man and woman and look at every rabbit. By two o'clock my face was stiff from smiling and making polite speeches. But they were really dears, especially Wrodzinski, the Minister of Health. The men were mostly American-trained and the Rockefeller Institute had helped them to put up a fine building, the first effort of the new government. I got a deep impression of their eagerness to make their country fine and the equal of others, to do all the things that civilized countries do but that Russia never let them do. They were struggling with such overwhelming problems, with malaria and tuberculosis, which had never even been studied in Poland, and typhus on the Russian border, and typhoid in Lodz, where with half a million people there was no sewage system, and only wells and rain water.

Dr. Wrodzinski offered us his rattling old Cadillac, left behind I believe by the American Army, to take us and the Quakers to a place about twenty miles away — where the Bolshevists were driven back from Warsaw in 1921 — to visit a normal school where peasant girls were being trained as teachers for peasant children. We rattled along over uneven cobblestones between squalid houses, with the untidy country sprawling on all sides. I felt better about the Poles in America, thinking that nothing they found in Pittsburgh or

South Chicago or Cleveland was uglier and bleaker than what they had had at home. The very cows were wretched, and because the grass was so scanty a child must watch them all day long to see that they did not stray beyond the narrow little strip of grass allotted them. Maybe some of the children went to school but we saw lots of little goose girls, looking like German picture postcards, and little boy goatherds. The bigger girls were the cowherds and shepherds.

But the school was charming, a hundred and eighty girls, many of them in their peasant costumes. They were under a delightfully pretty little headmistress who spoke good French. She gave us dinner in a low-vaulted white room with deep windows and a sanded floor and white scrubbed table and chairs. We had sour soup with bits of cucumbers in it, and more cucumbers dressed with whipped cream, and pickled mushrooms, as well as chicken and potatoes and delicious cauliflower. Then we went upstairs and the girls sang peasant songs, acting them out with gestures as stiff and convention-alized as the Japanese. It was both beautiful and strange. This school was started as soon as "Poland began," they said; that is, after the Armistice. Education was a passion with the Poles. One afternoon, at Dr. Radziwillowicz's, where we met a lot of ladies at tea, they told us that educated Polish women and young girls had always secretly taught children to read and write Polish, forbidden by both the Russians and the Germans, so that many of them could qualify as teachers to a certain extent. After they gained their freedom they threw themselves into teaching with much enthusiasm.

It took us a week in Warsaw to get our visas, so that we saw much of the city and something of the surrounding country. Poverty met us everywhere, not only in the country but in the city streets, especially in the almost incredible Jewish quarter, where one could see in stark realism the tragic Jewish problem, the effort of an alien race to find a home in a country and yet remain separate, apart, not modifying one of its customs or rituals under pressure from its neighbors. And the more primitive a people is, the more it resents differences. The Jews have their own feast days, the Poles have theirs, both of them sacred and important; the Jewish boys go to their own schools, they never play with the Polish boys; no Jew may eat in a Gentile house nor any Gentile in a Jewish house, and intermarriage is a horror to both. As I saw the Jews in Warsaw, so different in their clothing and manner of wearing their hair that one could distinguish them a block away, I thought what an impossible situation it was. Only the breaking down of the barriers between the two races would solve it and for that there must be a desire on both sides.

Perhaps it is only in a new country free from traditions that such a breakdown of barriers can occur. I remembered a Polish Jew I had known at Hull-House, a young man who had escaped a pogrom in which his mother and sister had died with their tongues nailed to the floor because they would not say the name of Christ. He told me that he too would have died rather than say that accursed name or swallow a bit of pork or uncover before the Crucifix. But when he reached this country, he found all his principles slipping away. Nobody cared whether or not he ate ham and he suddenly found he did not care either. He no longer bothered about kosher food and he had even been in Christian churches, taken his hat off, and risen and knelt with the congregation — and not cared at all. He was frankly puzzled at his own indifference to things which in Poland had been matters of life and death to him.

Warsaw was a trying place for Americans. For breakfast we had very poor coffee with milk, and rolls, and butter which we usually could not eat. By eleven o'clock we were hungry but we could not get a real meal before two, when apparently one was supposed to eat enough to last for the whole twenty-four hours. The food was abundant and delicious — but it did not last for twenty-four hours, and suppers were very late and unsatisfactory.

In the restaurant we frequented was a man who sat in the same corner each day and I could not help watching him. He had the face of one who has been through hell and bears the marks thereof, and I wondered what his life had been. So I was much interested when I met him at a coffee party in the house of one of our Polish acquaintances. He told me that he had been professor of astronomy in the University of Tiflis. One evening when he was working in the observatory he heard a tap on the window. He guessed that it was one of the political suspects whom he, like many of the intellectuals, often helped to hide. When he opened the door he found he was right. The man was a Georgian, swarthy, heavily built, secretive, asking for shelter for a short time but saying nothing about himself. He worked in the laboratory for a month, then disappeared as silently as he had come. "That was Dzugashvili, Stalin," the professor said. "Why then," I exclaimed, "if he is under such obligation to you, surely you can appeal to him and get permission to return to the university." He smiled and shook his head. "You do not know him," he said. "Nobody who knows Stalin would ever appeal to him on personal grounds or expect him to feel gratitude."

The professor had fled at the beginning of the Kerensky revolution, when the hordes of returning soldiers roamed through the country, pillaging and murdering. It was that experience, with its horrors which he would not speak of, that had left that look on his face.

When finally word came that our visas were in order and we might take the train for Moscow, we had only a few hours in which to get photographed and to make out pages of "protocol" in Russian. The photographer was almost hysterical when confronted with the job of producing ten prints of each of us in three hours' time and kept repeating, "This is not America. We do not work that way." The porter at the hotel undertook to make out our papers in Russian and that was a terrible job, for his English was not what he claimed it was. The greatest difficulty came with our fathers' Christian names — always a matter of such crucial importance in Europe. Louise Lewis's gave no trouble. Lawrence is a saint's name and known in all lands, but Edith Hilles's Allen, Mabel Kittredge's Abbott, and my Montgomery were too much for him and I don't know what he really wrote down. We made the train, however, and the next evening we reached the Russian border.

It is amusing to look back on that entrance into Russia, which was even more exciting and frightening than the visit to occupied Belgium in 1915 because it was much more unknown — none of us had ever been there, none of us could speak the language — and for the first time we would be outside the protection of our own government. There would be nobody to appeal to, nobody to defend us if we got into trouble — only the Quakers. We clung to the thought of the Quakers.

Russia in 1924 was so unlike the Russia under the Five-Year Plan and the Russia of today that in later years when I have heard returning travelers describe what they saw, I have felt that it was not the same country. At that time Russia was still suffering from the "imperialist" war, the civil wars, the war against Poland, and the great famine; it was struggling, not very efficiently, to start up industry and to get the people housed and fed, but everything was fairly chaotic and the Russians admitted it with a humility that was disarming.

They believed that, since we were Americans, we had never seen anything but the most highly mechanized processes, and when I said that in my Connecticut home oxen were still used to plow and harrow, they smiled incredulously and said I was very kind. They told us a humorous story that was going around Moscow, about the Commission for the Electrification of all Russia, which bore on its office door the notice, "Please knock. The electric bell does not work." Where I had expected defiance and a Martin Chuzzlewit kind of bragging, I met rarely anything but this engaging self-depreciation. Dr. William Thayer, who went over during the Kerensky regime, told me he had the same experience, but judging from the reports I have heard since then, all that has passed away.

When one lives with a Quaker relief group one does not "live soft." We were four in one fairly large room, with four army cots, one tin wash basin, and a great porcelain stove which served as chimney for the stove on the first floor and was always warmish so that one could thaw out one's hands against it and dry one's towel. Even in October Moscow was bleak and cold and I remember no sunny days. There was, however, one warm room, which served as living room and dining room, and there we could have an open fire of birchwood. All Moscow was heated with wood, we saw great piles of it around the buildings of the Kremlin. As for food, I can remember only that I was hungry a good deal of the time, that I got the most satisfaction out of the heavy, damp, strong-tasting black bread; that kasha, a queer sort of cereal, was rather horrid; but most of all, I remember that the tea was not tea and the coffee was not coffee.

Our host was a most likable young Englishman, Edward Balls, the only Quaker left in Moscow, though there were still a few in the famine districts beyond the Volga. Later on, Dr. Effie Graef, an American, came back from the Volga region and added much to our little household. Our house-keeper was a gracious lady of the old regime, who spoke of her position with great thankfulness and said nothing at all about any trials she had been through before she came to the Quakers. Mr. Balls, however, told us that she was just back from Siberia where she had gone to visit her exiled daughter. The girl, only eighteen years old, had been arrested because she was frequenting the British Trade Commission, going there on Sunday afternoons to tea dances to which the young men invited these girls of the former aristocracy. The charge against her was "unconscious espionage," which seems quite impossible to refute, and she was exiled to Siberia, to some village which must not have a school higher than a primary. This sort of sentence was quite common, apparently to guard against any contact with the intelligentsia. The poor mother could not share her daughter's exile, for they would have had nothing to live on, but her old peasant nurse went with the girl, back to her own Siberian village, where it would be easiest to look out for her.

That first evening we had two interesting visitors. One was a tall, distinguished-looking Englishman dressed in the very becoming Russian clothes which our host also had adopted, for comfort and ease: a Russian blouse of black velvet, buttoned high around the throat and belted at the waist, high leather boots, and a flowing cape instead of over-coat. His name was Wickstead and he was a passionate dev-otee of Soviet Russia. "It is the only country in which life is really free," he said. We gasped at that. Mr. Balls had just finished a long speech of caution, warning us that each would have her spy following and reporting; that careless words, even in English, might cause grave danger to others, if not to our-selves; that we must walk on eggs always.

"Oh well," said Mr. Wickstead, "if you are thinking of politics, all right, but I care nothing for politics. The Rus-sian mind is so open and free from inhibitions that talk about real things can be freer than anywhere. If I should go into my club in London and ask a member what he thought about immortality, for instance, he would simply stare at me and think me mad. Here you cannot get off a theory so preposter-ous that the Russian will reject it. He will say, 'Now that is strange. I have never heard of such a thing. Let's sit down and discuss it.' And look at the freedom of social life. If in Eng-land I am asked to dinner and accept I must remember to go that particular night whether I feel like it or not, and I must be on time. Here I can go or not and at the hour I please. Ten chances to one my hostess has forgotten she asked me, and the meal is never on time."

The other visitor was a Russian, a man who had worked with the Quakers during the famine, acting as interpreter and liaison man with the government. I asked him if he was a Party member. "Not at present," he said. "I have been ex-pelled but I hope to win my way back." "Should I be imperti-nent if I asked you why you were expelled?" "No, I can tell you that. It was for disobedience to orders. I was in the Volga region, at the height of the famine, when a summons came for me to return to Moscow. But the Quakers simply could

not spare me, few of them spoke any Russian, I was urgently
needed, so I disobeyed the order and for that I was expelled."
"Was the job in Moscow very urgent?" I asked. "Not at
all," he said. "The summons was just a bureaucratic blunder.
But," he went on very seriously, "you see I followed my own
judgment and that one must not do. One must bow always
to the decision of the Party." "Even if you believe it to be
wrong?" I asked. "Even then. Indeed a Communist must rejoice to sacrifice his own judgment and his own will to that
of the Party."

The days in Moscow were bewildering, exciting, exhausting.
Since neither Mr. Balls nor our Russian guides ever thought
of taking a cab — the funny little horse cabs with their bearded
istvostchiks in enormous overcoats were the only remnant left
of Czarist Russia — and since the streetcars were usually full
up, we tramped for hours over cobblestones slippery with
mud. The first thing that struck us in the streets was the contrast with Warsaw, for here in Moscow we saw neither wealth
nor abject poverty, except for the spectacular beggars, old
men and women looking as if they were made up for the stage.
The crowds were uniformly shabby, the women hatless, the
men in Russian blouses, but they were much more warmly
dressed than the poor in Poland and they looked well-fed.

We had come fully expecting to find everything topsy-
turvy, but all the same it was exciting to see the beautiful
Galitzin Palace turned into a Museum of Safety and the
great white marble Noblemen's Club housing the trade-
unions. We were taken to the Red Square and joined the
procession of the faithful who were worshiping at Lenin's
tomb, among them a crowd of awe-struck school children,
shepherded by their teachers. We visited schools and told

each other we must not be critical if much that we saw was crude and even ridiculous. To try to carry out John Dewey's theories with no equipment and with only ignorant young Bolshevists or bewildered elderly White Russians for teachers could not produce anything but a queer mess.

I felt, as I visited the schools, that I was witnessing the birth of a new religion. Everywhere, from kindergarten to medical school, each room must have its Lenin corner, containing usually a red-covered altar with a picture or bust of Lenin, and with various "Thus spake Lenin" texts on the wall. For the little children the altar had a picture of the child Lenin and often a vase of flowers standing before it. Under the Czar, children had been taken to church; now they were taken to Lenin's tomb, not once only but again and again.

I also saw the birth of a new aristocracy. We visited a school which formerly had taken only the daughters of the nobility; when we were there it took the children of Party members, and among them I found a ten-year-old girl whom I had known at Hull-House, the daughter of a very interesting Russian refugee. "How do you happen to be in this school, Sonya?" I asked. "They told me only Party members' children were admitted and your mother tells me she is not yet a member." "But I am an exception," replied Sonya. "You see, Mother was a hard-labor convict; she assassinated the Governor, so I can come to the school without waiting for her to be admitted to the Party." After all, the basis for this new aristocracy is not essentially different from that of the old regime. It is only more recent.

Moscow was terribly overcrowded. There were no new buildings to house the great influx of people since the Revolution, and though the houses and apartments of the Whites had been taken over and divided among the workers there were not nearly enough, and the government was rationing space very strictly. A commissar came to measure our bedroom — characteristically he did it with a tape measure instead of a yardstick — and if he had found it too large for four, we should have been obliged to put in a fifth cot for Dasha, our heavy-footed housemaid. Luckily he found we had a little less space than we were entitled to. In a way it was curiously satisfactory to be able to feel, for the first — and last — time in my life, that I was no better off than anyone else.

We kept reminding ourselves that we must compare what we saw not with America but with Czarist Russia. I had heard a description of the housing of the poor from a clergyman's wife in Boston, Mrs. G. L. Parker, whose husband served several years as incumbent in the English Church in St. Petersburg. When winter came, Mrs. Parker joined a charitable association of Russian ladies and went with them to visit the poor. She said she found families living in cellars under the street, two or even three stories down. There were children there who never came up to the surface all winter long for want of warm clothes, and she said that as she looked at them in that dim, underground light, she could think of nothing but big white worms. A woman we met in Moscow, the daughter of the chief leather manufacturer in Russia, told us that her father, who was of German descent, built for his workers big barracks, each to hold twelve families. There were no partitions, only one huge room, with stove and sink at one end, yet the other manufacturers blamed him bitterly for coddling his people and spreading discontent.

The Minister of Health, Semaschko, was a big, ruddy, pleasant-mannered Russian. He knew no word of any language but his own, and he passed me on to two German-trained and German-speaking Jewish doctors, Guelman and Gilewitch, who were very good to me and showed me hospitals and factories. There were not many of the latter to interest me, but I saw some excellent, newly equipped rubber and electrical works, and some old, primitive textile mills. Pottery, felt hats, paint grinding, were still largely home industries carried on by peasants during the winter months, and there was no eagerness to show me that sort of work. The most impressive sight was the Institute Obuch, the first hospital in the world devoted to occupational diseases only, with seventy-five beds, five laboratories, and a staff of thirteen physicians. They told me that Leningrad and Kharkov had similar institutions. Indeed, it seemed to me that there was more industrial hygiene in Russia than industry.

My guides were deeply absorbed in their work and enthusiastic over it. As we tramped over the cobbles or sat in tramcars I learned a good deal about the life of a physician in Russia. They were both frankly shabby — Dr. Gilewitch's overcoat was fastened with a safety pin and he was literally "on his uppers." But he had what an American doctor does not have, independence of money, for in Russia money does not spell success. The Russian doctor has no need to sacrifice the research work he loves and go into practice in order to make more money for his family; he does not need to have an office on a good street, drive an expensive car, send his children to private schools, carry a heavy life insurance — he is free from all those compulsions. And though he lives in scant comfort, he knows that if he breaks down, or his wife or child is ill, the best sanatoria and rest homes in the country are open to him. Above all, he is free from the drive of competition.

I looked with a little envy at the women doctors, for never before had I been in a country where men and women in

medicine are absolutely equal. The head of the best hospital
in Moscow, the one devoted primarily to textile workers, was
a tall, blonde woman who had a mixed staff under her. The
Medical School was full of girl students and I have been told
since then that some 70 per cent of the graduates now are
women. The Russians say women are readier to take up the
hard life in the villages than men, and that they are for the
most part interested in practical medicine, not research. Russia needs practising physicians far more than pure scientists.

The Obuch Institute had already begun to make routine
examinations of groups of workers exposed to certain dangers
and at that time they happened to be working on the men in a
rubber factory who handled benzol. The men would pass the
night in the hospital so that all the tests could be made without any interruption of their work. I was reminded of an
interesting incident in a rubber factory during the Czarist days
which was related by a Russian doctor, Dworetsky, in 1914
in a German medical journal, since he was forbidden to publish it in Russia. He tells of a mysterious outbreak of illness
among women working with a rubber solution in a large factory in St. Petersburg. A new solvent had been introduced
and, soon after, many of the women began to complain of
headache, dizziness, nervousness, some were greatly excited,
some fainted, others had epileptoid convulsions. The foremen
evidently did nothing sensible about it and by the end of four
days 231 had been affected. The tale spread and with it the
rumor that the employers were starting a wholesale murder of
the workers, so then the sickness spread to the women in
chocolate and tobacco factories. The employers lost their
tempers and declared a lockout, whereupon the Duma voted
an emergency fund for the thousands thus turned out in the
depth of winter. Naturally the doctors were much interested

and eager to discover whether this was really an instance of intoxication by a volatile solvent or only mass hysteria, but they were not allowed to find out, for the chief of police stepped in, declared that it was all the work of radical agitators, forbade any discussion of the subject by a group larger than three, and refused to let the Duma distribute any relief. The factories were reopened after the workers had been brought to a proper state of meekness, and the incident was closed. About the same time a similar situation developed in rubber works in Moscow and in Riga, where a quiet investigation revealed the illness to be acute benzol intoxication, for the new cement had been made with almost pure benzol. The illness in the chocolate and tobacco factories was undoubtedly hysterical.

This was certainly a striking contrast to the Russia of 1924. Another contrast, not so dramatic, came to my mind, an incident which had happened just before I left home on this trip. Some cases of severe benzol poisoning had occurred in a Massachusetts city, in men applying a coating to patent leather. I was very keen to study them, to discover just what conditions had caused the trouble, but it was impossible. The employer was hurt and indignant at the implication that his plant was at fault, the company doctor was secretive. The hospital, which at first was eager to help me, suddenly drew back after being notified by the insurance company that if any information was given out, their cases would thereafter be sent to another hospital. In Russia, worker, employer, doctor, insurance carrier, all were responsible to the government only.

Madame Rykova, the wife of the then Premier, took me to see some of the eighteen centers for the treatment of tuberculosis. It was the only time I traveled in a really good automobile in Russia. Dr. Guelman once drove me in a patched-up Ford, the two front doors of which were tied together with a clothesline to keep them shut. The tuberculosis dispensaries were excellent; they deserved to be copied widely. They were for ambulatory patients, men and women still able to work, who would come during the two-hour midday pause customary in Russia. There they had a nourishing meal and a siesta, well wrapped up, on an open porch, and then again at night they came for a good meal and a bath. They slept in great white bearskin sleeping bags in a ward with open windows.

Moscow's industries were for the most part more interesting to the student of personnel management and general factory hygiene than to a specialist in poisons, and my friends found a great many things to interest them while I was hunting for lead and benzol. It was a surprise to us all to find that the piece-work system was in force everywhere, more than in capitalist countries. We were told frankly that if he were paid by the day, the Russian would not work. Probably now it is quite different, but in those days Russian factories had none of the ordinary comforts one expects to find — proper seats for women at work, rest rooms, a pause for lunch in the seven-hour day. When we spoke of this last, we were told that no break in the working day was needed; the women did not get tired as they would under a capitalistic system, for they were working for their own benefit.

Our evenings we spent at the opera, or ballet, or theater. Lunacharsky was keeping up the Czarist traditions in the arts and we saw beautiful ballets and heard good music. We might have seen the Moscow Art Theatre but chose instead Meyer-holt's, as something we could not hope to see at home. They were giving Revolutionary plays, most hilarious for us, though the audience took them seriously. There was much satire about the bourgeois nations who were repeatedly taken off, especially the Poles and the Americans. The former would be shown in medieval costume, bowing and kissing the ring of a prelate, or reciting poems with great fervor to ladies who swooned with emotion. Our countrymen were instantly recognizable; they wore tortoise-shell spectacles and high, shining collars, and were constantly having their shoes shined by little bootblacks. They sat in enormous rocking chairs with a telephone in each hand, and plotted the destruction of Soviet Russia. The women tilted across the stage in high-heeled slippers and rifled the men's pockets.

The most amusing play was *The Lake of Lull*, a fictitious place in the United States where there are great mines on an island, most conveniently situated for the capitalist owner who can shut off supplies when he chooses and starve the miners into submission. Here we saw a peculiarly dreadful lot of American capitalists who bribe the young hero to betray the workers by promising to make him Minister of Foreign Affairs. He thinks that then he will make the United States recognize Soviet Russia and all will be forgiven. But his sweetheart discovers his criminal purpose and — heroic Bolshevist that she is — shoots him dead, then plays the Judith part with the American general who, dressed in Buffalo Bill costume, has come to break the strike. She shoots him while he is kissing her. The finale comes when the Red Army marches on the stage and the miners and soldiers and the noble girl join in the "*Internationale*." It was explained that the army had marched through a tunnel, leading from Leningrad to New York. The audience took it with solemn enthusiasm.

We saw a good deal of Anna Louise Strong and were impressed by her unwavering faith in all things Russian. She was living in a half-dismantled hotel, cooking her meals in the squalidest kitchen I ever saw, the hotel kitchen, used by a dozen or more families, none of them responsible for cleaning anything but their own pots and pans, which then had to be carried up to the bedrooms — or they would be stolen. She was most cheerful about it all. We had as housemates for part of the time William Henry Chamberlin and his Russian wife. Later on, when I met him in Cambridge, after the famine of 1930 and the liquidation of the kulaks, he was deeply disillusioned about Russia, but at that time he still had great hopes for the future and sympathy with the present difficulties. We were disappointed not to meet Walter Duranty, who was in the Crimea.

One American woman who came to see us several times made a rather dreadful impression on me. She was the first one of that class of American Communists whom I came to know later at home, who are ready to go to any lengths for the sake of "the Cause." One evening we got to discussing the universal espionage and I said Russia could never hope to have a united people till she got rid of it and restored people's trust in each other, that mutual suspicion and mutual betrayal spoiled human relations. She insisted it was necessary. "But," I said, "don't you value at all a sense of honor, respect for truth-telling, loyalty?" She smiled in a pitying way. "Petty bourgeois ideology," she said.

"And you are not revolted at all by the cruelty, the midnight arrests, the shooting without real trials, of hundreds?"

"Certainly not," she said. "The one question I ask is, 'Does that help the Party?' If it does, it is right; if not, it is wrong." She was a beautiful creature, with gold-red hair and a profile like Duse's, but I found her a horror.

After a fortnight we decided that we must see more of the country than only Moscow, so we separated. Louise Lewis and Edith Hilles went with the Chamberlins to Leningrad and Kiev, while Mabel Kittredge and I accepted Mr. Balls's offer to pilot us to the Quaker stations near the Siberian border. I shall quote from the description I wrote at the time.

We left with Mr. Balls at noon, and I was a little disconcerted to find that we three were in one compartment with two lower berths and two which could be made into uppers, but Mabel Kittredge said she had often traveled that way in France during the war and it was perfectly easy, and I must say that it was. Of course it was not what we should call a real sleeper. It was "traveling soft" — that is, the seats were cushioned, but nothing else and not much of that. There was a filthy little table which was also a stepladder for the upper berth, and a box for a candle which was lighted about an hour after dark and went out some time after midnight. We had a lunch basket, well stocked by Dr. Graef in Moscow, and every now and then when the train stopped we would pile out with all the others and run to a hot water spout and fill our teapot and drink more tasteless Russian tea. We spread our food on a clean towel and used the remainder of the tea for dishwater. It was squalid but nothing to the squalor of the toilet room. I thought of the grand Institute of Sanitary Hygiene where they were doing research on germs and wished they would tackle some simpler and more immediate problem.

When night came Mr. Balls climbed up on the upper berth and Mabel and I spread sheets (Quaker sheets) over the straw-stuffed cushions and lay down under rugs, with a holdall and a softish suitcase for pillows. The journey was really delightful. Once we had left Moscow we were out on the steppes and for hours we would travel without a sign of human habitation — just the endless plain, sodden with rain, brown plowed fields or blue-green from the sprouting rye. The sky hung dark over it all, and rain fell most of the time. As we jogged on, not fast but steadily, it seemed like crossing the ocean, it seemed as if it might go on for-

ever, so unchanging, so endless it was. Now and then a village
would appear, little brown huts, rarely a town, but most of the
time we looked out on fields and nothing else. It was dreadful to
think of the miles the peasants must walk to their work, and the
miles back. Through the night I would wake and look out and
always it was the same. The next afternoon we came to the Volga,
yellow and wind-tossed, not so wide as the Connecticut at Lyme
Bridge, with one bank very low and the other higher. This, we
were told, is true of all the rivers in Russia, and they gave this
reason for it, that the earth as it turns does not pull the water with
it as fast as it goes, the water lags behind and drags back, piling up
the earth behind it.

At eleven o'clock that night we reached Buzuluk, the center for
the Quaker famine work, and Mr. Balls left us, for it had been
arranged that we should keep on three hours more to one of the
villages, where Alice Davis was keeping open one of the Quaker
centers. I had not felt so young and timid in almost half a century
as I did when he left us and two young Red soldiers came in to
occupy the other two berths. They were nice boys and went to sleep
at once, but we spent a rather long three hours, trying not to
wonder what we should do if Alice Davis had not got the telegram
and was not there to meet us. I kept dozing off and waking in
a panic thinking I had forgotten the name of the town, which is
none too easy, Sorotchinskoi, with the accent on the "rot."

The conductor, however, came to put us off and there on the
platform with a lantern was Alice Davis in a great fur coat and
cap. She explained that her Ford was out of order but she had
brought the cart. She piloted us out to a country cart filled with
straw covered with burlap and we swung ourselves up and sat flat,
with our feet out, and bounced along to the village, two miles
away, a scattering of brown mounds with a vast space which was
called a street. Presently we drove into a courtyard, a door opened,
and we entered a lovely little house — clean and white and empty
and warm and sweet, after dark, stuffy, crowded, untidy Moscow.

The big white stove was warm and a samovar was humming and Alice Davis's Russian friend and housemate, Nadezhda Victorovna Danilewska, was there. She was of the old regime, and had her own tragic story, which I heard later. They gave us tea and we went to bed in narrow wooden beds, with ropes for springs, but heavenly comfortable after the shelves in the train. The wind howled all night and I kept dreaming of wolves, for there are many around these villages and it seemed just the night for them.

The next morning we had breakfast at a white deal table scrubbed till the surface was silver, and we drank real coffee, wonderful after the roasted wheat we had in Moscow. As we ate, the village priest was shown in, a gentle man who came to get help to send a blind child to Orenburg for operation. Alice Davis promised it to him. She worked with all of them — with the Soviet, giving a ration of fats to the hospital and of food and clothing to the children's home, with the Central Health Department by maintaining the malaria clinic, and even with the Tartars, for she found them worshiping in a mosque where all the windows were broken during the famine. She gave them new ones because the poor things got pneumonia or a relapse of malaria, and they had to pray. She had a dozen villages under her, where she supervised malaria work, and she raised cabbages and carrots and potatoes for her child feeding. She ran three tractors. A fourth tractor she had had harnessed to mill machinery which cleaned millet and ground sunflower seed for the villages.

She took us to the children's home, where we found a sickly-looking youth with fanatic blue eyes instructing the youngsters in "political knowledge." He was a young Communist and as such his duty was to go to schools and orphanages and teach Bolshevist doctrine. Then we went to the school, across mud such as I have never seen. It was black, soft on top, greasy and slippery underneath, so that all one's mind had to be concentrated on one's footing for fear of being precipitated into the awful filth. The school was small and all of the children were crowded into one room watching a rehearsal of a play, to be given on the great day, November 7. It had been sent from Moscow and the teachers were ordered to train the children to perform it. Mrs. Danilewska murmured a translation to us as we watched.

We saw a peasant family, parents, grandparents, children, and we saw the conflict between the rigidly orthodox and superstitious old people and the cheeky young generation boasting of the new Science learned in school and ridiculing the old beliefs, while father and mother looked on in bewilderment, not knowing which was right. At last the old man gave up. "Well," he said, "I can see it is time for us old ones to turn our faces to the wall and die. There is no place left for us." And on that note the play ended. Later we heard some children singing in the street and their song was: "Get out of the way, you old folks. There's no place for you but the grave."

It was indeed at that time the avowed policy of the Kremlin to do everything possible to break up family ties and get the children away from parental influence into the pure air of Bolshevist doctrine. The ideal was to bring all children up in great communal homes, but this could not be realized at once; it cost too much. If one suggested that it would be hard to substitute loyalty to an abstraction for love of one's own family and that impersonal discipline would be less effective than a father's authority, one was smiled upon. Youthful delinquency, one was told, was the product of capitalism, there would never be any need for juvenile courts in Soviet Russia.

Some thirteen years later, a friend of mine who is a passionate admirer of Soviet Russia came back from one of her many visits there and told me that she had been bewildered to find a complete *volte-face* on the part of the governmental attitude toward children and the family. Now all the stress was laid on the close relation between parent and child, even to the point of sentimentality. She had never heard so many songs about mother love and home, sweet home. Evidently the ruling group had seen during those years that there were causes for youthful delinquency which could not be brought under the head of capitalism and, as dictators can do, they declared a new policy, discipline and order in the family and in the school, loyalty and obedience to individuals, not to an abstraction.

The meeting in celebration of the November Revolution was held that evening in Sorotchinskoi, and it was impressive. There was much oratory, which was not worth translating, but it was well worth while to watch the faces of the men and women gathered there, so clearly filled with a sense of their new dignity and importance. When they rose and sang the *"Internationale"* I was much moved. It is far more thrilling than the "Star-Spangled Banner" or "God Save the King," but less so than the *"Marseillaise."* Mrs. Danilewska said that before the war a holiday in that village meant simply a church service and then mad drunkenness, ending in fights or wife beating.

We went back to a most luxurious dinner of cabbage soup with a big spoonful of thick sour cream in it, fresh rye bread, and homemade sweet butter, roast chicken and baked apples, and then to bed for a long sleep. The next morning was clear and cold. The mud had frozen hard and for the first time I could really see the village as I walked through it. The streets were ridiculously wide, it seemed to me that one could run from twelve to sixteen trolley lines through them and have plenty of room. It reminded me a little of a town on the border of New Mexico, Alamosa, where I once spent a night, a village with wide streets out of all proportion to the little houses and stores, and beyond it the desert, stretching in all directions. The steppe is so like the desert. The houses were of adobe too, like those in New Mexico, but with thatched roofs, the windows tiny with irregular panes of glass, and the walls very thick, making charming deep window recesses. More pretentious ones would have the clay covered with boards, which gave them the cold, thin look of frame houses. Some had a heavy basketwork woven out of birch branches with clay piled between it and the wall, so as to have more protection against the cold. Sheds and barns ran in a square connecting with the house and making a courtyard inside. All along the street at short intervals were wells with long well-sweeps such as one sees still in New England.

We made rounds with the visiting nurse, who had been trained in Moscow, making calls in peasant houses, the poorest of the poor, people who had survived the famine but had lost many of their family in it. But even in those houses it was not squalid, never close and odorous, not even in one where the woman was washing clothes in a big trough in front of the stove, her two little boys peering down from the top at us, and a little brown calf tethered beside her and a little white pig sitting in front. I thought of the heavy, human odor in Chicago tenements. If people are to be poor, there is an advantage in living in the country. We went into one Tartar house, beautifully clean, where we saw a pretty young girl, dressed in burlap, which had been carefully sewed into a full skirt and scant waist, and with a clean kerchief on her head. Her father explained to the nurse that he hoped to sell her soon, for tea, sugar, and rye, a good deal of rye. We told the nurse to beg him to find a good man for her — she was quite unmoved throughout the conversation — but he said there were no good men left since the war.

We took a Maxim Gorky to Buzuluk, a three-hour journey. That is a fourth-class car, or rather an accommodation train with third-class seats. They call it a Maxim Gorky, some say because it turns everyone into pessimists à la Gorky, some say because he wrote so much about such trains. Along one side of the car runs a long bench and opposite are rows of shelves, three deep, placed at right angles to the car. You can climb up to the top or to the middle one and lie there all day, if you like, but if you choose the bottom one you must be prepared to let your upper neighbors come down and sit with you sometimes. Our car was full and quite dark, except for a candle at one end. The train burned wood and ran slowly but very steadily, not wasting time at stations. One gets a little hypnotized by the slow, steady jogging and the endless plain outside. There seems no reason why it should ever stop or why one should ever get out. The men were eagerly curious about us, after we had shaken our heads and said "Amerikansky," and I did long to talk to them. It is missing half of the interest of a country not to be able to talk the language.

Buzuluk is a town, but not radically different in appearance for the most part from a village. The Quaker headquarters were large and comfortable, in charge of an American, Mabel Phillips, with two White Russian ladies, one of them with an adorable six-year-old daughter. There we had our first experience of a Russian bath. The household had just completed theirs, having gone into the big shed in two groups, first the women, then the men. It was still hot and we eagerly accepted the invitation to use it. We found it cloudy with steam from a great caldron into which hot stones had been put and then water poured over them. You sit on a bench and soap yourself thoroughly, then you wash with dipper after dipper of hot

water, and then you sit and steam a long time and then repeat
the process. I wondered if it was not this weekly soaking that
explained the surprising sweetness of the air in the peasant
houses. The day ended with a lovely church service, to which
we went by bright moonlight, making me think of the description in Tolstoy's *Resurrection*. Little Natucha adopted me
and chattered Russian without caring at all to have me answer.
We walked together to church and once there she edified
me by her crossings and bowings and prostrations, though the
last did make me squirm, the church floor was so dirty for a
nice little child's face.

The train for Moscow left at half-past three in the morning,
but it was an hour late, which meant an uneasy night for us
and for our hostess. Then we could not be sure till it came
whether we could get on, for they only sell a ticket if there is
a vacant place. As a matter of fact there was only one vacant,
but they let us on. Mabel and I stretched out, feet to head,
on the single lower berth of a two-berth compartment, and
the man in the upper left us at Samara, at nine the next morning. It was a long journey, till six of the following evening, but
I never tired of it. A snowstorm came up and the steppe and
the villages were altogether different from those we had seen
on our way east. The carts now were low sleds, making a
wonderful background for the scarlet skirts of the women;
the villages were white blobs; the rivers were dark green; the
few pine forests were like fairyland. We got very expert in
taking care of ourselves, running for hot water, buying little
loaves of rye bread and chunks of roast chicken which the
peasant women were selling.

When we reached Moscow we heard, a week late, that
Coolidge had been elected. In Sorotchinskoi, at the November 7 celebration, we had been told that the United States

would be the next country to go Bolshevist, for the workers would no longer endure capitalistic oppression.

Our last week, as I remember, was not filled with officially planned visits and we were free to go our own way, so we managed to see a number of White Russians and hear their stories. To me they are as pitiful a group as the world has seen and when I think of the sympathy that was lavished on the victims of the French Revolution and on our Southerners after the Civil War, I wonder why these people have met with little but indifference. Alexandra Tolstoy, who was a neighbor of mine in Connecticut for several years, let herself go on this subject once, comparing the widespread indignation against Hitler for his persecution of the Jews and the generous help poured out for them with the way the White Russians had been allowed to die of privations and starvation with none to care. I suppose it was because there were no influential and wealthy Russians in other lands to take up their cause, as the Jewish cause has been taken up by Jews all over the world.

A visit to a prison was one of our most exciting experiences. A Tolstoy follower — the younger Tchertkoff — the son of Tolstoy's closest friend, came to ask me if I would request permission to visit a prison in which one of the conscientious objecters had recently been placed. He was a physician, a Tolstoyan, and he refused to do military service. While Lenin lived such men were exempt if they succeeded in convincing a jury that they were sincere in their belief, but after his death the military authorities took things in hand and refused exemption to doctors. Tchertkoff had heard that the doctor was to be sent to an agricultural colony to do farm work instead of practising his profession. So we went to the Prison Department to get a permit. That was the only government service which shocked me profoundly. The chief, named

Korngold, looked like a gorilla; his neck was thicker than his head and there was almost nothing of a head above his eyes. Even worse was a woman who came in and stared at us. She also had no forehead, she was cross-eyed, her hair streaked down over her cheeks and her mouth was half open. I thought her an idiot but Korngold presented her as chief psychiatrist for the prison system.

We got our permits and Dr. Graef, Mabel Kittredge, and I went to the prison, escorted by a young official and two doctors. Of course it was a fairly good prison or we could not have seen it, and most of the politicals were not there. The lack of ventilation and of cleanliness would make most Americans think it a dreadful place, but what struck me most was the informality and humanness of it all. I would far rather be there than in any of our prisons I have seen. The men were all working except those who were practising for a concert, but not one was in uniform, nor were the guards, so that we could not tell guards from convicts. They were allowed to talk to each other and when we came in they would all stop work and cluster around us, together with their guards, and chatter eagerly. They were allowed to smoke, too. We went into one of the cells, a big one, with fifteen squalid cots, a clay stove with the inevitable teakettle on it, a long table, books, checkers and chess. I met the doctor and found that he was practising his profession there and also allowed to abstract medical articles. He was in for five years but at the end of half the time he might petition for release, if he had a good record.

On our last evening Mr. Wickstead came in. I was much worked up over the plight of a young Prince Galitzin whom we had talked to that afternoon. "Suppose," I said, "he should go to Lunacharsky and tell him that, because he is an aristocrat, he cannot get work, nor can he finish at the University, nor can he leave the country, and what do they want him to do? What could Lunacharsky say?" "Probably he wouldn't bother to say anything," Mr. Wickstead replied. "You must remember that in Russia the individual does not count. In England, and I suppose in the United States, if you want to rouse people against a social wrong, you always speak of some individual case. 'This child is ill-treated.' 'Look at this picture of a woman in a sweat-shop.' But the Russian is Asiatic in some ways and one case does not impress him. He shrugs and says, 'But there are so many starving aristocrats, what does one matter?' " I am thankful to say that the young man soon after succeeded in escaping over the Finnish border.

Some of these helpless people brought me letters they dared not mail. Dr. Kalina had offered to wrap up and seal, with a government seal, all the pamphlets I had accumulated, and some of our party thought the best thing to do with the letters was to slip them inside, then they would be safe. But my instinct was against that and I made a tight little package of them and put it inside the bosom of my dress, which was lucky, for at the border the Red Guards were so intrigued by the government seal that they broke it and searched carefully through the pamphlets.

We crossed into Poland with a feeling of indescribable relief, and that is an experience which many travelers have since told me they also had, even when, as has been true now for many years, they were carefully shielded throughout their stay in Russia from any contact with people of the old regime. But there is for many people, as there was for us, a sense of underlying terror which they cannot explain, not fear of any danger to themselves but a sense of mysterious and dreadful things going on under the surface. It was exactly the way I felt when in 1915 I crossed the border from German-occupied Belgium into free Holland — that at last I could draw a long breath, at last I could speak without whispering and looking over my shoulder and feel free from a hundred vague fears and dreads. We used to laugh these away sometimes, when we had seen some specially fine piece of work — such as Kalinina's reception station for the waifs — but always something brought them back.

Russia is such a strange mixture; I felt as I looked back that I could never generalize about it because one thing contradicts another. I had shuddered over the cruelty to the people of the old regime, but it seemed unfair to dwell too much on that because in the Revolution of 1905 the Whites had been quite as cruel. Even the aristocrats in Moscow took it for granted that if the Whites had won they would have exterminated the Reds so far as they could, and they told me that, in the matter of brutality, of killing prisoners and hostages, of torturing and the rest, there was nothing to choose between the two. One woman of the aristocracy, who was a Red Cross nurse under both sides, said that she blamed the Whites more, because they were the highest in the land and one expected more of them than of the lowest. But to say that the Czarists would have been as bad was not to defend the Bolshevists. They were planning for a land where justice and security and mutual trust would prevail, but they were sowing the seeds for a harvest which was just the reverse. We found that there was less free speech and free press than under the Tsar, for absolutely nothing was allowed to be said or printed that was not orthodox Bolshevism. Even so humble an organization as the Fellowship of Reconciliation was not permitted and Tchertkoff's copy of the *World Tomorrow* was confiscated.

Chamberlin had told us that when he and his wife were traveling in the country and spending the nights in villages, they always inquired if there was a Baptist in the village, for they knew that they would find in a Baptist house cleanliness and sobriety. But before we left Moscow the head of the Baptist mission told us he expected to be expelled and he soon was.

We did not sense this at first — we were meeting officials and people like Anna Louise Strong, Gertrude H——, Marie Y——, who were enthusiastically loyal to the Soviet — but little by little the other world began to come up to the surface, through interpreters, people I met in the laboratories, teachers, and intellectuals the others met, and the women who stole in to talk to us after seeing our names in the papers. The stories were heartrending, there is nothing worse in George Kennan's book; and it was not only isolated instances, but a whole class. One felt it was more than fear that prompted the persecution, it was in part the joy of the underdog, now on top, to repay the kicks he got when he was down. It seemed to me that a government that could hold its own only by denying the people all freedom, that made opinion a crime, was wrong no matter what its theoretical aims. Soviet Russia made me think of Spain under the Inquisition — it was no more confident of its wisdom and infallibility than Spain was. But if it succeeded in lasting, it would be only at the expense of its intellectual life, as was so in Spain. It was quite true that the ruling class lived simply and did not grow rich, but men care far more for power than for money and their power was unlimited. The convinced Bolshevists among our friends kept on by losing themselves in work, very necessary work, and not thinking of anything else; so did the Quakers. But to people only looking on, as we were, it seemed a terrifying land, and we were thankful to be back in unenlightened Poland, free from spies.

In Paris I delivered my letters, one of them to Prince Yussoupoff, the assassin of Rasputin, a tall distinguished-looking man, whose great hands I looked at with fascination, seeing them in imagination doing their work on that powerful peasant. Paris was a great contrast to Moscow but, as I wrote Miss Addams, "though I love to see gayety again and to have comfort and ease, there are lots of things in Moscow that are finer. It is fine to see people all alike plain and shabby, never to see a flapper or a woman with a made-up face (the Russian girls with their knitted scarfs are far more attractive than Paris women in fashionable hats), to see no rich people and few abjectly poor. But certainly a soft bed and warmth and light and delicious food are delightful."

The aftermath of my Russian visit was a meeting of the Foreign Policy Association in Boston where I spoke, together with Maurice Hindus, Father Edmund Walsh, Donald Stevens, and James M. Landis, then a Research Fellow at Harvard Law School. I remember the meeting vividly for it is the only time I was ever hissed. The papers made a good deal of the hissing but it was really not very bad, only it gives one a strange feeling. I had said that modern history had seen three great revolutions and in every case there was one country that underwent the greatest upheaval and one country that succeeded in remaining untouched by it. First came the intellectual revolution, the Protestant Reformation. Germany was torn by it, Spain shut it out. Then came the political. France was torn by it, Russia shut it out. Now we had the economic revolution, with Russia the seat of the greatest upheaval. Was our country to follow the example of Spain and of Czarist Russia and refuse to let any influence from that movement reach our land?

If we did might we not come to the same fate as those two backward nations? There was some hissing then but more when I quoted the *Magnificat:* "He hath put down the mighty from their seats, and exalted them of low degree. He hath filled the hungry with good things; and the rich he hath sent empty away." Clearly one must not bring communistic sentiments in the Bible to bear on modern life.

XIX

The Lawrence Strike

My BOSTON life covered the years of prosperity, the affluent twenties, but as I look back I do not see a picture of easy living, extravagant spending, perhaps because my job at Harvard kept me there only for half the college year and I continued my explorations into industry. So I saw the "deflation of labor" which came suddenly in 1921, with widespread unemployment and a quick abandonment of all the "frills" which employers had thought necessary to adopt in the nervous period of 1919. For two years industrialists had been willing to go to any expense to keep labor satisfied; those were the days of personnel directors and of so-called industrial psychologists who knew just how to combat Bolshevism from within. They were also the days of the industrial doctors, who were in demand as never before. Industry expected a huge market for all sorts of goods in a stripped and hungry Europe. But when it appeared that Europe could not buy our goods, no matter how much she needed them, there was a sudden drop in production, which meant discharge of workers, closing down of medical departments and of "welfare work."

Gradually employment came back and wages rose in most industries, but curiously enough not in one which held my interest for many years, the textile industry of New England, especially the woolen mills in Lawrence, not far from Boston. During all the period of high wages before the great depression, Lawrence's wages never went up. The contrast between their lot and that of more fortunate workers caused great discontent among the Italian and French-Canadian textile workers and there was a succession of strikes in Lawrence, I cannot remember how many. Mrs. Glendower Evans and Mrs. William Z. Ripley drew me into them and I remember, especially in connection with the strike of 1931–1932, dramatic mass meetings in that drab city of mills, and many talks with young labor leaders, Rivière, the French Canadian, and Robert Watt, the Scotchman, who has since gone to the top in labor circles.

The habit of careful inquiry before forming conclusions which Ann Arbor and Hopkins and the Memorial Institute had inculcated made me probe as deeply as I could into the causes for Lawrence's backwardness, and I still have a file of correspondence with the textile companies, with labor leaders, and with statisticians and financial authorities. I wrote at the time an account of it which has never been published, and as I now read over that manuscript I know that though the indignation it reveals is emotional, it is founded on cold facts. I think I must quote it in part: —

The woolen-goods industry in the United States is the beneficiary of a high tariff which the American people have granted to it in order to protect it against the competition of "the pauper industries of Europe" and to enable it to thrive and to pay good wages so that its employees may enjoy a high standard of living.

To achieve such excellent results we have had to consent to very considerable sacrifices. If we are unpatriotic enough to bring back lovely pure woolen sweaters and coats and scarfs from Europe we must submit to a heavy fine in the Customhouse, and we must not rebel if we are too poor to pay the duty on foreign wool or to pay the high prices asked for woolen goods here. We may look with envy at Irish turf cutters in Connemara, or shepherds in the Dalmatian mountains, who can go clad from head to foot in soft, warm, waterproof woolen clothing, such as we Americans of the middle class cannot afford to buy, and we know that our own working people must content themselves with shoddy clothes and heavy, soggy cotton blankets and coverlets. It does seem a pity that peasant women of Europe can have their hands always busy with knitting when they sit gossiping on their doorsteps and their children can wear warm stockings in winter, but when they emigrate to this country, though they would gladly keep on knitting, their hands are idle for they cannot buy the wool and their children must wear cotton stockings.

Yes, we make quite severe sacrifices in order to help the American Woolen Company, but we are told that we should make them willingly, for the sake of the mill hands, to guarantee to them the sort of life we want for our countrymen. Contentment and prosperity in the mill towns will be our reward and who shall say the price is too high?

Then something happens to shake our faith in the results of this beneficent tariff. Twenty-three thousand men and women in Lawrence, the seat of the largest of the American Woolen Company's mills, strike and that at a time when unemployment is rife and winter coming on. It is true that the strike is short-lived, the workers go back to the mills — those who can get their jobs back — at the new wage cut, the city of Lawrence, which suffers such disasters with a frequency hard to understand when one thinks that all her industries are tariff-protected, draws a long sigh of relief and the public accepts the outcome as only reasonable; since the cost of living has fallen, wages must fall too.

But some of us cannot accept the outcome so easily, we are skeptical and insist on looking more closely at the reasons for the strike, feeling that there must have been strong motives to drive an unorganized army of workers to an act so mad. And when we look we discover widespread destitution that has continued for years, a low wage scale that was kept up even during the period of prosperity. For Lawrence mill hands did not share in the fat years when wages in other industries mounted and mounted, nor is it true that this last wage cut only met the fall in the cost of living. The wages of Lawrence mill workers were cut in the depression after the war and from that time on they were kept low. The U. S. Census of Manufactures issued by the Department of Commerce has tables showing that, in a list of sixteen industrial groups, textile workers were the lowest paid during the prosperous years of 1923 to 1929. Why should there be a low wage scale in these mills? What has become of the arguments we heard when duties were put on woolen goods, and then raised, and then raised again? After all we have done for the industry, why is it that the workers are not getting a good life either in the lean years or the fat years? Surely we have a right to ask an explanation. When an industry goes to Washington and demands a public subsidy, asserts that it cannot live without help, then it would seem that the public that grants the help it asks is justified in insisting that the industry live up to its side of the bargain.

Possibly the American Woolen Company will concede that it has failed to provide a wage sufficient for an American standard of living, but it will certainly insist that through the beneficent working of the tariff, Lawrence mill hands are better off than foreign workers. Suppose we compare the lot of the Lawrence man with that of his English brother and see what are the evils from which the tariff has protected him. Grant that his money wage is higher — I do not know what the English wage is — certainly it should be considerably higher since industries in this country with no tariff protection pay higher wages than are given in England. But there are important factors in a mill hand's life besides his pay envelope. There is the question of provision against three great fears which haunt every wage earner — fear of sickness, fear of unemployment, and fear of old age. In Lawrence the mill worker faces them alone, in England he knows that a measure of security is guaranteed to him. One does not like to think about Lawrence just now, with thousands not yet taken back into the mills, no savings left, no help against sickness and hunger and cold except private charity. And Lawrence, suffering always from the fact that she is the seat of a low-wage industry, plagued by recurrent outbursts of industrial war, is not in a position to supply from the pockets of her citizens the help that the English mill hand receives as a right from his government.

There are other ways in which a comparison between the pauper worker of England and the tariff-protected Lawrence mill hand seems to work out to the advantage of the former. After all, man does not live by bread alone, self-respect and a sense of human dignity are essential to us all. Those of us who visited Lawrence during the strike felt that much of the bitterness on the part of the strikers came from their sense of being treated as beneath the notice of those absentee financiers who had assumed charge of the strike from their offices in New York and who would not condescend even to answer a communication from them. For this strike was conducted by the Textile Committee, which represented all the mill owners of Lawrence, in the old way, approved in the eighties and nineties. Again we saw the employers welded into a strong organization which acted through a small committee, facing a mixed group of men and women, poorly organized, who were not allowed to do that same thing, to choose a committee to act for them in dealing with the other side. They were expected to go one by one and treat as individuals with that powerful organization. Whatever people may think of trade-unions, they cannot fail to see the injustice of such a method, which gives to the side already the stronger, the side with money and influence, the right of combination and denies it to the side that has so many handicaps.

The English mill hand is a member of a strong trade-union. No radical change can be made in the conduct of the mill without his voice being heard. When wage cuts are proposed there must be a joint conference, such as we have seen in our own country between the strongly organized railway men and the road executives. The mill hands must be treated as men and women who can be reasoned with and who have sense enough to accept the inevitable. English textile men do not issue ukases, the age of industrial feudalism is past in that country. If the tariff is designed to bring to the American workman benefits which his foreign competitor cannot hope for, how is it that the latter has so much more self-respecting a position than the American?

Even compared with workers in other American industries, the Lawrence mill hand is at a disadvantage. For while the last twenty-five years have seen a great advance in co-operation and mutual respect in the relations between employers and employed, the woolen manufacturers and their feebly organized workers have continued to maintain relations based on autocracy on the one hand and futile efforts at revolt on the other.

As for the attitude of the mill owners toward the public to which they are indebted for tariff favors, that too harks back to an earlier time. It is true that employers do not nowadays say, "The public be damned" — that is outmoded. But the conduct of the Textile Committee during the strike was one suggestive of contempt for the public rather than respect. They consented to deal with a citizens' committee in Lawrence to the extent of telling it what they meant to do. Offers of mediation, suggestion of an impartial committee to inquire into the necessity of a wage cut, were not even answered, yet it would seem that if a cut was unavoidable, that fact could have been made clear to the public. But apparently the Textile Committee felt that the public had no concern in the matter except to furnish a police force to carry out their will. It is difficult to understand this haughty aloofness on their part, in view of their conspicuous failure to do what they had assured us the tariff would enable them to do. A spirit of apology, if not of humility, would seem rather more appropriate.

Not only in Lawrence but in Chicago I saw in the twenties a picture completely inconsistent with the one generally accepted, for there was plenty of unemployment in those glittering years, and old age and sickness still were burdens to be borne by the sufferer himself, unless charity could help. Then came the crash of 1929 and the clouds thickening all over the land, over all classes, not only the poor, till they culminated in the spring of 1933. So that, when I went to Germany in April of that year it was not a journey from a victorious, rich, prosperous country to a vanquished, impoverished land which had been driven into the mad course of Hitlerism by its intolerable sufferings. I saw no sign in Germany of suffering which could not be duplicated again and again in my own country; instead I saw many benefits which had been bestowed on the poor by the Weimar Republic but which the Republic of the United States had never dreamed of providing for its poor. So I could not accept that easy explanation for the rise of Hitlerism in Germany.

XX

Germany, 1933

THE Oberlaender Trust, a branch of the Carl Schurz
Foundation, had as part of its program an exchange of American and German "fellowships," under which plan Americans
were sent to Germany to study conditions there and Germans
came over to this country for the same purpose. It was one of
the many postwar efforts to increase mutual understanding and
friendship between the two countries, efforts made with
apparent success, until they were swept away like straw before
the waters of a bursting dam. Wilbur Thomas, whom I had
known through the Quaker feeding missions in Germany
and Austria, was the executive secretary of the Foundation in
the thirties and in 1932 he invited me to accept one of these
fellowships for travel in Germany. It was a very tempting offer
but I was not able to accept it until the spring of 1933. By
then Hitler had risen to all but supreme power and the Jewish
boycott had been proclaimed. However, this only increased
my eagerness to go and see for myself what was happening to
the country I knew so well, but I was reluctant to go alone
and Mr. Thomas willingly acceded to my request to have
Clara Landsberg go with me. She knew Germany even more
intimately than I and her German is perfect; mine is fluent
enough but otherwise deplorable.

American newspapers were full of tales of atrocities against
the Jews, and even against American citizens if they failed to
give the Nazi salute. My sister Edith was very loath to have us

face these possible dangers, which might grow worse while we were on the way over, and she made me promise to leave the German ship at Cherbourg and go first to Paris where we could see an American Consul and find out just what was happening, since the ship's radio news would certainly tell us nothing. In Paris I decided that a newspaper correspondent would probably know more than anyone else, so we went to see Paul Scott Mowrer whom Miss Addams and I had met in 1919. It so happened that he was waiting for his daily telephone call from his brother, Edgar Ansel Mowrer, in Berlin and the call came in while we were there. It began with the words, "I am quite sure this wire is being tapped," which, Paul said, was the way Edgar always started his daily report. After the conversation was ended Paul told us that Edgar had said there was no possible reason for us to hesitate, we should be perfectly safe if we used ordinary prudence. I had felt all along that with our diplomatic service there to be appealed to there was nothing to worry about.

We went by way of Cologne to Berlin and called at once on Consul General Messersmith, whom we found informed, sympathetic, intensely interesting, and willing to give us a lot of time. Later we dined with him and Mrs. Messersmith and had another long talk. Professor Dodd had been appointed to the Ambassadorship but had not yet arrived, so matters were largely in Messersmith's hands. We talked also with John Elliott, of the *Herald Tribune*, and told him about an ardent Nazi woman on our ship, who had insisted all the American correspondents in Berlin were Jews. "And that John Elliott, he is the worst Jew of them all." Edgar Mowrer and his wife invited us to their home and gave us a most vivid picture of the changes that had come already in every phase of German life.

Germany was not my first experience of a country under
tyranny. I had been in Belgium in 1915, in Russia in 1924.
Both those countries had taught me what life is like under the
terror but neither had affected me as poignantly as did the
Germany of April 1933. After all, the Belgians knew that most
of the world — all of the world that they really cared about —
was full of sympathy and trying to help them, and furthermore
they were united in suffering, in resistance, and in hope. The
White Russians were pitiful but they were a poor, weak lot,
most of them — nobody could possibly wish them back in
power; and though the Reds were cruel, it was a primitive
savagery, not cold-blooded, and not nearly so thorough and
systematic. Moreover, in Russia I felt something new and
great developing, something far better than that which had
been.

But in Germany I did not feel that. It is true that I heard
much about the new spirit of hope, of religious devotion to
the Leader and to the Fatherland, especially in the young
generation. But it was impossible to rejoice over this spiritual
revival when one heard of the uses to which the leaders put
their youthful followers. Many were the tales we heard of
deliberate terrorization by the Brown Shirts, midnight in-
vasions of private houses, not by any means only of Jews, to
bully and intimidate old men, women and children; many tales
of physical cruelty of the meanest type, a group of strong
young men making a massed attack on one man, sometimes an
old and feeble one, leaving him for dead and marching on
singing the "Horst Wessel" song. The Germany I had known
had had its faults — arrogance, worship of authority, contempt
for women and weaker nations — but it had also many virtues.
It seemed to me that Hitler's Germany had kept the old faults
and had lost the old virtues — respect for order and discipline

and integrity, kindliness, and a great capacity for gayety, for the enjoyment of simple things. In Hitler's Germany there was neither gayety nor kindliness, and not even the most rudimentary function of government, the protection of the weak against unauthorized violence. And of course all that had made Germany a leader in certain intellectual fields was being deliberately destroyed.

We were told that we must not forget that this was a revolution, and revolutions are always bloody. But what had been a quite valid excuse in Russia could not be accepted in Germany where there had been no attempt at armed resistance. All the violence from January 1933 on had been on one side only.

Yet I did not see Germany at its worst by any means, for though the changes were coming very fast they did not reach their peak till after June 1934. In April 1933, it is true, it seemed as if everything, from the legal profession to the ping-pong clubs, had already been swallowed by *Gleichschaltung*, which is usually translated "co-ordination," but "switching onto the same track" is perhaps nearer the real meaning.

Those first days were crowded with vivid and astonishing impressions, for although I had read tales of what was happening as Germany set her clock back, it is one thing to read and quite another to see and hear.

One of those early happenings is etched very sharply on my memory. We were dining at the home of a young Jew we had met on the steamer coming over. Conversation at the table was very discreet, but when we were in the drawing room and the servants had disappeared, it became free. I sat next an attractive young man, a Gentile but an intimate friend of our Jewish host. It was from him that I had the first vivid description of the plight of the German intellectuals, which reminded me of Moscow in 1924 where I was told that mathematics and physics and astronomy might be taught as before, but that history, geography, economics, and even biology must be revamped in accordance with Marxian dialectics. In Russia that was bad enough, in Germany it was tragic. This young man was professor extraordinary (equivalent to our "associate") in history and he had just received instructions as to how from then on he must handle his subject. It meant that instead of being a conscientious historian he must become a mouthpiece for Goebbels's propaganda. I have seldom felt sorrier for anyone than I did for him.

"I know I ought to resign," he said, "but it would mean perhaps prison and certainly starvation for my wife and my two little girls. And there is not much satisfaction in being a martyr when nobody knows anything about it; one is not allowed to bear witness. After all, an auto-da-fé did proclaim to the world the courage and steadfastness of the heretic, but I should simply drop into oblivion. The newspapers are no longer permitted to publish dismissals from the faculties, because there has been such an outcry in the outside world. And," he added rather wistfully, "perhaps I can manage to keep my intellectual integrity, to avoid telling actual lies." I wondered if he could, with Brown Shirts among his students, eager to detect and denounce the slightest heresy, but I could not blame him for trying. It was not courageous, but then what impressed me most in all my stay in Germany was the lack of any sign of courageous protest, to say nothing of resistance.

We had supper one evening with the loveliest woman I met in Germany. She was the Christian wife of a half-Jew who had held an important position in the city government, and had been responsible for outstanding work in prevention of tuberculosis. Their apartment was that of prosperous people with taste and education. She was gentle, with a stillness that was full of thought and strength. Her husband, a nervous, tense, talkative man, was called to see someone in his office and in his absence she spoke freely to us.

"My father is a Lutheran minister in the Rhineland," she said, "and my husband made no objection to my bringing up the children in the Christian faith. Just this Easter, Hedwig — she is twelve — led the procession when her confirmation class marched into the church. Now it is impossible for her to go to school. I cannot force her to sit and listen to the talk the teacher is obliged to give, on Jews as subhuman beings, detestable in looks and in all their acts, responsible for every harm Germany has suffered. She is at the most sensitive age and now she sees herself suddenly changed from a popular, leading member of the class to a pariah. I do not know what it would do to her if we stayed here, or what it would do to my husband, who takes such things almost as hard as Hedwig does. We must leave this city. We have a summer cottage in Bavaria and we will go there. Fortunately the two youngest are too little to sense the change. The saddest thing about this new regime to me is that it divides people violently into the despisers and the despised, people who up to now were friends, bound together by many ties. Do you remember Tolstoy's saying, 'The things that men have in common are much stronger, more fundamental, than the things that separate them'?"

Her husband came back then, bringing in an elderly man whom they introduced as a professor of the university. Herr P——'s face was radiant, he seemed a different man, and when his guest departed he said, "Well, at least we have one friend left." Frau P—— said, "Yes, the only one who has been under our roof since the blow fell."

That gave me furiously to think. Are Germans, then, such cowards that they desert a friend the moment he is in danger? For such a thing could not happen in America, friends would rally around the unfortunate man and protest against his unjust treatment. But in Germany I heard again and again of cases like this and, though the fellow members of the university faculty or the medical or legal profession might deplore it in private, the only instance I heard of an open protest was made by Professor Wolfgang Kohler, who not only published an article on intellectual freedom but refused to discharge his Jewish assistants. Because of the sensation his article had made in England and America, the government let him alone till 1935, then again ordered him to discharge his Jewish assistants. Kohler refused again, left Germany with his Jewish colleagues, and is now teaching in Swarthmore. But this seemed to be the one courageous exception. It was not easy to discuss this with Germans, but once I did express my bewilderment to a professor who is half English, and more than half in his attitude toward life.

"You see," he said, "Germans are not used to acting together, to joining in a spontaneous movement for a cause, especially if it involves a conflict with the authorities. In Anglo-Saxon countries that is the sort of thing that happens all the time. But not here. The protest of a single man would do no good and it would be impossible to get a large group to take any such action."

"But the students," I said — "students are a rebellious lot in any country. We are always reading about student demonstrations."

"Oh, we have them too," he answered, "but only of one side, the side that is on top. In the University of Berlin, Wolf, the most popular professor in the law faculty, was shouted down by a group of half a dozen young Nazi students and had to announce that he would not lecture this term. There were some three hundred students who had registered for his course. They are furious that they cannot have him but they dared not throw out the half-dozen Nazis, for that would have meant mobs breaking into their homes and no hope of protection by the police. The Nazis would have gone to the university office and copied the names of all who had registered for Wolf's course and then taken their revenge on the students or their families. Nobody can protest now, only wait."

All the same I wager three hundred American students would not have meekly waited.

I was especially keen to learn what had happened to labor, to the famous trade-unions which had been able to secure the eight-hour day for steelworkers long before it was grudgingly granted, in response to President Harding's plea, to American steelworkers. They told us that all would be made clear on May Day when Hitler would speak to Labor. We were in Berlin then and we spent much of the day in the streets, sitting for a couple of hours on the base of the Brandenburger Thor to watch the great procession of men and women, boys and girls, who marched by singing as only Germans can sing. The marchers were on their way to Tempelhof where they gathered to hear Hitler speak, the largest audience ever assembled in Germany till then. We listened to the speech over the radio, together with two delightful young people who took us in charge that day, Betty Ripley, William Z. Ripley's daughter, and Monica Ratcliffe, S. K.'s daughter, both of them students in Germany and intensely interested in the strange metamorphosis that was taking place before their eyes. The speech was more than disappointing, it was frankly what a disrespectful American would call ballyhoo. It was the sort of speech that used to be made before a Civic Federation audience or a Manufacturers' Association: flowery sentiments about the brotherhood of workers with brawn and workers with brain, about commonweal instead of individual profit, about a united country where employer and employee march hand in hand for the Fatherland. There was nothing that could be called a program, a definite plan, and our little group of Americans marveled that Hitler would dare so to disappoint his waiting followers.

But the next day his real plan was carried out without warning. The trade-unions were dissolved, a leader of labor was appointed (the Ley whom the labor representatives in the International Labor Office in Geneva later refused to recognize), the "principle of leadership" was substituted for democratic majority rule, the funds and properties of the unions were taken over. Nothing was said of course of the notorious agreement between the Nazi Party and the great industrialists whereby the latter promised to finance the movement on condition that the unions be wiped out.

An amusing incident happened when I went into a little shop to buy a cleverly made figure of Hitler with a joint in the right arm so it could give the *Heil Hitler* salute. My accent betrayed me and the woman who kept the shop asked where I came from. She was much interested to hear that I was an American and wanted to know how the Nazi movement was progressing over there. "We have no Nazi movement," I said firmly. "Oh yes you have," she insisted. "We hear about it every day over the radio." A man at the back of the store put in, "What is the matter with you Americans that you have no man of your own good enough to be President so you have to take a Hollander?" "Why, Roosevelt is not a Hollander," I tried to explain. "Of course all of us came originally from some country." But another man cut me off with, "Ah, he is no Hollander, he is a Jew. His real name is Rosenfeld."

A few days after we arrived, there was a great assembly of Lutheran clergymen and I read the newspaper reports of the meetings with eagerness, feeling sure that some protest against the persecution of the Jews would be made by these Christians. But not a word. An English Quaker, Bertha Bray, whom I met in Cologne, was amused at my astonishment. She told me that since Luther's day, the Church in Germany has held itself aloof from all public life, has felt in no way responsible for anything the government might do. The duty of the Church is to deal with the soul of the individual. Only if its spiritual functions are interfered with will it protest and resist. She gave me a letter to Professor Spira, the man who was regarded as the greatest of the mystics after Karl Barth (who, being a Swiss, had uttered his protest and been expelled from Bonn University), and I had an interesting interview with him. He was clearly unhappy but he would utter no word of censure against the Nazi regime. I spoke of the Jews. Yes, their suffering was terrible, but suffering ennobles, purifies. They would emerge, cleansed as by fire. "But what of the effect on their persecutors?" I asked. "You must have Brown Shirts in your classes, Herr Professor. What do you say to them?" A look of suffering passed over his face as he answered, "I tell them that love, pity, humility, are the Christian virtues."

I felt sure that his attitude could not be that of the greater number of German clergymen and I wanted very much to have a talk with one of them, to learn what was the general feeling toward the new regime. This became possible when we received an invitation from a young Lutheran pastor, whose mother and brother I knew, to visit his country parish in eastern Pomerania. He could house us in his largest village (his parish consists of four villages) and we would be quite comfortable. We were indeed; the house of the village carpenter was spotless and we had the parlor, with a huge bed piled with feather beds, made from real Pomeranian goose feathers, as our hostess told us. She was plump and smiling and blue-eyed and she had four plump and smiling and blue-eyed children, three of them girls with blonde braids wound round their heads, all of them looking as if they had just stepped out of a German Christmas card. Frau Vollner was enthusiastic about the Herr Pastor. "He is wonderful to us," she said. "Only think, he stands at the church door after service and shakes hands with all of us." "Did not the old pastor do that?" I asked. "Oh no, not us common people. The Herr Baron and the doctor and the teacher and the apothecary, but nobody else."

I repeated this to the pastor as we sat over our lunch in his bleak and comfortless parsonage. The lunch was bleak too. It was brought in a basket by the two oldest of the little Vollner girls and was cold when it got to us. We began with a thick gray soup, which I afterwards learned was made by boiling stale rye bread to a paste and adding a little milk. Then there were some cold boiled veal and plain boiled potatoes and no salt. But the Herr Pastor had no idea what he was eating. He was absorbed in his endeavor to make us understand the attitude of the "German Christians," for, to our surprise, we found he belonged to that (in our eyes) unchristian group.

He said, when I told him of my conversation with the

carpenter's wife, "That is exactly one of the things we German Christians are fighting against, that aloofness of the clergy from real life, from all that has to do with government, politics, world affairs, as well as their aloofness from the lives of common people. In Anglo-Saxon countries the clergy mingle in all public movements, often initiate them; in Germany we are expected to deal only with the individual soul. We young German Christians are determined to put an end to that. We claim our part in the great movement to satisfy Germany's century-old longing for a national religion, a national church."

Then he also spoke of the new spirit of equality which National Socialism had brought about. "This May Day for the very first time all the people in the village marched together to the village square to listen to the Führer over the radio — peasant, independent farmer and squire, schoolmaster, merchant and laborer, doctor and minister. Always before the educated class has held itself aloof from the common people. Hitlerism wipes out class distinctions and it drives out the Communists and silences their press. Since 1918 there had come a cleavage in every village between the devoutly religious, conservative, old-time people and the new, freethinking Socialists and Communists. They were opposed to each other in every way. I could not speak in a public meeting without the dread of being interrupted by some scoffing radical. Now the leaders are gone and the followers are slipping quietly back into the community. You Americans are all for liberalism, but liberalism is simply materialism. The greatest thing in the world is obedience; that lies at the foundation of any good State — obedience, it does not much matter to what, but it must be a yielding to the will of something greater than oneself."

I think that what struck me most forcibly in the talk of this young man was his assumption that it was right to have his opponents removed by the strong hand of the law. His American brother would assume that, if he could not win over the scoffer, then he must submit to the annoyance. But not so the German. This stressing of the importance of obedience and of the old-fashioned discipline which Hitler had restored to Germany was evident in the talk of many others. One wise man, a Catholic (we found the Catholics on the whole far saner than the Protestants, probably because their church is universal, not narrowly national), said, "The Nazis dream of unity, but they attempt to achieve it not by the persuasion of a great ideal, but by the ruthless beating down of opposition." Perhaps that is because of something in the German temperament that loves authority, perhaps it is because Hitler's movement is a movement of youth as was Mussolini's, of youth with its hero worship, its devotion to a great cause which will give dignity and meaning to life, and youth with its intolerance of criticism and dissent, its gang instinct and its capacity for unimaginative cruelty.

But he was an admirable fellow, this unchristian Christian minister. He was responsible for four villages, miles apart, and he had only a bicycle to carry him. He lived as ascetic a life as any monk and a far more exhausting one. We saw, under his guidance, the life of a typical Pomeranian village. He took us to afternoon coffee at the house of the local nobleman, a descendant of the Teutonic Knights of the thirteenth century. The Herr Baron is an excellent farmer and we were much impressed by his little kingdom of 130 *Instleute*, tenant farmers with a much more feudal relation to their lord than ours have. It was a largely self-sustaining unit, with a carpenter shop, a machine shop, a lumber yard, a flour mill, an electric light and power plant, horses, cattle, pigs, sheep, poultry, grain, potatoes, vegetables. They built and repaired the houses themselves and made the stone walls. The peasant got his house, usually three-roomed, solid, well built, his electric light and his fuel, a strip of land for a garden, seed, a cow, a pig, fodder and rye. Just what money wages he got I was not told but it represented one third of his earnings; the rest was payment in kind. It struck me as far better than our form of feudalism, the share-cropping system in the South.

We had Sunday supper at the home of an independent peasant whose family came there in 1750. He showed us with pride a wonderful parchment all covered with seals, which attested the freedom his ancestor won in 1805. This was not freedom to go elsewhere or to sell his land except by permission of his lord, but he was no longer a serf, the land was his to work as he pleased. I thought of our farmers in 1805. No wonder it is hard for us to understand the Germans, when our background, our traditions, are so different. At the time when serfdom still flourished in Germany, Americans had thrown off a yoke far lighter than that and self-government was already a tradition among us.

The farmer had accepted National Socialism, not with enthusiasm but as far better than the Republic. He had hated the bureaucracy of the latter, city people coming and bossing the farmers and messing up everything; tales of big salaries and of graft, while the farmers were so desperately poor. Hitler would stop all that.

We asked the Herr Pastor if the Jewish boycott had reached as far as his villages and he said, yes, orders had come from Berlin and Brown Shirts had been stationed in front of the two or three little shops run by Jews. "Our people did not like it," he said. "They have always had friendly relations with these Jewish families who are really fine people. Why, that day they, the Jews, felt so sorry for the Brown Shirts who had to stand all day long in front of the shops that they carried some chairs out for them. But, of course, when commands come from above they must be obeyed."

When we returned from Pomerania to Berlin we were given a reception by a large group of women who belonged to the old women's-rights movement, the *Frauenbewegung* which had had great influence under the Republic and which was still holding together and refusing to oust its Jewish members. Not long after, the organization was given the choice between joining the Nazi women's union and disbanding and, to their honor, they chose the latter. We happened to say to some women at this tea that we planned to visit East Prussia and Upper and Lower Silesia, to get some picture of the Polish-German situation. One of the ladies, a Gräfin Finkenstein, said at once that she lived in East Prussia and hoped we would stop with her, at Castle Schönberg, and another said that if we wanted our journey made easy we must go to the *Wirtschaftspolitische Gesellschaft* and let them plan it for us.

This proved to be an excellent suggestion, for the very competent lady in charge of this propaganda office made out a detailed program to cover Danzig, East Prussia, and Silesia and arranged to have us met by Nazi officials, entertained by Nazi hostesses, lectured to by Nazi professors, in short subjected for a whole fortnight to the most orthodox influences. We welcomed the experience, knowing that up to that moment we had heard much more from the other side than from the Nazis. And so we left Berlin for Stettin, then the Polish Corridor, Danzig, Königsberg, the western and southern parts of East Prussia, back across Poland again, to Upper Silesia, which is like the Pittsburgh region only without mountains, to Breslau, with excursions into Lower Silesia. Everywhere we were met by assiduous guides and hosts till we began to wonder whether we were not being mistaken for really important people.

As I look back on it I still wonder at the pains they took with us, the amount of trouble they went to, giving us official lunches and dinners, taking us on long motor rides to *Sehenswürdigkeiten* such as Marienburg and Marienwerder and Zoppot, the seashore resort near Danzig. But always the trips were planned for our instruction, always we were shown the iniquities of the Versailles *Diktat* and the stupidity of the Poles. We were taken to wonderful museums — I remember the one in Danzig as the most fascinating — to listen to discourses by learned curators proving that that particular spot (Danzig, Königsberg, Breslau) had been Teutonic since the Stone Age, and outlining in contrast the despicable history of the Poles. Again and again we would be driven to the Polish border and told of the hatefulness of the Poles.

And indeed the conditions along the border were hateful but it was not by any means all Polish hate. Both sides kept up a system of petty irritations and did everything to fan hostility. I can see now the outskirts of one of the steel cities, Hindenburg, which lay right on the boundary. On the German side were miners' houses and children were playing in the only place they had, a stretch of cinders from the mills, while just across a barbed-wire fence lay the green meadows of Poland. One of the women told us that they had to watch all the time to keep the children from crawling under the wire to play in the grass and be caught by the Polish sentries and held sometimes for days before the distracted parents could get them back. At another point, near Marienwerder, we saw the boundary, a narrow stream, with children on either side, making faces at each other and throwing stones. There they told us that if a German cow strayed across the creek, the Poles confiscated her. But, later on, our Consul in Breslau told us that the German restrictions were just as hard on the Poles as they could make them. The boundary the Germans resented most was what they called the Japanese line. This was in Lower Silesia. The story ran that the Boundary Commission consisted of a Frenchman, who wanted to give everything to the Poles, an Englishman who wanted to be fair, and a Japanese who was so bored by the discussions that finally he took a ruler and drew a straight line, and that was the line that we saw.

The Versailles Treaty was for all our guides the King Charles's head which could not be kept out of their talk. Every disaster was attributed to it. I could not help thinking what a comfort it was to have a foreign scapegoat in 1933 when we at home were forced to face our own mistakes and take the responsibility for the great depression. In Gleiwitz, one of the Pittsburghs of Upper Silesia, our guide pointed to the smokeless chimneys of the great steelworks and said that the output then was less than one third of what it had been under the Germans. "But that situation is world-wide," I said. "When I left home our steel production was much lower than that." But of course he was convinced that it was all due to the *Diktat* of Versailles. We did see many stupidities that the Treaty was responsible for, not only the Japanese line. In Breslau we were taken to the Museum and in one room was a wonderful collection of firearms, from the time gunpowder came to Europe up to the latest model of 1918. And the curator showed us how every single one had been mutilated by an Allied commission, under a Treaty clause which required the total disarming of Germany. Even the centuries-old ones had not escaped. It was so utterly stupid, to do something at once useless and humiliating.

Surrounded as we were by good Nazis we had opportunity to hear their doctrine expounded from all sides. There was a fine, upstanding, blond young man in Königsberg who told us cheerfully that he owed his health and strength to the Quakers, for he had been fed by the Quaker mission after the war. It was he who took us to see the burning of the books in a public square on a cold rainy evening. To him it was a wonderful, inspiring spectacle, to us it was almost as strange as a voodoo ceremony would be. A great fire, fed continually with heaps of books brought in carts and barrows by eager students, a crowd of silent, awe-struck people looking on. Some weeks later, when I was in Würzburg, I ventured to ask an old friend what he had thought of that performance which had been enacted that same night in every large city in Germany. He was K. B. Lehmann, professor and *Geheimrat*, a famous toxicologist whom I had for many years regarded as my teacher. To my amazement the burning of the books met with his enthusiastic approval, it had been to him a solemn and beautiful experience. He said, "I stood for two hours in the square watching the leaping flames and the crowd of silent worshipers. To all of us it was a symbolic act, a renunciation of the religion of class hatred and conflict, of sexual looseness and of scoffing at all that was old and revered, a freeing of the people from all the decadence that followed the war. And to me it was also a purification of the spot where, in the fall of 1918, I witnessed a Communist attack, a mob of the most degraded people I ever saw, who swooped down on the city, nobody knew from where, and took possession of the public buildings. As I watched the flames that night I felt that at last that crime was wiped out."

When we returned from that strange ceremony to our Königsberg hotel we were accompanied by a little group of university students, friends of our young guide, all of them filled with a sort of religious ecstasy. They spoke of the new order with its repudiation of intellectualism, of humanism and liberalism, the devilish trio which had destroyed the German soul. Apparently scientific search for objective truth was Jewish and Marxist, the German soul must attain to truth through blood and race and soil. The revolution belonged to youth and, under Hitler, youth would guide it to a glorious future. I asked a girl sitting next me what she had planned to do and she said that she was studying architecture. "What if the professions and even the universities are closed to women, as seems probable, and all girls sent back to domestic life?" I asked, and she answered proudly, "If the Fatherland asks that sacrifice of me, I am ready."

Our visit to the Countess Finkenstein in Schönberg Castle was an experience which delighted us. The castle dates back to the fourteenth century, to the Teutonic Knights; it is simply one's dream of a medieval castle — towers, walls, moat, drawbridge, portcullis, everything. But the Countess herself is far from a medieval chatelaine, she is a trained "agronome"; she rules a community of five hundred souls and manages the raising of cattle, sheep, fowl of all kinds, pigs, even fur-bearing animals. We longed to go over the castle but instead we followed her through fields and barns and styes, we saw the brood houses for chicks and the paddocks for colts and calves, and we heard about the responsibilities of the *Junker* class toward their "people" (*Instleute*), who may never be discharged no matter how unsatisfactory they are and must be cared for in sickness and old age. At dinner that night we met the young Count, a brother-in-law of the Countess, who

is a widow, and the Dowager Countess, her mother-in-law,
and a Countess von Keyserling. The Dowager Countess was
of a family of old Kurland nobility which was driven out by
the Lettish revolution following the war and Countess von
Keyserling was from Esthonia, whence she also had had to flee
before the Bolshevist revolution. Both had lost homes, land,
everything. They spoke of the noble families still left there,
the sons and daughters working on what land was left to them
as farmhands and dairy maids, to the anguish of their parents,
who see all culture and gentle ways being lost. But the young
are very plucky; they work hard and then once in a long while
they come together and sing and dance till dawn, just like
peasants.

It took me back to Russia as I heard them tell of their
perilous escape over the border into East Prussia and as I
heard Countess Finkenstein speak of the relief from fear that
had come with Hitler's rise to power. "You can hardly realize,"
she said, "how helpless I felt during these last years. At the
Castle gates there are more than a hundred families of our
people. I knew that a Communist cell had been formed in the
village but I did not know just who had joined or whom I
still could trust. And the nearest neighbor of our class is twenty
miles away and if my telephone line were cut, I should be
at the mercy of the mob."

The next morning I had a talk with the young Count, who
revealed himself, surprisingly, as an ardent Nazi. He told me
that, like many others, he had come to it through Socialism.
"Yes, I was a Social Democrat, a passionate adherent of that
party, but as the years went on I became disillusioned by the
greed and smugness and personal ambition of those on top
from whom one had expected self-sacrifice for the common
good, and the increasing class hatred at the bottom where

one had expected brotherhood. The Nazis are for a return to the old German probity, for a new freedom from all class distinctions, and for a Germany united in faith and in deed."

"You are an intellectual," I said, "what do you think of the treatment of the universities? Remember what happened to the intellectual life of Spain and of Russia when freedom of teaching was suppressed."

"Yes, we are driving out many of our intellectuals, but you cannot frighten us by pointing to the experience of Spain, for we do not want that kind of intellectualism. We have been misled for a decade by a cold, sterile worship of science, which leads to materialism and kills the true German spirit. The German is not a materialist as is the American, who thinks only of money and what he can buy with it."

"Were you ever in America?" I asked.

"No, but I know all about Americans, we all do. We have read Sinclair Lewis. But the German is altogether different, he cares for the things of the spirit. The industrial revolution brought much evil with it. I trace the beginning of modern materialism back to about 1850, when the worship of wealth and luxury began. But that is over now and so is the corruption of spirit that went with it in these latter days when one could not read a book or pick up a newspaper or go to the theater or to an exhibition without having all one revered held up to ridicule and all that was revolting and degenerate presented for admiration. We have abolished all that, no longer will such outrages be permitted. You do not realize that this is a revolution. It is like the Reformation, and of course there are excesses, cruelties, intolerance. But this stage will pass."

"You believe, then, in dictatorship, in the suppression of all individual liberty. You do not think that a government needs a vigorous opposition, as we do,"

"Well, I understand what you mean by that and later on we will permit a healthy opposition to be formed, but now it is too early, all must stand together till the enemy is routed."

The Polish Corridor controversy ran through all our excursions, for our guides seemed to think that their first duty was to send us home convinced that that injustice must be done away with. I grew a little tired of the endless insistence on the sufferings of the German minority in Poland, and one day, when we were being seen to our train by an assiduous Nazi, who begged us to tell our countrymen of these outrages, I suddenly turned on him.

"No," I said, "I do not think I will. Because I am quite sure Americans would feel no sympathy for the German minority in Poland so long as Germans are treating their Jewish minority so shockingly." He started as if I had struck him, turned on his heel and hurried away, but when we entered the train he was waiting there and he whispered to me that he did not approve of the persecution of the Jews, it was a concession to popular feeling and a frightful mistake. One should not fight intellectual battles with force.

It always embarrassed our Nazi acquaintances when I brought up the Jewish question, but I never failed to do so in every city we visited. The most naïve explanation was given me by a woman in a little shop in Rothenburg who answered my question about the Jewish boycott thus: "Yes, the boycott against the Jews was ordered because Jews had spread lies in other countries about Germany — none of it was true, nothing happened to any Jew in all Germany — and, because of these lies, foreign Jews were attacking German Christians and throwing them into prison. So the boycott was ordered, and then the foreign countries stopped persecuting Germans and let them out of prison." Usually I would get what I came to call a "radio answer," for the same statements would be made in almost the same words and I felt sure it was Goebbels talking.

Now and then I would venture to argue with someone who seemed reasonable and capable of normal thinking, but usually with little success. For instance, when a very attractive and unmilitary ex-officer told me that the Jews must be driven out of the learned professions, journalism, art, and music, because they had invaded all these fields and occupied them, so that the Gentile had no chance, I asked how that had been possible — had the Jews secured university positions, had they been made judges, theater managers, newspaper editors, by bribery? "Oh no," he said, "we have never had your American corruption in government. No, they got their positions fairly enough, in a way."

"Then," I said, "it means that 65,000,000 Germans have been submerged, choked, by 570,000 Jews, and since there is no hope of the Germans winning the battle by intellectual weapons, physical force alone will work. Do you know, it is staggering to me to hear such talk in a country whose intellectual achievements I have held in such high esteem. And you do not even seem to feel humiliated by such a confession of inferiority."

"It is not inferiority," he retorted. "It is the opposite. Cannot you see that we are engaged in a holy war to purify Germany, to make our land Nordic again? The Jew is alien to us, he is a critic, a scoffer, a satirist. Nothing is holy to him, his intellectualism sears and withers the poetical, dreaming German spirit."

Here again, as so often, I heard a German defending the use of force to put down ideas he disliked. Germany had had her postwar decadent movement in literature, art, the drama, but so had America and England and France. Many of us detested the cheap debunking, the straining at a startling originality, and what Renoir once called "sentimentalized harlotry," but we were ready to wait till the pendulum swung back, as it did. Only Germans felt it right to crush with an iron fist what they disliked.

A more practical explanation for the treatment of Jewish intellectuals was given me by a university professor who, when he talked to me, was still lecturing but who has since lost his place on the ground that he "is unfitted to instruct German youth." "Germany is an overcrowded country which has no possible outlet. The overcrowding affects not only labor but the professions. There are more young people studying medicine in Germany than in the United States and where are they to find work? Germany's colonies are gone; they were never the most valuable parts of Africa, the best pickings were already snapped up, but they did furnish opportunity for young engineers, physicians, pharmacists, teachers, officials, and that they attracted first-class men was shown by the medical and sanitary work done in Germany's East Africa, which was admitted by the Health Organization of the League of Nations to be far superior to that of any other colonial power in Africa. In earlier days Germany could also have poured some of her surplus into North and South America; now those doors are closed. This means that competition in universities is fierce and ruthless, it is a struggle for existence. Our faculties are full of espionage and intrigue and none of us feels safe, even if we are pure Aryans, for a denunciation on the ground of 'an un-German spirit' made by a covetous assistant may mean ruin to the best of us."

During the last ten days of our stay in Germany, we watched

the clouds thicken, the suspense increase, and finally we saw the dreaded blow fall on friend after friend; that which had only been threatened in May became a reality in June; those who escaped the first flood and hoped they were safe were caught by the rising waters. Even then we could see only increasing disaster; we were convinced that so long as Hitler rules Germany there can be no place there for the independent thinker.

Our last German city was Hamburg, which always seems only partly German, more cosmopolitan, more English even, than other German cities. It is a beautiful city with its two great waterways, the inner and the outer Alster, which reminded me of the Charles River Basin between Boston and Cambridge except that in Hamburg the outer Alster especially was crowded with little craft of all kinds. We had supper at an open-air restaurant and as dark came on an orchestra struck up and the rowboats and canoes and little sailboats came crowding up until the water all around us was solid with them. Now and then voices would catch the strain and sing an accompaniment to the instruments. Somehow I could not imagine such a scene on the Charles River Basin, but maybe some day Americans will come to love music and outdoor life as Germans do.

We had letters from the Kirchweys to friends in Hamburg and I remember a lunch on a roof terrace of a charming house, where we met some women doctors, for our hostess was a doctor of medicine. One of these women told us of the instructions which they had all just received from the government, as to what a physician must say with regard to marriage between Jew and Gentile. "We must tell the man or woman who is contemplating a mixed marriage that the offspring of such a marriage will be a mental and physical monstrosity," she said. "And are you ready to obey that order," I asked, "to repeat such an absurd and cruel lie?" She shrugged her shoulders. "If I want to keep on practising, I must. Don't you see that spies will be sent to our offices, pretending to consult us and reporting what we say?"

Our friends drove us outside the city one evening, through Altona, to a popular restaurant which they assured us would be very gay and give us a cheerful memory to carry away with us. But they were dismayed to find all the gayety vanished. It was full of people, but so quiet one could not believe that it was in Germany, where boisterous gayety used always to go with crowds and beer and music. In our room there was a group of a dozen or so, all young people, who dropped into silence when we came in and then resumed their talk in whispers. After this depressing experience we had a melancholy drive back to the city, past great estates with beautiful houses, empty since the war or turned into sanatoria.

It was with the greatest relief that we boarded our steamer and left Germany behind us, the same relief that I had felt when I crossed the border from conquered Belgium into Holland, and from Soviet Russia into Poland. The oppression of spirit that an American suffers under a tyrannical government must be experienced, it cannot be logically explained. But we soon realized that we had not altogether left Germany so long as we were on a German boat, for we met on board Charles Beard's daughter Miriam, whose father and mother were old friends of mine, and her husband, Alfred Vagts, then still a German subject. Miriam was sure that the ship was full of spies and that her husband's imprudent tongue would get him into trouble and Clara Landsberg felt the same way about me, regardless of my American standing, so they made us uncautious ones promise to speak of Hitler (they knew we could not be prevented from mentioning him) as Herr Lehmann. We kept our promise and it led to an amusing but rather startling incident. The Vagts' little son, a charming youngster of four years, was a great friend of the waiters and one day at lunch he suddenly turned to one of them and said in German, "Did you know? There is a wild man in Berlin. His name is Lehmann." We had never imagined that he was listening to our talk, but we did realize then that our precaution had saved Dr. Vagts from a disastrous experience.

XXI

Viscose Rayon

MY LAST detailed study of a poisonous trade was made in 1937–1938, when after many fruitless attempts I found it possible to explore an important but little-known industry — little-known in this country only, to the rest of the industrial world it had long been familiar. Along in the early thirties I began to be very uneasy about a new industry which was using an old poison, a poison whose effect was well known in Europe and which I had myself encountered in 1914 when I studied the manufacture of rubber goods. This was carbon disulphide, a poison to the central nervous system, which causes mental disease and sometimes loss of vision, sometimes motor paralysis. It had been studied abroad since 1856 when a Frenchman, Payen, first described this new form of occupational disease of which he had seen twenty-four cases in rubber workers, and after that reports came from other countries, all from the rubber industry. Laudenheimer, a German psychiatrist, published records of fifty cases of carbon disulphide insanity, from the rubber works in Leipzig. In England, Oliver wrote of a raincoat factory where the windows of the vulcanizing department were protected with bars to prevent men who suddenly were taken with maniacal delirium from leaping out. As early as 1886 twenty-four cases of carbon disulphide blindness were reported in a British medical journal.

In this country we used far less carbon disulphide in the rubber industry because Americans have always preferred the method of vulcanization which depends on heat and pressure. Vulcanization means incorporating sulphur in the rubber and it may be done by treating the rubber with carbon disulphide, which is known as the "vapor" or "acid" or "cold cure," or by mixing flowers of sulphur with the rubber and heating it under pressure, which is known as the "heat cure." Even in 1914 when I investigated rubber manufacture I found the so-called "acid cure" used only for splicing inner tubes and vulcanizing thin rubber goods. Still I did find some cases of typical carbon disulphide poisoning and a few more were published by others. But as I have continued to visit rubber works I have found less and less carbon disulphide, it has almost completely disappeared from this industry.

Then, as so often happens, it reappeared in a new industry, artificial silk or, as we now call it, viscose rayon. This is not an American invention; it came to us from France, Switzerland, and England, and spread rapidly here and over Europe and the Orient. Most of the European countries had brought their rubber factories under strict control and carbon disulphide poisoning had almost ceased to appear, but there was a rapid and serious outbreak of cases when the rayon industry started. The medical journals were full of reports, from Italy especially, but from all over Europe and even from Japan. Not from the United States. In 1904 two cases were reported in rayon manufacture, in 1905 one, in 1914 I published two. Then for over ten years, during which time the viscose industry in our country grew enormously, no American report of damage from this poison appeared. Foreign literature was full of detailed descriptions, but I doubt if any American medical student ever heard a word on the subject.

The second poison encountered in making viscose rayon, hydrogen sulphide, is a very powerful asphyxiating poison, but in viscose spinning it is present in such a small amount that it causes only inflammation of the eyes, not severe enough to do lasting damage.

There are three kinds of rayon made in this country: one called celanese or acetate rayon, whose manufacture does not require the use of any dangerous poison; Bemberg, which is even more innocuous; and viscose rayon, which must be produced with the aid of carbon disulphide, and in the course of this production, fumes of hydrogen sulphide are given off. Viscose rayon is pure cellulose, purer than the silk produced by the silkworm. What the silkworm achieves by digesting mulberry leaves, the viscose manufacturer achieves by treating wood pulp or cotton fibers with chemicals, of which carbon disulphide is the most important. This last process is carried on in great revolving barrels, called "barattes" or "churns." From these churns comes the yellow, rubbery "cellulose xanthate" which is dissolved to form a thick syrup, and this is forced through spinnerets, tiny nozzles with tiny holes, the threads of syrup being hardened in an acid bath and then wound on bobbins. These two departments, churning and spinning, are the danger spots, because of carbon disulphide fumes in both and of hydrogen sulphide in spinning.

There are few industrial diseases which move one's sympathy more than does carbon disulphide poisoning. The first two cases I saw, one of slowly developing paralysis of the legs, the other of rapidly developing manic-depressive insanity, made a deep impression on me, and as the years went on I could not help wondering what was happening in all those plants that were increasing in size and in number every year, especially after the war. As always, I found it impossible to believe that an industry which in the countries of its origin was looked on as a dangerous trade was perfectly harmless over here, since we were using the same processes as the Europeans and the Japanese. Again and again I had heard that claim made in connection with some industrial poison but always it proved to be quite unfounded. So I was not surprised when stories began coming to me of acute insanity in churn-room men and spinners in viscose plants.

For instance, a young woman physician sent me histories of thirteen cases of maniacal delirium, with hallucinations, with homicidal or suicidal impulses, leading to asylum care which sometimes lasted several years, though usually the man was discharged after some six to twelve months, more or less a nervous wreck, but sane. While he was incapacitated, his wife and children went on public charity, for the employer was not held responsible. Most of the cases were milder — the men suffered from an emotional change, they were excitable, hysterical, easily angered, unable to sleep, or disturbed by terrifying dreams. One of the worst features of the state of things that then prevailed was that a man who had actually been declared insane was allowed, when he returned from the asylum, to go back to his old job. This always resulted in a relapse worse than his first attack.

Other histories came to me from Estelle Lauder, of the Philadelphia Consumers' League, but I had no way of checking up on these stories, of confirming them by expert medical examination without which one dare not quote a case, no matter how convinced one is of its authenticity. The usual physician knew absolutely nothing about this form of occupational disease and even when the victims reached asylums for the insane and were examined by specialists, the cause was not revealed, for carbon disulphide insanity simply was not recognized as a clinical entity by American psychiatrists. There must have been company doctors who knew, but they kept the secret. This prolonged neglect, both by the medical profession and by state governmental officials, can be explained only by the fact that the most important plants were situated in states where labor laws and labor inspection were practically nonexistent or very imperfectly administered, and where, no matter what sickness the worker contracted, he could claim no compensation from the company employing him. Under such circumstances it is always easy for the employer to take refuge behind an ignorance which has been encouraged by the very men whose duty it is to enlighten him. It was true that in viscose rayon manufacture, as in other dangerous trades, there were some shining exceptions. One of the largest companies, and two other less large but important, voluntarily put physicians in charge to look for early symptoms and engineers to see to it that the exposure to dangerous fumes was kept down as much as possible.

But the neglect in other plants persisted and it seemed impossible to bring about a change, or even to collect evidence sufficient to arouse public opinion, because of the widespread secrecy. For instance, I received a telegram, back in the early thirties, from an industrial nurse in a state which has practically no factory-inspection service. She wired: "Epidemic of insanity has broken out in rayon plant. Doctors do not understand. Can you help?" I answered at once, with a full description of carbon disulphide and an offer of my services. I also begged for more detailed information. No answer came to that or to my other inquiries, for I wrote to physicians and to the nearest insane asylum. The veil of secrecy dropped and was never lifted, nor have I ever been allowed to visit that plant even after all these years. Once I was on the verge of being admitted. It so happened that I sat next to the president of that company at a dinner in Washington and got from him a cordial invitation to visit the plant as soon as some alterations were completed, but when the time came I received a formal, impersonal letter from the company saying that it had adopted the policy of not admitting outsiders. This was after there had been some newspaper comments on an investigation of carbon disulphide poisoning in another state.

My efforts to interest state and federal authorities in this question failed, because I had not enough incontrovertible evidence to be convincing, and it was plain that if I were to get anywhere I must arm myself with such evidence, I must make at least a preliminary exploration of the field myself. This was not the sort of work the Department of Labor was supposed to do but when I put the situation up to Secretary Perkins and V. A. Zimmer, head of her Division of Labor Standards, they agreed to let me do it, provided I could get the co-operation of the state Departments of Labor. This was in 1937 and under Governor Earle's administration in Pennsylvania the State Labor Comissioner was Ralph Bashore. I met him in Washington and he entered into the plan with enthusiasm, promising me all the help I needed.

The study started in Pennsylvania and we secured the help of specialists from the University Medical School to make the indispensable medical examinations. This group was under Dr. F. H. Lewey of Berlin, who was chief physician of the Neurological Institute of that city till Hitler's rise to power made him a refugee. Dr. Lewey had studied carbon disulphide psychosis and palsy in German rayon workers. We had also the invaluable help of Lillian Erskine, with whom I had worked during the war, and who visited the homes of the churn men and spinners, encouraged them to talk to her and helped them to come in secret to the doctors' headquarters for examination, a procedure they and their wives believed meant the loss of a job if it were discovered. Mr. Bashore lent us two state cars to carry the men to the places of examination. The state labels were removed from the cars and they were parked at a distance from the plant, so the men could enter them unobserved. Even so, Miss Erskine failed to get some of the severer cases; the men were too nervous and frightened to run what they thought was the risk.

I talked with a number of men who had only the lighter forms of carbon disulphide psychosis but even so they were very pitiable. They knew that a distressing change had come over them, one they could not control. It spoiled life for them, it ruined their homes, it broke up friendships, it antagonized foreman and fellow workers, and it made day and night miserable. They knew it was the job that caused it but neither doctors nor employer would admit that and their bitterness and anger over this injustice was great.

The story of this investigation is all too recent history to recite in detail, for it is not a pretty history and it was curiously bound up with a not very creditable political situation. It will be enough to say that the publication of the medical findings, together with the passage, at long last, of a law granting compensation for occupational disease in Pennsylvania, resulted in a radical reform in that state and was greatly influential in other states. For the first time it was made clear to Americans that the production of viscose rayon was a dangerous trade and that carbon disulphide was a poison.

My study then was extended to the other rayon-producing states, Massachusetts, Rhode Island, Connecticut, New York, Ohio, Virginia, West Virginia, North Carolina, Tennessee. There was the widest variety of conditions, and of employer attitude — from excellent, intelligent management to ignorance and indifference. But during the following three years changes in this industry came more rapidly and completely than any in my previous experience. New methods have been devised by engineers to prevent the escape of fumes, and now it is the general custom to have routine tests of the air made by the chemists to see whether the amount of carbon disulphide or of hydrogen sulphide is nearing the danger point. In all the large plants and in many of the smaller ones there is regular medical examination of those men who work in the dangerous departments so that the very earliest signs of poisoning can be discovered. The control of this dangerous trade was slow in coming but when it came it was astonishingly rapid and complete. It is safe to say now that no large viscose rayon works is a dangerous place to work in and probably few of the smallest ones.

XXII

Germany in 1938

MY LAST sight of Hitler's Germany was in the fall of 1938, during what we now call the "Munich week." It was a meeting of the International Congress of Occupational Accidents and Diseases that sent me over to Germany, a meeting to be held in Frankfurt am Main from September 26 to October first. It was a poor choice for an international meeting; it meant that no Jews would be there — and many industrial physicians in Europe were Jews — no Russians, no Czechs. We missed therefore some of the faces we were accustomed to meet at such gatherings, men whom we had looked up to as leaders in this field. As for the women, I was the solitary member of my sex. I went as a representative of the Department of Labor with a "diplomatic" passport which impressed me deeply but whose chief value I discovered was to expedite my passage through our Customs Office when I returned.

The first impression of Germany, which I had not seen for five years, was confirmed every day of my stay there. It was the impression of a deep change in the people as one saw them on the streets. The whole tempo of life was changed. In the old days when I had come back home from Germany I had felt the sharp contrast between tense, hurrying New York and the easy-going, pleasant atmosphere I had left behind. But now Stuttgart, my first stop, and then Frankfurt were like New York only more so. People hurried along the street with that abstracted, strained look that comes from constant worry. Nowhere was there a sign of gayety and relaxation and the enjoyment of heavy food and drink out in the open air with music, all of which had been so universal a feature in the Germany I used to know, and which had not all disappeared in 1933.

My first night was spent in Stuttgart, where I had an appointment with a would-be refugee for whom a place in the United States had been secured, provided he could succeed in getting out of Germany. Having some hours to fill I went to visit the great building which houses an important organization, the *Deutschtum im Ausland*, whose task it is to keep hold of or win back the Germans living in other countries. There I found displayed in the public room maps showing the German population in cities from Shanghai to Milwaukee and statistics, amazingly complete, about these *Auslandsdeutsche*. There was a pamphlet dealing with the United States, which even went so far as to estimate how many Germans had Americanized their names, changing Schmidt to Smith, Braun to Brown, and so on.

It was Saturday, September 24, when I reached Frankfurt. Chamberlain had gone to Godesberg on the twenty-second and was still there.

On the way over we had had American radio news and we knew that the situation between Germany and Czechoslovakia, Germany and France and England, was growing daily more threatening. As soon as I reached Stuttgart I bought papers — all German, an English paper was very hard to find — and read them eagerly but with increasing bewilderment. Apparently at the Godesberg conference those two great statesmen, Chamberlain and Hitler, were devoting themselves to the task of keeping war from Europe, a war which only Czechoslovakia wanted because the Czechs hoped that if there were another world war, they would emerge bigger and richer, as Serbia did. The papers were full of the Czech "terror" in the Sudetenland and the illustrated ones had most pitiful pictures of mothers and babies fleeing from death at the hands of Czech mobs. Germany longed only for peace but it must be peace with honor and for all Germans. The democracies had been misled by Beneš's lying propaganda.

I went on an exploring tour the afternoon I arrived in Frankfurt. The Frankfurter Hof, where we were lodged, is on one of the grand streets of the city, with elegant shops. There was a striking change in the department stores — the show windows had nothing a well-to-do woman would care to buy — and the food shops were deplorable. I went into a fruit and vegetable shop, just across the way from the hotel, to see what sort of food people with money could buy. There were — in September — no vegetables except three kinds of cabbage, carrots, potatoes, and a few little tomatoes; no fruit except white grapes and some small plums. Even stranger were the bakeshops, with bread only — no *tortes*, no pastry, no whipped cream or chocolate icing. No wonder the Germans were depressed and unnatural. One had the impression of being surrounded by silent, frightened people, waiting helplessly to hear what was to be their fate.

That evening I had supper with Tilly Edinger, the daughter of my old friends, now a well-known paleontologist. Though Jewish she was still able to work in her laboratory and to publish her reports in Swedish scientific journals. A number of friends came in for supper and we all tried to persuade her to leave Germany while she still could, but she refused. "So long as they leave me alone I will stay. After all, Frankfurt is my home, my mother's family has been here since 1560,

I was born in this house. And I promise you they will never get me into a concentration camp. I always carry with me a fatal dose of veronal." One of the guests told a story of quite senseless and brutal treatment she had undergone in a railway station, with a policeman looking on. "Didn't you appeal to him for protection?" I asked. The guests smiled at me pityingly. "Don't you know," answered a former judge, "that for Jews there is no protection and no justice?" I looked around the table and realized that in that room I was the only person who knew security, who could face the world with the confidence civilized people expect in an ordered state. To lose that is to lose one's very foundations, to feel as I felt the only time I experienced an earthquake, a very mild one, when my world seemed to be slipping from under me.

The Congress opened the next day, in a great hall where the usual formal speeches were made — welcoming speeches by the mayor, the rector of the university, and the dean. I was delighted to learn what I had never known before, that the rector is called His Magnificence and the dean His Spectability (*Spektabilität*). At this first meeting we began to sense the curious spirit that was to dominate the proceedings. Heretofore, at one of these international gatherings, everything was done to make it as international as possible, the hostess country keeping itself in the background, but not so in Hitler's Germany. There were six speeches in addition to the welcoming addresses, and two were by Germans, four by Italians. The program of the meetings included 97 papers (many of them read by title only), but of these 79 were by Germans and Italians, leaving 18 for English, American, French, Swiss, Belgian, and the three Scandinavian countries.

We were a little group of Americans at the Frankfurter Hof. Dr. R. R. Sayers of the Public Health Service was there

with Mrs. Sayers and their young daughter; Dr. Robert Legge
of the University of California, Mrs. Legge, and their son;
Dr. Halbert L. Dunn, Chief Statistician of the Census Bureau,
and Dr. H. H. Kessler of New Jersey, a specialist in industrial
medicine.

An official lunch at the Frankfurter Hof followed this meeting. Usually on such an occasion the foreign guests are treated
with special courtesy, and if one is not only a foreigner but
the only woman present, the attention is likely to be embar-
rassingly assiduous. Not so in Hitler's Germany. Dr. Sayers
was shown to a table but the rest of us must shift for ourselves,
and I was glad to find a seat with Dr. Dunn in a remote corner
with an Egyptian as my other neighbor. Fortunately he could
speak French. This curious opening day was topped by a still
more extraordinary evening performance. The Congress was
invited to a "Gala Abend" at the Palmengarten, a charming
amusement place on the edge of the city, where we were promised music, dancing, and a cold supper. We went, to find a
solemn, silent crowd, waiting in the great beer hall for the
radio to begin the broadcast of Hitler's speech in the Sport-
palast. It started soon and kept on for an hour and forty minutes, during which the crowd, most of them Germans, sat
listening with eyes cast down, motionless, expressionless. There
was not a sign of emotion in all the room. It was the first time
I had heard what afterwards came to be familiar to all of us —
that high-pitched strident voice, rising sometimes to a hysterical shriek but never falling to a quiet, convincing level, keeping
on without a break except that now and then a roar of "*Sieg
Heils*," like the roar of a menagerie, would interrupt it for a
moment.

It was to me a dreadful thing to see those Germans, educated, civilized human beings, listening with no sign of re-

vulsion to the most hateful outpouring of abuse it has ever been my misfortune to hear. The Czechs — Hitler spat out the word — were depicted as the lowest scum of the earth, outside the pale, brutes, not human beings; Beneš was a liar and a traitor. I thought suddenly of Lincoln's Second Inaugural. Our country was already at war then, but where in any peacetime utterance can one find a spirit gentler, more magnanimous? And Americans accepted it then and have revered it ever since. Germany was not at war, Czechoslovakia had not harmed her, but not only was Hitler dripping with bitterness, his people were ready to follow him, to give their allegiance to a man utterly devoid of generosity, magnanimity, chivalry, integrity, and pity. In all that speech, as in all of *Mein Kampf*, there was not one noble, lofty idea, only hate, hate and lies, which he knew were lies. Yet the Germans worshiped him.

When at last the shrieking voice stopped there seemed nothing to do but to go back to the hotel; certainly none of us foreigners was in the mood for music and dancing. That speech meant war, we all thought, for Hitler had said he would have Sudetenland by October first and we did not believe France would desert the Czechs or England desert France. But we could learn nothing definite and all Tuesday the apprehension grew. The scientific meetings of the Congress began that morning in an atmosphere of suppressed excitement and nervousness which did not make for concentrated attention to scientific papers, to say nothing of discussion of those papers, usually the most valuable part of such a meeting. This tension, suspense, this preoccupation with questions not at all related to the subject of the meeting, increased as the days went on, and made me cling to my fellow countrymen as I never had before. That afternoon I went again to Dr. Edinger's and listened with her to the English broadcast of Chamberlain's short speech on his return from the Godesberg meeting. Even then it was rather risky to listen in on a foreign broadcast, but many people did it.

I went back to the hotel more uneasy than ever and on Wednesday morning uneasiness changed to alarm when we discovered that the French and British members had quietly slipped away, and the Swiss and Dutch and Belgians were planning an early departure. Our German hosts were more jittery than before; the meetings had degenerated into a perfunctory putting through of a program which interested nobody. Late in the afternoon I went back to Dr. Edinger's and as we sat talking one of her neighbors burst in, calling us to come and hear the English broadcast; there was to be no war, Hitler and Mussolini were to meet Chamberlain and Daladier in Munich on the twenty-ninth and all would be settled peaceably.

People who were not in Germany at that time, who had been able to follow hour by hour what was actually happening, cannot realize what the "good news" of Munich meant to me who had had little to go on except Goebbels's statements. I rejoiced with the Germans that the threat of war was lifted, my taxi driver and I congratulated each other, the hotel personnel beamed on me, the heavy silence of the last days was lifted. But then I found that the exodus of foreigners was continuing and that my American friends had decided to depart also, while the frontier was still open, for they did not feel much confidence in the outcome of the Munich conference. Dr. Sayers kindly offered me a seat in his car to the Dutch border, since the trains to France were crowded. My only reluctance over this early departure came from my strong wish to read at least the title and a brief abstract of my paper before the Congress and I had been put on the Friday program. However, Dr. Sayers found that the chairman was only too glad to move me to an early place on the Thursday morning program and I was able to announce that my paper, which would be published in full, was based on studies of carbon disulphide poisoning in viscose rayon production, carried out under the leadership of Dr. F. H. Lewey, formerly Director of the Neurological Institute of the University of Berlin, now in the University of Pennsylvania. I was determined to get that across before I left, for I wanted the Germans to know that a man they had driven out was holding an honored place in America.

As we drove north we grew more doubtful over the success of the Munich conference, for all along the Rhineland troop trains were moving south, and so were lines of infantry with tanks. In the towns the squares were full of soldiers, in the country old men, women, and children were harvesting the beets and potatoes. At the Dutch border we had a demonstration of German efficiency, of their amazing attention to detail. The frontier guards asked us what had brought us to Germany and when we mentioned the Congress they produced a list of all the members from outside Germany and checked our names on it.

Holland was like a breath of fresh air, and the day after our arrival we had the news of the Munich agreement, the full significance of which I did not grasp till much later. All I then realized was that the threat of war had been lifted, that it would be "peace in our time," that 1914 was not coming back. But there was no apparent rejoicing in Holland; indeed we soon realized how close war was to that peaceful country. All the bridges were mined, soldiers were everywhere, we were told where the breaches could be made to flood the country. But the people we met in The Hague had little hope of making any real defense against an invading army. They hoped that strict neutrality might protect them as it did in the first World War, but if it did not then there was no hope. It was only then that we learned that the British fleet had been mobilized, that Londoners were digging trenches in the parks, and that France had called up her army, for no word of any of that had been permitted to reach the German people.

I took advantage of my stop in Holland to visit two factories producing viscose rayon, for that was the industry I was studying at the time. Dr. Legge and I were taken to them by a very pleasant Hollander whom we had met at the Frankfurt Congress, Dr. P. van Luijt, the Chief Medical Inspector of Factories. We drove first to Arnhem, a pleasant town, one of those bombed in the 1940 invasion of Holland, so I suppose that beautiful factory is no more. It belonged, as did the one in Eedem which we saw that afternoon, to the Enka Company, whose plant in North Carolina I had visited and admired. No factories in any country come quite up to the Dutch standard of cleanliness. The Dutch know how to take care of foreign visitors to their factories. They served us coffee and biscuits on our arrival, they gave us an excellent lunch, and before we departed we had tea. We found them very pessimistic about Munich, believing that it meant only a temporary respite, six months at the outside, which was a pretty shrewd guess, for it was just about six months later that Hitler entered Prague. Hitler, they said, had shown plainly that war was what he wished, what he had been planning for years; he could not give it up without completely dislocating German industry and throwing so many out of work that his regime would be threatened. They hoped he would turn on Russia, the only country strong enough to offer a real resistance.

I left my companions in The Hague and went on into France, to join my sister Norah, who was in Brittany. I found Paris jubilant; Chamberlain was acclaimed as a peace-bringer, his umbrella would become a symbol and would be perpetuated in marble. In Rochefort-en-Terre, Norah's lovely Breton town, the young men who had been mobilized were returning home and all was rejoicing. We could only rejoice with them. It would take a spirit more heroic than mine to face with anything but horror the prospect of actual war in a peaceful, friendly countryside. It was not till I came home and could think again in abstractions — "France," "Italy," "Germany," "England" — that I was able to share the indignation of Americans over the Munich betrayal of Czechoslovakia, for as long as I was in France I read nothing in the papers to show that the Munich agreement was a betrayal, no word of shame over the broken alliance with Czechoslovakia, nor any account of the behavior of the invading German Army. It did make me rather uneasy to find no mention of the British-French Commission, which the Dutch and English papers had assured us was to supervise the transfer of Sudetenland to Germany and see to it that the Czechs got fair play. That commission seemed to have vanished into thin air, which was very disquieting. But at least there was no war and we went down to the Riviera for a wonderful month, making Menton our headquarters, with excursions up into the mountains, to Vence, St. Paul, Cagnes, Greolières, Gourdon, Sospel, Castillar. The heights, we were told, were covered with hidden gun emplacements and the same was true of the Italian heights facing them, but in Menton French and Italians were living together in amity, trading, intermarrying. I have never felt the blessings of peace so keenly as I did during those weeks in France.

XXIII

Hadlyme

IN 1935 Harvard made me a Professor Emeritus, which is
a great honor and pleasantly ignores my sex. It meant leaving
Boston, except for yearly visits, and making my home in Hadlyme, Connecticut, where I had already spent some eighteen
happy summers. After the home in Fort Wayne was sold
we sisters longed for a place which would be home for all
the year round, especially for the time when we should be
old and no longer working, and I wanted to get it soon, so
that when that time came we should have struck our roots
deep and retiring from professional life would not be a bewildering shock but a release to a home that had grown very
dear. So in 1916 I began to look about for a place in New England, not too far from Baltimore and not too solitary for our
old age. Katharine Ludington found it for me at Hadlyme
Ferry, some twelve miles from her family home in Old Lyme.
I knew the country for I had come many times to Katharine's
house parties, which she assembled each autumn and of which
Felix Frankfurter and I were charter members in 1912. I used
to meet many interesting people there, Walter Lippmann and
Francis Hackett and Herbert Croly, all of the *New Republic,*
Harold Laski, Lord Eustace Percy, Graham Wallas, Manley
Hudson, Charles and Mary Beard, the Henry Goddard
Leaches, and a host of others.

Hadlyme is not even a village; it has no legal existence except that we are allowed a fourth-class post office in the store

at Brockway's Four Corners. It is a loose collection of groups of houses, at the Ferry where we live, at the Center, at the Four Corners, and at Town Street, a long road with scattered houses and Hadlyme Church. It seems that in the old days of bad roads and primitive vehicles, the people of this region found it almost impossible to get to church either in Lyme to the south or in Haddam to the north, so they petitioned the Ecclesiastical Society for permission to have a church of their own. This was granted and the new community was given a name made up from the names of the two old ones.

The house where Margaret and I live is one of the old Brockway houses. It was lived in for many years by Mrs. Samantha Brockway Comstock, who is still vividly remembered by my older neighbors as a lady of strong will, some eccentricities, and a great love of flowers. We still have dozens of her white trilliums which we are told must be more than fifty years old. The house is lovely, spacious and dignified, built by people who loved beauty and were ready to take a lot of trouble to achieve it. All around the house there is wonderful stonework, paths and steps, terraces, which we call "off-sets," and, to provide protection against floods, the house itself stands on a high terrace faced with granite blocks. These blocks came from a quarry which is up at the top of our hill, now overgrown with tall trees but still showing the marks of blasting and the track down which the stone was rolled to the shore.

The Comstocks were not farmers; Captain Henry followed the sea, coming back from the West Indies with Jamaica rum and molasses which he landed at his own dock. There seems to have been also a certain amount of shipbuilding here and the place was called the "India docks." Zebulon Brockway, the father of the Brockway of Elmira Reformatory, who was a famous pioneer in prison work, kept a little ship chandlery opposite the house, now turned into living quarters downstairs and Norah's studio upstairs. We have no meadows, only a terraced hill behind the house that runs back to end in granite cliffs, dropping down steeply to Whalebone Creek, which flows into the river and forms one of our boundaries while the Connecticut River itself forms another. When we bought the place we found that it was described as "fifteen acres more or less." I said that that description would fit the whole American continent and anyway I did not believe it was a bit over six acres. "If you flattened it out, it would cover fifteen," I was told, and doubtless that is true.

When one climbs to the top of the cliff one sees a wide stretch of the river with its deeply wooded banks, and the dark, winding creek, bordered with blue pickerel weed and rosy-purple loosestrife. That creek is as lovely as any little "river" which English poets have sung. You can go up it with the inflowing tide, swinging gently around the curves, between banks where the wild rice grows high and the birds come in flocks to feed on it, where white goose-neck and scarlet cardinal flower and the hardier joe-pye weed and white boneset make vivid patches close to the stream. The marsh, covered with wild rice, spreads out on both sides and the creek takes a winding, wandering course through it. High tide is the best time to go, for at low water the muddy banks show, and if you linger long enough for the turn to come, you can float silently out with only now and then a touch of the oars to keep her headed right.

Then there is the River. On the creek a motorboat is sacrilege, but the River is wide enough to stand the chugging of the engine and you can go up to Chapman's Pond for white waterlilies or, better still, you can slip into Selden's Cove at high tide (at low tide you can enter only if you get out and wade, pushing the boat through the shallow channel), go through the long, lovely stretch of Selden's Creek, out again to the River and to the great granite rocks at Brockway's Landing. Here you can build your fire and cook your supper and watch the sunset, then return softly up the River in the gathering darkness.

The River is our joy and our terror. Three times in our twenty-five years we have been flooded, in the fall of 1927, in the great flood of 1936 and the almost equally disastrous one of 1938 when a tidal wave followed the hurricane. Thanks to the foresight of the builders, the house itself has always escaped, but its cellars and the little "store" have suffered the kind of damage which is peculiar to floods. A fire does destroy, but it leaves you clean; a flood leaves you unspeakably filthy. We were in Spain in 1936 when the great flood came and when we returned some three months after, kind neighbors had cleared away most of the mess. When the hurricane came in September of 1938, I was on my way to Germany but Margaret was in the house, with an invalid friend, a schoolgirl of fifteen, and a colored maid. She watched that night the water creeping up the cellar stairs and the waves breaking against the wall of the ell, and when day came she resolved to leave the house to its fate and take refuge with our cousins in Deep River far above flood water. Even if the waters had receded she could not have stayed, for one of the first things that happens is the seeping of the flood into the well, polluting the drinking water. Of course electric pump and electric lights went literally with the wind in that hurricane. Margaret piloted her charges along the terraces to the top of the valley, where a neighbor met her and drove her by devious and long detours over the hill roads to safety. So, though we love the

River there are times, in the spring freshets, when we watch the lapping waters creep nearer and nearer with a fear born of experience.

To Midwestern eyes Hadlyme and the neighboring villages are surprisingly attractive, with their old houses, so generously built and so well-kept. One wonders why, on a small and rocky farm, there should stand a large, dignified, sometimes almost stately house. In Indiana and Illinois the farms are vast and fertile but the houses are nothing like so fine and big. Yet much of the Middle West was settled from New England. It is as if the first settlers came over from England with the English tradition of founding an estate which would go down through the generations, but when the restless descendants broke away and emigrated west they had lost the sense of permanence and did not build homes to last for all time.

A great deal of nonsense has been written about the drabness and dreariness of life under the New England Puritans who are supposed to have crushed all love of beauty from men's minds. A single hour spent in such a village as Essex across the river from Old Lyme, looking at the old houses and especially the porticoes, would be enough to upset that theory. These houses were built by people who had excellent taste and skill and were willing to take endless trouble to achieve the result they wanted. They seem to have adopted instinctively one of the first rules of decoration, "nothing too much." There is never a touch of display; the ornamentation, if it is there, is delicate and restrained. And they must also have had an instinct for proportion, the rooms are so pleasantly and simply shaped. Nowhere else except in the Southwest have I seen rooms with so many doors. Our dining room has no less than nine, and each room on the ground floor has at least one door leading out to the yard.

The people who live in these dignified houses are proud of them and almost never does one see a house neglected and squalid. When new ones are built they reproduce the old, in style, not in size, for the big house is now a burden — compactness, convenience, comfort, are what we want now. These people, our neighbors, are many of them of old New England families. Across Whalebone Creek is the old Selden homestead, the finest house in our countryside, where you may be shown the original deed of purchase, dated 1695, and it is still in Selden hands. Scattered through the village are many Bartman houses and the Bartmans claim descent from the Indian Chief who once owned all that land. When we first came, twenty-five years ago, there were few "outsiders" (in spite of our quarter of a century we are still and always shall be outsiders), but of late many new people have come for the same reasons that brought us and have made their permanent homes here — artists, writers, architects, tired businessmen. For the most part, they fit easily into the community; there is, to my eyes, none of the gulf between them and the old Hadlymites that one sees in summer vacation places. We have neither Greenwich Villagers nor quaint and picturesque natives.

By far the most beloved outsider who ever came to Hadlyme was William Gillette, the actor. He did not think of himself as an outsider, belonging as he did to some of the founding families of Hartford, and he loved the neighborhood and we all loved him. When we first came here he was living on his houseboat, the *Aunt Polly*, out in midstream, while his granite castle was building on the first of the Seven Sister hills which shut in our narrow valley. In winter it towers over us most impressively, but gloomily, for it is empty now. Mr. Gillette was a man of unusually charming and winning personality, and with a kind of shyness that was amusing in a famous actor. He would not come and call on us unless he was sure we would be alone, but if we invited him to a big neighborhood party he would come and make himself the center of it. And he was endlessly hospitable, but it seemed that he could not endure being taken by surprise. I have known him to dodge behind a tree when I came on him unexpectedly as I walked through his woods. We have never ceased to miss him and to miss the warm welcome of the castle with its lofty living room and great fireplace.

When I was a girl in Farmington John Fiske, huge and bearded, used to come and lecture to us on colonial history, and one whole evening was devoted to the New England town meeting. I wonder why when the New Englanders moved west they did not take this very democratic measure with them. Our town meets regularly twice a year and every now and then there comes a call for an emergency meeting. Everybody goes; we would not miss it for anything. Naturally there are some who never "speak up" and there are others who never fail to do so. There is the town humorist, and we are all disappointed if he fails to set us laughing; there is the town wastrel who makes thundering speeches about his constitutional right to do as he pleases on his ancestral acres. We know he does not own a foot of land and that the neighbors built the house he lives in, but we listen indulgently and then get back to business, road building chiefly, for in the country a dirt road spells imprisonment for much of the year, a tarred road spells liberation. Then there are bridges to be repaired or rebuilt, there are the school budget, the tax rate for the year, the question of poor relief and the ever-recurring problem of fire-fighting equipment, because what good is a fire engine if there is only a well or a tiny creek to pump from. And to sink emergency wells is so costly. This thrashing out of every detail of town government in a meeting where everyone has equal standing is self-government at its best.

Our town has a little less than eight hundred inhabitants, but we send as many representatives to the Capitol as do the towns of Bridgeport, New Haven, and Hartford, for when Connecticut framed her constitution, all the towns were given equal rights, and this "rotten borough" system has never been changed. When I asked one of my neighbors if he thought it quite fair, he said, "Well, but we New England country people can't let those city foreigners run our affairs." The contrast, I find, is between Yankee, Protestant, Republican country, and foreign, Catholic, Democratic city. Margaret once told one of the ferrymen that he really should vote for the re-election of Governor Cross. He admitted that the Governor was a good man but "I don't know as I could ever bring myself to vote for a Democrat."

One of the very best things about our town government is the way we treat the poor. It is all done in an individual, very human way. Tramps and hoboes, for instance. We have no police station, the nearest jail is in Haddam way off across the River, but of course a tramp must be sheltered and fed, so the Selectman is required to provide him a bed and supper and breakfast, for which the town allows him a dollar. Some of the hoboes come through at regular times of the year and present themselves at the Selectman's house as at a hotel. Then there are our poor, mostly old men and women. We have no poorhouse, so we leave them in their own homes, give them food and fuel and doctor's care till they die, then take over the property and sell it to reimburse the town. If there is anything left over after this, it goes to the heirs. When the old man has no house of his own, he is boarded out in somebody's home and the neighbors would know it if he were not well treated.

The great flood and the hurricane showed that the pioneer tradition of mutual aid is still strong in this old community. We were the recipients of all sorts of services in both those emergencies and nobody would take any pay; neighbors expect to come to the rescue in a disaster and those that live on high ground naturally look after the flood sufferers down by the River. I have known the people to come together to raise a barn after one had burned down, to shingle a roof, or to help buy a yoke of oxen to replace two killed by lightning.

The love of reading is not peculiar to New England but it is certainly widespread in our neighborhood. The Rathbone Library in East Haddam plays a large part in our lives, especially in winter. When we meet, it is not long before we are discussing the latest books the library has bought and whether or not we agree with the reviews of them we have seen in the papers.

Connecticut seems to me an autumn country, at its loveliest when the year is coming to its close and the beauty of blue haze and golden and crimson leaves has that touch of impermanence which makes it what Wordsworth called "an aching joy." Spring is excitingly charming, each day brings something new and lovely; the loveliest, perhaps, the sudden flowering all over the hills of the dogwood. Summer is steady, deep green, little change except when the south wind with its soft purple hazes gives way to the north wind and crystal clearness. Most changeable of all is winter, for nothing else can so transform the scene overnight as can a fall of snow.

In winter the granite cliffs come out, one can see the very bones of the land when their soft green covering is gone, and then the pines and hemlocks come into their own, no longer green but a purple black. The marsh is a frozen lake, the River is an intense blue, filled with ice cakes which go swinging up and down with the tides. Life becomes something of an adventure in winter, when roads are icy or deep in mud and the nearest chain grocery store some fifteen miles away. But nothing in summer can be as purely delightful as a snowy walk against the north wind, coming back to the welcome of a cup of tea before an open fire.

This home of my declining years is a place for meditation on many things, for looking back and for looking forward. It is not that I think my years have brought me wisdom; my thoughts about labor and government and war are of value only as they are based on an experience which goes back to a time now so remote and different that it might be a century ago. That experience gives a background, a yardstick, a basis of comparison to my meditations on the world as it is today. Let me touch on only a few aspects of our life; first my own special interest, workers in our industrial system.

As I look back over the history of labor during the years which followed my discovery at Hull-House that there was a labor question, I can see an advance that is truly amazing. For I can call up pictures of what were really the dark ages: of Mother Jones, that valiant old champion of the soft-coal miners, telling us how, during a strike in the West Virginia mines, she had had to wade along the bed of a stream to reach one of the villages, because all the land and even the highway belonged to the company and was patrolled by its police; of a Catholic priest from a coal town in western Pennsylvania describing the plight of his mining village during a strike when the water supply — owned by the company — was shut off and, had it not been for the priest's own well, the village would have gone waterless. As for the tales of violence on the part of company police and of the Pennsylvania State Constabulary, they were too numerous to count. We have come a long way since then. And yet the so-called Memorial Day Massacre in South Chicago, only a few years ago, serves to remind us that there are still Americans in high places who believe that "ruthless brutality," to use Hitler's favorite phrase, is the only way to deal with a rebellious mob.

In my own field, the dangerous trades, I have already shown repeatedly in the course of these chapters that the reforms already great are continuing. Moreover we have developed a method of dealing with new industrial dangers which is peculiarly American and which works very well in a country composed of forty-eight independent states, a method entirely without legal compulsion. Let me cite two striking instances. The first came in 1923–1924 when newspapers carried stories of a number of cases of severe poisoning among chemists and workmen who had been exposed to a new poison, tetraethyl lead, which was being produced by one large company and used by several for blending with gasoline. This is a very dangerous form of lead, it is more quickly absorbed than any of those ordinarily used in industry and concentrates in the central nervous system, causing insomnia, excitement, twitching muscles, hallucinations like those of delirium tremens, even maniacal attacks and convulsions, and death. The *New York World* took up the crusade against this dangerous poison; there was widespread panic lest the use of the blended gasoline involve risk to the public; several states hastily prohibited the sale of "ethyl gasoline" and foreign countries threatened to forbid its import. There were even questions in Parliament on the subject. The emergency was met by Surgeon General Cumming, who called a conference in May 1925 at which industrialists, chemists, labor representatives, and physicians agreed to entrust the problem to a small group of experts who should decide on the nature of the danger and on whether prohibition or control was needed. Meantime the manufacturers promised not to sell ethyl gasoline until the report of the experts had been made. The committee found that the hazard to producers and blenders could be wholly prevented by mechanical devices and that the danger to garage workers was slight and to users none at all, unless gasoline was used for cleaning textiles. To obviate this small element of risk warnings were to be put on all supply pipes and the blended gasoline was to be colored.

Another instance, very similar to this, occurred in connection with the making of luminous figures on watches and clocks. Here too a new, almost unknown poison was involved, radium (using this term to cover radioactive bodies); the effects of the poison were peculiarly terrible; the public was aroused by newspaper stories of women dying after months of suffering (again it was the *New York World* that led the crusade) and a demand was made for some governmental action. This was provided by the same method, a conference called by the Surgeon General, an expert committee appointed by him, and the manufacturers voluntarily pledging themselves to abide by its decision.

I was a member of both those committees and it was to me both surprising and heartening to see men of such widely separated backgrounds and interests — manufacturers and their chemists and research workers on one side, trade-union officials, independent physicians, and toxicologists on the other — meet in a spirit of reasonableness and a genuine desire to get at the real facts and deal practically with the problem.

In connection with both ethyl gasoline and luminous paint,

close watch is still kept to detect possible cases, but the precautions worked out in these occupations seem thus far to be so adequate that we do not fear any serious injury to the people employed in them.

Finally this same method is being applied to that new-old industrial disease, silicosis, the dust disease which threatens men employed in work exposing them to dust containing free silica. Since Roman days it has been known that dusty work caused a wasting disease of the lungs. "Grinders' rot" and "potters' rot" are ancient terms in England. Silica dust is a slow, insidious poison (though not usually classed as a poison it has a toxic action), and while the employer finds himself confronted with responsibility for a sickness he never heard of before, the employee finds himself faced with the prospect of losing his job because of a sickness he has known about all his life but which he is willing to risk rather than lose his status as a skilled workman and sink to the level of the common laborer or of the unemployed. Obviously the way to attack silicosis is to prevent the formation and escape of dust, and it is in this direction that efforts are now being made by an expert committee appointed by the Division of Labor Standards of the Federal Department of Labor.[1]

Even if we reach a point at which all poisons and harmful

---

[1] Since the autumn of 1935 I have been attached to Secretary Perkins's Department as Medical Consultant, and I have no hesitation in saying that this Department, especially the Division of Labor Standards under V. A. Zimmer, should be given a large share of credit for the improvement now seen in the dangerous trades. The public does not realize how greatly the Labor Department has expanded and developed under Secretary Perkins, but I, who have known it since its foundation in 1912, have seen it pass through a promising childhood and a troublesome adolescence, to its present capable adult self. The careful, steady spadework carried on in the different states, all of them sovereign states with their own standards or lack of standards, is the least spectacular but I think the most rewarding part of the campaign against industrial accidents and diseases.

dusts have been brought under control we shall still have to deal with that much more baffling and widespread industrial evil, fatigue of "mind, body and soul." Fatigue is a problem that increases in importance with the increase in mechanized industry. A typical modern factory impresses the visitor with its spacious workrooms, its good lighting and ventilation, cleanliness, rest rooms, generous provision of washrooms and showers, sometimes as good as those in a country club. Some factories provide a dance hall, a baseball field, or a bowling alley for their employees. And yet, if you linger in a factory long enough to get a real impression of what is going on, you begin to wonder whether it would not have been better to devote all that money to one thing — to slowing up the speed of production. Once you begin to look for what we call speeding up, the rest becomes of minor importance. I have walked through a roomful of women and girls in a shoe factory and seen hardly one of them lift her head from her machine to look at this woman from outside, to see what sort of hat she was wearing. I have seen men building rubber tires working with an intensity of speed which it seemed impossible to keep up for even one hour.

Neither of these jobs was on the assembly line. When work is on the assembly line the workers cannot time their motions, the machine determines that. They cannot change, vary the routine, let up for a little, then speed up again, for they must fit accurately into the machine. The strain of keeping up a fixed pace for hours with no change, no letup, no control on the part of the workers, brings about a weariness that is out of proportion to the muscular strain, because it is emotional as well as physical. This is the field of increasing importance now for the industrial hygienist and it will grow more and more important as industry becomes more and more mechanized.

But no matter what new dangers may be brought about by new methods of manufacture, they can be controlled and they will be. Even if, after this war is over, a wave of reaction sets in as it did after the first World War, even if, as an investment counselor said to me the other day, "We shall be in a position to put labor back in its proper place," even then the setback will not be so serious nor will it last so long. The medical profession will never again neglect industrial diseases, the employer will never again refuse to assume responsibility toward them. Our progress in this field has been great and it will keep on.

America is supposed to be the paradise of women. It is far from that. In many ways women do not hold as respected a position here as they do in other countries. Frenchwomen have not the vote but they have an important place in the business world. In the first World War, the Scottish Women Doctors' unit was recognized by the British Army and did valiant service, caring for the wounded. We sent over to France a women's medical unit but they were allowed to care for civilians only. They opened a hospital near Belleau Wood and after the battle there they offered their services to the military authorities. But though the army hospital was so crowded that wounded men had to be laid on the grass to wait for a bed, the offer was refused. The Army could not recognize women surgeons. This war bids fair to break down that barrier, as well as many others that have been built up through the ages to keep women in a separate class.

As for the field of industrial medicine, it has been very

largely closed to women and this is a great pity, for many women graduates have wished to enter it. There are several reasons for this, one a very valid reason. If an employer needs only one physician he knows that both men and women workers will be content to have a man, but he is by no means sure that the men would accept a woman doctor. Even if there were not this objection there would still be the half-unconscious attitude of most industrialists toward women, that their place in the industrial world is a strictly subordinate one; they are acceptable as secretaries, typists, filing clerks, but not in a position of importance and authority. Russia admits women to industry on an equality with men and therefore it is natural for her to accept women as doctors in charge of the health of the workers. It may be, however, that the scarcity of men doctors brought about by the war will compel industry to turn to women. I feel sure that, once they have found a way in, they will not only make good but will remain as an essential part of the system.

Perhaps the greatest change in American ways I have seen in my lifetime is in the relative importance of the individual and the state. At the beginning of 1900 one of the Hull-House residents, Elizabeth Thomas, a Socialist, made a journey to Russia. We were all excited over her adventure, which began with the securing of a passport, a document none of us had even seen before and which only Czar-ruled Russia demanded. When Miss Thomas came back she was full of interesting tales but the one I remember most clearly concerned her entrance into Russia, for she was detained overnight at the frontier by the Russian police who searched through her luggage and confiscated two books on Socialism. This was an incredible and even ridiculous procedure to our American eyes, some forty years ago. It was not till after the war that "subversive

literature" and even "dangerous thoughts" began to be matters for governmental control. We had no Lusk Committees,
no Red Network, no Spider Web, no Dies Committees; all
that is of more recent growth. We have traveled a long way
since 1914 and not only under the compulsion of war;
indeed the attacks on the freedom of the individual were
bitterest during the peaceful and prosperous period of the
twenties.

All these attacks have called forth protests from large and
influential groups and the protests have often been successful;
no one would say that our loss of individual liberty increases
steadily. But that there has been such a loss in the last forty
years cannot be denied. It has its good side certainly, in the
control of anti-social practices by big business, but there is
one department of life where I believe the authority over the
individual is not justified. That the state should presume to
dictate to a man's conscience in matters of religious practice
where this harms nobody is certainly a new thing in our
country, and it is strange that the Christian Churches have
not protested against it more vigorously. The Supreme Court's
decision in the Macintosh case in 1930 upheld the government
in refusing citizenship to Professor Macintosh, a Canadian
teaching at Yale, to Mme. Rosika Schwimmer, a Hungarian
refugee, and to a third applicant, who was, I think, a French-
Canadian trained nurse, all on the ground of their having
refused to promise to take up arms if the country should go to
war. This was twelve years ago but just lately the decision of
the Court against Jehovah's Witnesses in the famous flag-
saluting case shows that our government still holds that the
individual conscience must yield to the dictates of the state.
To me it seems not a question of the rightness or wrongness of
pacifism or of refusal to honor the flag, but a question of the

right of the state to dictate to the religious convictions of citizens and would-be citizens. One of the favorite "Sunday books" of my childhood was Foxe's *Book of Martyrs*, and, as I remember those heroic histories, the victims were all upholders of the authority of their own consciences against the authority of the state. The invasion of this field by the Federal government seems to me far more dangerous than any of the moves toward state socialism.

Throughout the first World War I was a pacifist and opposed to our entering it. The Kaiser's Germany did not seem to me a menace terrible enough to cause a world war, especially since Czarist Russia was on the Allied side and it was impossible to close one's eyes to the fact that both Britain and France had carried on ruthless wars of conquest in Asia and Africa and, if they now condemned such excesses, still they insisted on holding onto the spoils. Then, too, I dreaded the change I felt sure would come over us as a people, the intolerance of any dissent, the violent suppression of minorities, the deliberately fostered hatred of all things German, and indeed what really did happen was worse than anything I dreaded. Then, for the next twenty years I never wavered in my attitude toward war, yet now, in the third year of this most terrible of all wars, I am among those who believe we are right in taking up arms on the side of the United Nations. As has so often happened to me, the change in my views has come slowly and almost unconsciously.

As I followed our national policy after the last war I could find little to accept, much to deplore. We were so unbearably smug in those days. President Harding told us that we had "shirked no duty which comes of sympathy or fraternity or highest fellowship among nations." President Coolidge told us that we had never engaged in a war which was not prompted by the most unselfish idealism (conveniently forgetting the Mexican War), and he told Soviet Russia that she must first bring forth fruits meet for repentance before we could recognize her. Even President Hoover, in his first Thanksgiving address, assured us that our riches were the reward of our peculiar national virtues. Apparently people believed it. To label anything un-American was condemnation enough, to label it American was to make it a cloak to cover the narrowest and most selfish nationalism.

Our refusal to sign the Treaty of Versailles did not seem to me wrong. I had come back from Europe too deeply impressed with its injustices, but as time went on I was forced to admit that our motive was not a generous one, it was not because we wanted more justice for Germany. Our refusal to enter the League and our almost complete withdrawal from the tangled mess in Europe were indeed deeply disappointing, and the more I read and listened to the arguments against our joining in the World Court the more deplorable seemed our national attitude. Then came the Smoot-Hawley tariff, which I knew was a terrible mistake though I did not know how terrible it would really prove to be. And then the successive disarmament conferences which I followed with eagerness and with an increasing sense of shame, for our country, safe and rich and free from deep-seated, inherited hatreds, gave no help to the cause of peace among the nations; we sent over to represent us military experts to haggle about six-inch, eight-inch, ten-inch guns. And the scandal that broke finally, the revelation of the part played by a hired representative of our munition makers, added shame to our sense of failure.

All through the twenties we refused every suggestion of co-operation for the maintenance of world peace: [2] we would not pledge ourselves not to sell munitions to a nation which, unprovoked, broke the Kellogg Pact; we would not even promise to consult with other nations in such a case; we refused to commit ourselves in any way to join an international effort for the prevention of war.

And we entered early on a program of active and intensive preparation for war. I need not go into the figures which show the enormous increase in our army and navy budgets during the twenties, the increasing militarization of our schools — all that is familiar to everyone. There was strong opposition to this program on the part of the peace societies and I used to be called on often to speak against it. Some of my speeches lie before me now. The one I used oftenest compared war with disease. I used to say that the arguments in defense of war could be applied to disease also. Every doctor knows that suffering sometimes brings out heroic qualities, but he knows that this is rare, that by and large suffering withers and stunts. And certainly our postwar periods, the Grant and the Harding administrations, showed that the unselfish devotion which war calls forth does not last long. War, I would say, is supposed to be inevitable, given human nature. Well, certainly no doctor expects that disease and death will ever be banished from the world, but all the same he is ready to devote his life to the prevention of disease and death. Only when statesmen, I used to say, come to detest war as genuinely as physicians detest disease shall we do away with it. My closing sentence would be: —

---

[2] I cannot make an exception of the Kellogg Pact, which seemed to me only a characteristic American gesture — noble, high-sounding words with nothing behind them.

If we really believe that war is wholly evil and that an evil tree cannot bring forth good fruit — and surely the history of the world since 1919 proves that — then we will take the stand toward it that we take toward disease, that it is a menace from which we shall probably never be free but which we will oppose with all our powers, without compromise and without fatalistic acceptance.

But the years since 1938 have shown me that analogies are fallible tools in argument, the matter is not so simple as that. When preventive medicine breaks down and an epidemic rages through the land, there is no question as to what we must do; when war breaks forth it is not so clear. Still, I cannot feel guilty when I look back on those years of protests against military training in the schools, against huge appropriations for the Navy, against the fortification of Guam. Nowadays to have held such ideas is taken to be proof that a man is unfit for public office. But it is not the group of anti-militarists and internationalists in any country that has brought us to the state we are in now, it is the group of narrow nationalists and militarists, the believers in force and in empire and in racial superiority, those that refused to help the weak and struggling German Republic but were willing to do business with Hitler, those that insisted on insulting Japan with the Oriental Exclusion Act but were glad to furnish her with munitions to fight China. Now that they have had their way all over the world, now that the fire has been kindled, it is no longer possible to go on striving for our program of prevention, for war is here.

Together with almost all my pacifist friends I found myself in the fall of 1939 bewildered. My clean-cut principles no longer seemed to apply, I must think it through again. And as the war clouds thickened and our country moved nearer and nearer to the conflict I began to feel that if we chose to keep out, it would be at a great cost. For the anti-war movement seemed to me narrow and nationalistic and I felt that if we as a country remained aloof from the disaster which was spreading over Europe, it would not be for generous motives but for selfish ones, and that would be very bad for our national soul. To watch Norway, Holland, Belgium, France, fall under a foreign yoke, to watch the unspeakable horrors of the conquest of Poland and Jugoslavia, and to tell ourselves that it was not our business, that only this hemisphere concerned us, would be to stifle some of the finest qualities in our nation. It is no defense of war as a means of settling disputes to say that when once war has been started by greed for power and helped on by blindness and selfishness we cannot save the world by saving our own selves, we must get down into the arena and throw our strength on the side we think the right one. After all, we are far from guiltless ourselves of the blunders which led up to the war, we too have clung desperately to privilege and fought change, we have been almost as narrow and selfish as those we criticize.

America has gone into this war in a spirit very different from that of 1917. Among Christians it is an attitude essentially penitent even when it is determined and aggressive. There is little of the sort of talk we heard in 1917, when the war was idealized by churchmen as a crusade. Now it is an evil brought on us by our own un-Christlike actions since the last war, a hideous struggle in which we are forced to engage because to stand aloof would be to abandon our brothers to a fate they have deserved no more than we have, and to permit the sway of a system we believe would bring about for the civilized world a second Dark Ages. Many Christians say that this world catastrophe is a punishment for the world's sin; in other words it is the natural consequence of the policies followed by Europe and America during the last twenty years.

It is this changed attitude toward the war which gives me hope for the peace. Not that I believe we shall emerge from the long-drawn-out conflict with a spirit of sweet reasonableness. We shall surely have to pass through the stage of weary reaction against self-sacrifice, of longing to return to our own comfortable ways, that followed the last war, but I do not believe it will last for years as it did then. There has been too much soul-searching, too much deep probing into the causes of this war and into the ways we must take to prevent another. It will not be possible for us to draw back into our own shell, nor do I believe we shall wish to. Mankind does not of a sudden become sinless, but he knows little of history who thinks that our progress is downhill, not up. We do swing down sometimes but not as far as we swung the last time, and when we swing up again it is to go higher than we went before. I do not believe I shall live long enough to see that upswing but I know it will come.

INDEX